Detoxification

All you need to know
to recharge, renew
and rejuvenate
your body,
mind and
spirit!

by
Linda Page, N.D., Ph.D.

Detoxification is the oldest and most
effective healing method
known to man.

Hippocrates, "the Father of Medicine,"
Galen, Paracelsus and other
great physicians throughout history
prescribed detoxification — it was
practiced by Plato and Socrates
and was thought to help people attain
"mental and physical efficiency."

In this book
you will learn all you need to know about
detoxification and cleansing so you can awaken
"the healer within."

The information in this book is intended solely for information
and educational purposes and not as medical advice.

Published by
Healthy Healing Publications
PO Box 436, Carmel Valley, CA 93924

ISBN: 1-884334-54-7

Do you have natural health questions?
Call the Natural Health
Information Service
1-900-903-5885, Monday through Friday,
9 AM to 5 PM Pacific Time.

Visit Healthy Healing Publications
on the web: www.healthyhealing.com

Cover design by Barbara Howard

Linda Page, N.D., Ph.D.

Long before natural foods and herbal formulas became a "chic," widely accepted method for healing, Dr. Linda Page was sharing her extensive knowledge with those who dared to listen.

During the late seventies, she opened and operated the Rainbow Kitchen, a natural food restaurant, and became a working partner in Sonora, California's Country Store, a natural foods store.

Through what some would call an accident of fate but she calls a blessing, she was compelled to research alternative avenues of healing. Sequestered in a hospital with a life-threatening illness, watching her 5-foot frame wither to 69 pounds, her hair drop out, and her skin peel off, doctors told her they had no cure. With only a cursory knowledge of herbs, she began a frantic research process of testing herbal formulas and healing food combinations on herself.

She read voraciously about herbal healing. Good friends shopped for herbs and she began to formulate the many compounds which would eventually save her life, revitalize her health and restore beautiful new hair and skin. It was that incident that led her to seek her degrees in Naturopathy and Nutrition.

A prolific author and education, Dr. Page has sold over a million books including **Healthy Healing, Cooking For Your Own Herbal Pharmacist, Party Lights** and a popular series of 20 library books which address specific healing therapies for topics like menopause, male and female energy, colds and flu, and cancer. Her book **Healthy Healing** is a textbook for courses at UCLA, The Institute of Educational Therapy, and Clayton College of Natural Health. Dr. Page also formulates over 250 herbal formulas for Crystal Star Herbal Nutrition of Earth City, Missouri. She received one of the first herbal patents in the United States for her formulas that help balance hormones to ease meno-pausal symptoms.

Dr. Page is an Adjunct Professor at Clayton College of Natural Health. She is also the executive editor of a monthly national natural health newsletter, *Dr. Linda Page's Natural Healing Report,* published by Weiss Research of Palm Beach Gardens, Florida.

Dr. Page appears weekly on a CBS television station with a report on natural healing; she is featured with CBS fitness reporter Bonnie Kaye on national CBS television; she is principle speaker at national health symposiums and conventions; she is featured regularly in national magazines; she appears on hundreds of radio and television programs.

Today, Dr. Page delights in having come full circle. "I feel I am living my dream. I am so grateful that knowledge of healing through herbal formulas and good foods is becoming so widespread. I see it as an opportunity for people to seize the power to heal themselves. Knowledge is power. Whether one chooses conventional medicine, alternative healing avenues, or combines them both in a complementary process, the real prescription for healing is knowledge."

*This book is dedicated to
those who are just beginning the journey;
who are taking the first deep,
cleansing breaths,
the first determined steps toward a measure
of control over their own wellness;
who are starting to hear the first
"cellular phone calls"
from the miraculous, self-healing body
in which they live.*

About This Book....

Detoxification is comprehensive. It addresses the reasons why body cleansing is so necessary in today's world, what a good body cleanse really does, and how to direct a cleanse for the best results. It comprehensively details every cleansing phase and detoxing agent for all types of cleansing, for each body system, as well as for the total body.

The book also covers detoxification from many modern ailments that are the direct result of body toxicity and compromised immunity. Most of them respond positively to body purification techniques. Simply consult the particular ailment chart for a complete cleansing program that is beneficial for the problem.

Body purification has been a part of mankind's rituals for health and well-being for over twenty thousand years. Cleansing is a rich tradition that has helped humans through all ages and cultures. Indeed, it is at the foundation of every great healing philosophy.

Detoxification examines the cleansing techniques of the five healing traditions that influence contemporary alternative health care — Ayurvedic, the Western European view, the Rainforest culture, the Native American legacy, and Traditional Chinese Medicine. Most of the techniques are still used effectively today, and this book offers them as additional choices for your body cleansing experience.

Detoxification procedures in America's alternative medicine detox programs draw on all of these systems, eclectically selecting methods and techniques for the individual, the problem and the goal. Step by step cleanses are provided for each ailment, each type of cleanse and each body area, with time frame monitoring so you determine when and what you might reasonably expect as results.

Dear reader, let me tell you a true story about detoxification....

I embrace things very enthusiastically. When I first heard about a cleansing diet in the 70's I thought it sounded like just the thing for me. I had fought my weight all my life. I was tired all the time (probably from all the crazy diets I went on to lose weight), and I felt "toxic," constantly getting fever blisters, urinary tract and yeast infections. I had dull hair, poor skin texture, peeling feet and breaking nails. Oh, I remember those days well.

Detoxification seemed like it would solve of lot of health problems. I thought I would be on a cleansing diet all my life.

The trouble was, I had almost no idea how to go about it. The 60's and 70's were the decades that the FDA had what amounted to a "gag order" on all books and information about alternative health methods, healing techniques and products. (You would not be reading this book now if the owner and employees of a very brave health food store in California had not finally challenged this regulation in the early 1980s in the courts and won, after many years and enormous expense.)

But I had a little knowledge and some enthusiastic friends who were detoxing, too, so I started on what was essentially a 5 food diet — cabbage, lettuce with a little salad dressing, apples, oranges, peanut butter (for protein), and a few whole wheat crackers occasionally. I was delighted with my weight loss (I averaged about 90 pounds for my 5 foot frame). I rarely ate other things; this went on for several years. I didn't realize it, but my body was going into major malnutrition decline.

Today, with all the information we have about nutrition, most people know this type of diet is not a cleansing diet. It's a prescription for terrible health. All I saw was that I was finally thin.

One week, in the winter of 1981, my energy had dropped so low that I couldn't make it to my job. I had just started working at the town's small health food store, and I loved my work, so this was very unusual.

I didn't realize it but I had already slipped into shock — the hours and days were slipping by like a dream. I lived alone with my dogs and cats, but my colleagues from work wondered why I wasn't there. Thankfully, one of them came to check up on me. He saved my life.

I had already collapsed, and was lying by my front screen door. He scooped me up and got me to the nearest emergency room. It was eight-thirty in the morning, at a very small Seventh Day Adventist hospital in a small California town. There were 12 people in the building. Everyone worked feverishly to save me, but my blood pressure dropped rapidly. The staff saw me slip into a coma — they thought they had lost me.

All I knew was that I was floating, above my body, the operating table and the doctors who were working on me. It was all very interesting. I saw all the frantic emergency room procedures — like a TV show.
And then...... I can see as clearly as when it happened, I floated to a top corner of the room. A million colors were swirling around me.
I saw a dark tunnel with a white pinpoint of light miles away at the end. I turned to go to it.... then everything when black, and I don't remember any more.

I was in a coma, and even though I didn't know it,
I had made it.

Eventually I regained consciousness, and woke up full of tubes and needles on a breathing machine. My blood was so toxic, the hospital had to have plasma flown in every 5 hours to give me a slow but complete transfusion. It kept me alive, but I wasn't regaining health, slipping back and forth into unconsciousness. The doctors wanted to MED-Evac me to Stanford for specialized treatment, but I knew that I would just become a number, so I wouldn't go.

One of the wonderful things about a Seventh Day Adventist hospital (especially in those days) was that they listened to the patient. I couldn't speak, of course, but I could write. So, I asked for green drinks from the health food store and the hospital staff allowed a small refrigerator in. It was like a miracle. Within hours I felt stronger; within days, they removed the respirator; within a few more, they removed all the tubes and needles. In a total of twelve days after I regained consciousness, I left the hospital, very very weak, weighing 69 pounds, and unable to walk because my legs would not support my weight.

I knew I had been given another chance at life and a tremendous challenge to regain my health. My hair had either fallen out or turned white; some of my veins has collapsed from the needles. I had pulled retinal tissue in one eye; my skin was peeling off at my fingertips. The hospital thought they might have to amputate my toes unless I regained circulation in my feet fast.

I started reading everything I could get my hands on about natural healing and herbal remedies. I started formulating herbal formulas to bring each part of my body back to health. It began to happen. I could see a new me emerging, with curly hair, and a better skin tone and texture (no wrinkles) than I had before the illness. My circulation came back (no toe amputations); my energy returned stronger than it had been in many years.

The experience and the healing changed my life. I saw that herbs are far more than remedies for colds and flu. They can bring your health back from serious illness.... literally from death's door. I was enormously impressed. I decided to devote my life to reaching out to others — to talk about the power of herbs, to write about their healing abilities, to return some of the essential universal knowledge that we've lost.

That early attempt at cleansing was almost fatally misguided. One of the reasons I wanted to write this book was to pass along all I've learned about how detoxification really works. Here's my cleansing diet today. It's nourishing, delicious, satisfying... and lean. I've lost ten extra pounds over the last year.

Salmon, fresh tuna and shrimp *for essential fatty acids, brain food, and protein*
A wide variety of sea vegetables *for minerals, vitamins, EFA's, protein, and antioxidants*
Sushi and sashimi *for B vitamins, protein and more of all of the above*
Fresh vegetable salads with tomatoes, peas, cucumbers, celery and plenty of lettuces *for minerals, vitamins, fiber, complex carbohydrates, antioxidants and system sweepers*
Apples, pineapples, grapes and oranges *for fiber, system cleansing and hydrating*
Steamed vegetables like green beans, broccoli and cauliflower *for vitamins and minerals, fiber, anticarcinogens, complex carbohydrates and stable nerves*
Brown rice, cous cous, brown rice crackers and rice cakes *for B vitamins, fiber and protein*
Miso soup *for immune enhancers, and thyroid boosters*
Green tea every morning *for antioxidants and detoxifiers*
Plenty of herbs and natural spices *for thermogenesis, circulation and immune response*

To your best health,

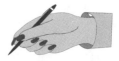

Linda

Table of Contents

Today is a very important day.
You are exchanging today
   for a day of
   your life.

You can waste it.... or use it for good.

When tomorrow comes,
   today will be gone forever,
   leaving in its place what
   you have traded it for.

Use it for gain and not loss,
   for good and not evil,
   for right and not wrong,
   for success and not failure.

Use it for the best that is in you
   so that you will never regret
   the price you have paid
   for this day.

Your worth is not determined by....
   the number of pounds you weigh,
   the amount of money you have,
   the color of your skin,
   the branches on your family tree,
   the size of the hill you can ski,
   the points you can score, or
   the people you know.

Your worth is determined by....
   your ideals
   your values
   your dreams
   your passions
   your commitments
   your thoughts
   your words and
   your deeds.

Your worth is determined only by
   the way you live your life.

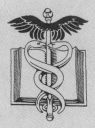

OTHER BOOKS BY

Linda Page, N.D., Ph.D.

Cooking For Healthy Healing

How To Be Your Own Herbal Pharmacist

Party Lights

(with restaurateur Doug Vanderberg)

AND

The Healthy Healing Library
Book Series

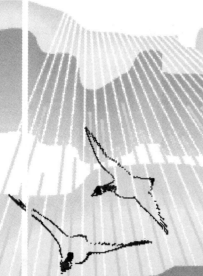

What is detoxification?

Why should you detoxify?

What body signs tell you that you need to detoxify?

What benefits can you expect from a good detox?

What are the steps in a good detox program?

Understanding Detoxification

What is detoxification?

Our bodies naturally do it every day. Detoxification is a normal body process of eliminating or neutralizing toxins through the colon, liver, kidneys, lungs, lymph and skin. In fact, internal detoxification is one of our body's most basic automatic functions. Just as our hearts beat nonstop and our lungs breathe continuously, so our metabolic processes continuously dispose of accumulated toxic matter. But in our world today, body systems and organs that were once capable of cleaning out unwanted substances are now completely overloaded; thus many unwanted substances stay in our tissues. Our bodies try to protect us from dangerous material by setting it aside, surrounding it with mucous or fat so it won't cause imbalance or trigger an immune reaction. (Your body stores foreign substances in its fatty deposits — a significant reason to keep your diet and body fat low. Some people carry around up to 15 extra pounds of mucous that harbors this waste!)

Ideally, we should live in a pollution-free environment, eat untainted foods and drink pure water. But, since humans are born with a "self-cleaning system," we know this has probably never been possible. Today, it isn't even practical, so the next best thing is to keep pollutants to a minimum and to periodically get rid of them through a detoxification program.

If our bodies can't cleanse us anymore, can we do it through a detox program?

Detoxification through special cleansing diets may be the missing link to disease prevention, especially for immune-compromised diseases like cancer, arthritis, diabetes and fatigue syndromes like candida albicans. Our chemicalized-food diet, with too much animal protein, too much fat, too much caffeine and alcohol radically alters our internal ecosystems. Even if your diet is good, a cleanse can restore body vitality against environmental toxins that pave the way for disease-bearing bacteria, viruses and parasites.

A detox program aims to remove the cause of disease before it makes us ill. It's a time-honored way to keep immune response high, elimination regular, circulation sound, and stress under control, so your body can handle the toxicity it encounters. In the past, detoxification was used either clinically for recovering alcoholics and drug addicts, or individually, as a once-a-year mild "spring cleaning" for general health maintenance. Today, a regular detox program two or three times a year makes a big difference not only for health, but for the quality of our lives.

Are detoxification and cleansing the same thing? After a detox, is my body purified? There is sometimes confusion about these terms because cleansing rituals are so ancient. In cultures like Native American, cleansing was regarded first as a religious practice, purifying the body as a living temple to God. In others, such as Chinese medicine, cleansing was part of preventive health care. Today, and in this book, the terms are used interchangeably.

Why should you detoxify?

Today, Americans are exposed to synthetic, often toxic chemicals on an unprecedented scale. Industrial chemicals and their pollutant run-offs in our water, pesticides, additives in our foods, heavy metals, anesthetics, residues from drugs, and environmental hormones are trapped within the human body in greater concentrations than at any other point in history. Every system of the body is affected, from tissue damage to sensory deterioration.

Many chemicals are so widespread that we are unaware of them. But they have worked their way into our bodies faster than they can be eliminated, and are causing allergies and addictions in record numbers. **More than 2 million synthetic substances are known, 25,000 are added each year, and over 30,000 are produced on a commercial scale.** Only a tiny fraction are ever tested for toxicity. A lot of them come to us from developing countries that have few safeguards in place. This doesn't even count the second-hand smoke, caffeine and alcohol overload, or daily stress that is an increasing part of our lives.

The molecular structure of many chemical carcinogens interacts with human DNA, so long term exposure may result in metabolic and genetic alteration that affects cell growth, and behavior. World Health Organization research implicates environmental chemicals in 60 to 80% of all cancers. Hormone-disrupting pesticides and pollutants are linked to hormone problems, psychological disorders, birth defects, still births and now breast cancer.

 As toxic matter saturates our tissues, antioxidants and minerals in vital body fluids are reduced, so immune defenses are thrown out of balance. Circumstances like this are the prime factor in today's immune compromised diseases like candidiasis, lupus, fibromyalgia, and chronic fatigue syndrome.

Chemical oxidation is the other process that allows disease. The oxygen that "rusts" and ages us also triggers free radical activity, a destructive cascade of incomplete molecules that damages DNA and other cell components. And if you didn't have a reason to reduce your animal fat intake before, here is a critical one: oxygen combines with animal fat in body storage cells and speeds up the free radical process.

Almost everyone can benefit from a cleanse. It's one of the best ways to remain healthy in a destructive environment. Not one of us is immune to environmental toxins, and most of us can't escape to a remote, unpolluted habitat. In the last few decades we have become dangerously able to harm the health of our entire planet, even to the point of making it uninhabitable for life. We must develop further and take even larger steps... those of cooperation and support. Mankind and the Earth must work together — to save it all for us all. It starts with us. We can take positive steps to keep our own body systems in good working order so that toxins are eliminated quickly.

We can also take a closer look at our own air, water and food, and keep an ever watchful eye on the politics that control our environment. Legislation on health and the environment follows two pathways in America today...the influence of business and profits, and the demands of the people for a healthy environment and responsible stewardship of the Earth. (See "Fluoridation - An unnecessary poison added to our drinking water," page 62).

Is your body becoming toxic?

Chemicals are polluting the earth's environment faster than the human organism can adapt to them. Toxins are building up and our bodies are becoming filters trapping the pollutants. The current level of chemicals in our air, food and water supply alters us at the most basic level - our enzymes, then spreads throughout every body function to lower our threshold of resistance to disease.

Besides coming into our bodies through every orifice and organ, prolonged mental stress and negative emotions can create internal poisons. A highly processed foods diet, a severely unbalanced diet, or simply too much food overburden elimination systems. Lack of exercise contributes to toxicity, too. The body's natural cleansing cycle of oxygen and vital nutrients depends upon exercise. A stagnant system encourages toxic build-up.

Do you need to detox? Ask yourself these questions:

- Do you feel congested from too much food or the wrong kinds of food?
- Do you feel lethargic, like you need a good spring cleaning?
- Do you need to eliminate drug residues? Or normalize after illness or hospital stay?
- Do you need a jump start for a healing program?
- Do you need a specific detox program for a serious health problem?
- Do you want to streamline your body processes for more energy?
- Do you need to remove toxins causing a health problem?
- Do you want to prevent disease? Or rest and rejuvenate your whole body?
- Do you want to assist weight loss? Do you want to clear up your skin?
- Do you want to slow aging and improve body flexibility?
- Do you want to improve fertility?

Note: Laboratory tests like stool, urine, blood or liver function, and hair analysis can also shed light on the need for detoxification.

Body signs can tell you that you need to detoxify.

We all have different "toxic tolerance" levels. Listen to your body when it starts giving you those "cellular phone calls." If you can keep the amount of toxins in your system below your toxic level, your body can usually adapt and rid itself of them.

Do you have:
- Frequent, unexplained headaches or back or joint pain, or arthritis?
- Chronic respiratory problems, sinus problems or asthma?
- Abnormal body odor, bad breath or coated tongue?
- Food allergies, poor digestion or chronic constipation with intestinal bloating or gas?
- Brittle nails and hair, psoriasis, adult acne, or unexplained weight gain over 10 pounds?
- Unusually poor memory, chronic insomnia, depression, irritability, chronic fatigue?
- Environmental sensitivities, especially to odors?

What benefits can you expect from a good detox?

A detox cleans out body waste deposits, so you aren't running with a dirty engine or driving with the brakes on. After a cleanse, the body starts rebalancing, energy levels rise physically, psychologically and sexually, and creativity begins to expand. You start feeling like a different person - because you are. Your outlook and attitude change, because through cleansing and improved diet, your actual cell make-up has changed.

1) Your digestive tract is cleansed of accumulated waste and fermenting bacteria.
2) Excess mucous and congestion is cleared from the body.
3) Liver, kidney and blood are purified, impossible under ordinary eating patterns.
4) Mental clarity is enhanced, impossible under chemical overload.
5) Dependency on habit-formers like sugar, caffeine, nicotine, alcohol or drugs is less.
6) Bad eating habits are often turned around; the stomach has a chance to reduce to normal size for weight control.
7) Cleansing also releases hormone secretions that coupled with essential fatty acids (EFAs), from fresh plant sources stimulate and strengthen the immune system.

What are the steps in a good detox program?

You've decided your body needs a cleanse. How long can you give out of your busy life-style to focus on a cleansing program so that all the processes can be completed? 24 hours, 2 or 3 days, or up to ten days? The time factor is important — you'll want to allot your time ahead of time, and prepare both your mind and your body for the experience ahead.

A good detox program is in 3 steps — cleansing, rebuilding and maintaining.

Years of experience with detoxification have convinced me that if you have a serious health problem, a brief 3 to 7 day juice cleanse is the best way to release toxins from the system. Shorter cleanses can't get to the root of a chronic problem. Longer cleanses upset body equilibrium more than most people are ready to deal with except in a controlled, clinical environment. A 3 to 7 day cleanse can "clean your pipes" of systemic sludge — excess mucous, old fecal matter, trapped cellular and non-food wastes, or inorganic mineral deposits that are part of arthritis.

An all-liquid diet is traditionally called a fast. It's not absolutely necessary to take only liquids, but a few days without solid food can be an enlightening experience about your lifestyle. A juice fast increases awareness and energy availability for elimination. Fresh juices literally pick up dead matter from the body and carry it away. Your body becomes easier to "hear," telling you what foods and diet are right for your needs via cravings — a desire for protein foods, or B vitamins or minerals, for example. This is natural biofeedback.

Fasting works by self-digestion. During a cleanse, the body decomposes and burns only the substances and tissues that are damaged, diseased or unneeded, such as abscesses, tumors, excess fat deposits, and congestive wastes. Even a relatively short fast accelerates elimination, often causing dramatic changes as masses of accumulated waste are expelled.

You will know your body is detoxing if you experience the short period of headaches, fatigue, body odor, bad breath, diarrhea or mouth sores that commonly accompany accelerated elimination. However, digestion usually improves right away as do many gland and nerve functions. Cleansing also helps release hormone secretions that stimulate immune response and encourages a disease-preventing environment.

What about a water fast? I don't recommend it. Here's why:

Leading nutritionists and detoxification experts agree that fresh vegetable and fruit juice cleansing is superior to water fasting. Indeed, juice cleansing is an evolution in detoxification methods. Fresh juices, broths and herb teas help deeply cleanse the body, rejuvenate the tissues and guide you to a faster recovery from health problems than water fasting.

A traditional water fast is harsh and demanding on your body, even in times before huge amounts of food and environmental toxins were part of the picture. Today, it can even be dangerous. Deeply buried pollutants and chemicals from our tissues are released into elimination channels too rapidly during a water fast. Your body is essentially "re-poisoned" as the chemicals move through the bloodstream all at once. Sometimes, the physical and emotional stress of a water fast even overrides the healing benefits.

Vegetable and fruit juices are alkalizing, so they neutralize uric acid and other inorganic acids, better than water, and increase the healing effects. Juices support better metabolic activity for fasting, too. Metabolic activity slows down during a water fast as the body attempts to conserve dwindling energy resources that further reduce productive cleansing. Juices are very easy on digestion - easily assimilated into the bloodstream. They don't disturb the detoxification process.

The first step of your cleanse is elimination. You'll be cleaning out mucous and toxins from the intestinal tract and major organs. Everything functions more effectively when toxins, obstructions and wastes are removed. Try to drink 8 glasses of water each day of your fast in addition to your juices.

The second step is rebuilding healthy tissue and restoring energy. With obstacles removed, your body's regulating powers are activated to rebuild at optimum levels. Eat only fresh and simply prepared foods during the rebuilding step. Your diet should be very low in fat, with little dairy (cottage cheese and yogurt are okay), and no fried foods. Avoid alcohol, caffeine, tobacco, and sugars. Avoid meats except fish and sea foods. Include supplements and herbal aids for your specific needs.

The final step is keeping your body clean and toxin-free—very important after all the hard work of detoxification. Modifying lifestyle habits is the key to a strong resistant body. A diet for health maintenance relies heavily on fresh fruits and vegetables for fiber, cooked vegetables, grains and seeds for strength and alkalinity, sea foods, soy foods, eggs and low fat cheeses as sources of protein, and lightly cooked sea foods and vegetables with a little dinner wine for circulatory health. A personalized group of supplements and herbal aids, as well as exercise and relaxation techniques, should be included.

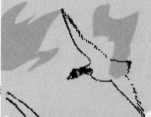

Body cleansing has many faces.

It's been a healing technique for 20,000 years!

Which detox techniques from around the world appeal to you?

Cleansing Around The World

Periodic body cleansing has been a part of human health care since mankind's ancient times. Obviously, it is a technique that works to keep our species vigorous. The following pages contain a short review of the world's traditional approaches to detoxification.

Ayurvedic Healing

Ayurvedic medicine is the world's oldest recorded healing system, in continuous use for over 5000 years. Originating on the Indian subcontinent in the practices of "Rishis," India's ancient holy men, Ayurvedic practitioners had astounding knowledge of the connections between anatomy, physiology, psychology, the use of herbs, minerals, exercise, even surgery. Their progress in the development of medicine and their success in healing reached around the ancient world, influencing the medical philosophies of the Chinese, Greeks and Romans. During India's colonial period under English rule, Ayurvedic practices were forbidden. Yet the healing knowledge was passed on and preserved. Today, once again, Ayurvedic medicine is a leading edge philosophy in world health care.

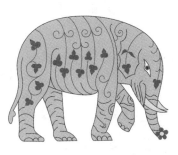

Ayurvedic healing is based on body balance for health and longevity, believing that imbalance and disharmony with the rhythms of nature are the foundation of illness.

Detoxification is a cornerstone of Ayurvedic medicine. It is believed that without proper digestion and elimination, toxins build up and disrupt body functions and body balance. There are two main forms of detoxification in Ayurveda. Both can be used in conjunction or alone for restoring health.

The first is called *Shamana*, a palliation therapy involving herbs, oils and therapeutic foods to stimulate digestion, reduce toxins, and return balance and function restoring health.

The second is *Pancha Karma*, a stronger method using massage and sweating therapy, is reserved for imbalances and diseases that are well established.

Ayurvedic practitioners use sign posts from nature to identify imbalances. Man is classified into prototypes or "doshas," based on the five natural elements of air, fire, water, earth and space (ether). The elements are believed to combine in pairs to form the doshas. Each person's emotional and body type is thought to correspond to one of the doshas.

There are three doshas:

— **Vata:** a combination of air and space elements, equated with circulation, the passage of food in the body, breathing and movement.

— **Pitta:** a combination of fire and water elements, equated with metabolism and the transformation and assimilation of nutrients.

— **Kapha:** a combination of the water and earth elements, equated to body structure like bones, tissue and muscle.

In seeking the cause and cure for an illness, an Ayurvedic healer first determines the dosha that best represents the patient's body and emotional type. While typing is not absolute, physical attributes like weight, body frame, complexion and behavior reflect the information for typing. For example: a vata type, governed by air, is thin, tall and wiry with prominent bone structure and a dull, darkish complexion. A pitta type, governed by fire, has a medium frame and weight with defined musculature and ruddy complexion. A kapha type, governed by water, is heavy to obese, with large frame and pale complexion.

However, since *"dosha"* means "that which changes," all the elements are believed to be continually balancing and changing each other. Making it even more complex, each element is also influenced by climates, seasons, stages of life, and one's thoughts and actions. A strong immune system is therefore the key to health in dealing with the constant flux of all the forces.

In Ayurvedic practice, toxins (ama) are deemed one of the main causes of disease, creating imbalances that must be resolved to restore health. When one's dosha becomes imbalanced, digestion, absorption and assimilation are disrupted. This causes the formation of ama or cellular debris which clogs cell functions and accelerates disease.

In a Pancha Karma detox, a popular spa method, five cleansing methods may be used depending on the type of imbalance to be normalized: 1) therapeutic vomiting, or emetic therapy to purge the stomach and lungs, or the use of expectorant herbs like pepper and ginger; 2) purgation, with herbs like senna and rhubarb; 3) medicated enemas, with herbs like fennel, ginger and licorice in sesame seed oil, flushed into the rectum to be absorbed through the colon and large intestine; 4) blood letting to eliminate toxic blood and stimulate production of new blood; 5) nasal and ear douching to cleanse the head and throat. Gotu kola or licorice oils in drops, cleanse and nourish the brain. Exercise, yoga, breathing techniques and meditation are highly recommended for every detox program.

In a self administered detox program, Ayurvedic practice begins with a fast of non-sweet vegetable juices — for vata types, 3 to 5 days, for pitta types, 5 to 7 days, and for kapha types, 1 to 2 weeks is recommended. Fruit juices and sweet vegetables juices like carrot juice are not used, since it is thought that sweetness increases waste deposits. Lemon juice mixed with ginger juice is a good choice. Herbal combinations like *"Trikuta,"* (black pepper, long pepper and dry ginger), or a tea of cardamom, cinnamon and ginger increase digestive fire.

Purgatives are included on the first day of the fast, and every three days following, to help clean the digestive system. Digestive bitters like rhubarb, neem, aloe vera and ginger are used. One of my favorite Ayurvedic formulas, "triphala," (a combo of amla, herada, and behera fruits), stimulates digestion gently and gradually and rejuvenates deep tissues. Steams medicated with mint or eucalyptus are used to cleanse the lungs. Diaphoretic herbs are sometimes used to promote sweating.

After the fast, a step 2 cleansing diet is begun, with fruits like lemons, grapefruits and cranberries, vegetables (except heavy roots like potatoes or sweet potatoes), and with grains like barley, or a blend of brown rice and split mung beans called *kicharee.* Oats, wheat and

other beans should be avoided. Vata types should limit the step 2 diet to one or two weeks, pitta types to three weeks, and kapha types to one to two months. Elderly, young, weak or anorexic people should avoid the step 2 diet.

After the cleansing diet is completed, a maintenance step 3 program, including a well-balanced nourishing diet, proper rest, exercise and tonifying herbs is established. The diet for this stage includes dairy products like ghee (clarified butter), butter, fruits and vegetables, beans, grains, oils like sesame, olive and avocado, and spices like garlic, pepper and curry to promote digestion. Step 3 maintenance herbs include ashwaganda (Indian ginseng), shatavari (asparagus), amla (high vitamin C berry), gotu kola (a nerve restorative) and triphala (see previous page).

Traditional Chinese Medicine

The first writings about Traditional Chinese Medicine (TCM) date back over 2000 years. The first known herbal materia medica was written during the Han dynasty between 206 B.C. and 5 A.D., and was said to be based on the emperor's personal knowledge of herbalism from nearly 2000 years before. The healing principles of TCM are bound up with the idea of yin and yang, opposing principles that represent both spiritually and physically the daily balance of universal order in Chinese philosophy. Yin and yang are thought to make up all things. Man, too is made up of yin and yang, composing his own balance of opposites for his proper place and function in the universal realm.

Chinese medicine characterizes the yin and yang opposites as harmony and disharmony in order to understand illness. When disharmony occurs, life energy cannot flow because the balance is upset. TCM assigns yin and yang designations to all body parts, essences and functions depending on their nature. Each designation is connected to an opposite organ or function by energy meridians. Between these flows the life force, or Be-Qi (chee). A TCM practitioner uses this philosophy to find the origin of an illness in order to treat it, rather than treating symptoms of the disease. Identifying the seat of the imbalance allows the TCM practitioner to use herbs and physical stimulation like acupuncture or accupressure to bring the opposites back into balance. Like Ayurveda, Chinese medicine has signposts, designating basic elements like earth, wind, fire and water to body parts, functions, and plants — then assigning qualities of heat and cold, damp and dry to help the practitioner recognize imbalances.

The Chinese belief of interconnectedness makes the TCM healing philosophy seem incredibly complex to the Western mind. Let me try to simplify it for clarity.

Yin and yang are opposites, darkness and light, hot and cold, male and female, yet elements of each are in the other. TCM identifies each vital body organ as yin or yang,

between which flows Qi or life force energy. The Qi flows are referred to as meridians and play an important part in maintaining balance in the body. The organs are influenced by the five basic elements — wood, fire, earth, metal and water. The Chinese assign a relationship of the vital organs in the body to the actions of the elements. Thus, the liver and gallbladder are connected to wood; the heart and small intestine are connected to fire; the spleen and stomach are connected to earth; the lung and large intestine are connected to metal; the kidney and bladder are connected to water. Each organ is also related to an emotion; the emotion affects the health of the organ and the organ affects the emotion.

For example, the liver is connected to anger. If a toxic condition exists in the liver it may manifest itself as anger or depression. Through the liver's meridian connection to the gall bladder, the gall bladder is adversely affected. The relationship between the elements is also compromised so that liver/wood that generates heart/fire becomes weak, jeopardizing the heart's ability to function. As imbalances become greater, farther and farther away from the original problem through their interconnection, more functions suffer.

The health and harmony connections go even further. In TCM, external conditions that cause disease are referred to as the Six Excesses, characterized as weather conditions — wind, cold, summer-heat, dampness, dryness and fire. Imbalances of these may cause immune response to weaken. For example, as spring moves into summer an unusual cold spell may hit; but the body has already geared up for warm conditions, so its resistance to cold is weak, allowing a "spring cold" virus to take hold.

The TCM practitioner has eight healing approaches to heal disease: 1) perspiration; 2) therapeutic emesis; 3) purgation; 4) neutralization; 5) stimulation; 6) heat-clearing; 7) reduction; and 8) tonic. For example, to reduce toxicity, a practitioner looks to herbs that take down inflammation and detoxify the blood or liver, reduce and move accumulated phlegm; then to tonic herbs, like ginsengs, for stagnant Qi energy, to nourish and restore balance.

When choosing herbs to treat illness, the TCM practitioner takes into account their "natures" (corresponding to the seasons — cold, hot, warm and cool), their "flavors" (describing the actions — sour, spicy, bitter, sweet and salty), and to their "directions" (movement within the body — rising, descending, floating and sinking), as well as the color and aroma of each herb. Besides their interconnectedness to the five elements and major organs, each herb has an affinity for a specific body organ that it moves and affects. Since the organs are interconnected by meridians, the opposing organ is also affected.

The idea in TCM is to achieve body balance through lifestyle means before an illness occurs — with herbs and food, physical stimulation, aroma and heat therapy, and meditation. For instance, overindulging in a particular food may cause "heat" in the body. A balancing, "cooling" food should be eaten to prevent disease.

Detox treatments provide another example — if toxicity causes heat to occur in the liver, herbs that generate cooling action are used to restore balance. Detoxification is not considered as cleansing, but rather as restoring.

In fact, the success of traditional Chinese medicine is the training its practitioners receive in recognizing symptoms before an illness occurs. Instead, prevention is the primary emphasis.

Western, science-based medicine has lost this personalized skill today, but illness symptoms may be diagnosed from changes in skin color or tone, tongue color or texture, pulse or thirst changes, unusual breath or body odor, behavior changes, etc. Diet, rest, stress, mental and spiritual health, seasons, climate and family history are also seen as major players in one's health. Time, too is a factor. Lifestyle corrections cannot take place without the time to correct lifestyle habits. Traditional Chinese Medicine sees an individual's life health as an ever-changing process of rebalancing. A TCM practitioner does not cure the symptoms to correct the cause of the illness. He is interested in how an illness acts rather than what it is, so that the origin of imbalance may be traced in order to restore harmony. Unless this process is considered, Chinese healers believe the illness will manifest again.

The Rainforest Culture

Rainforest medicine is a system largely based in shamanic tradition; much like Native American medicine, healing is interconnected with spiritual beliefs. Medicine in the rainforest is an herbally based art, not a formal system like Traditional Chinese Medicine or Ayurveda. Although there are vast areas of rainforest around the world, and herbs and beliefs vary widely, rainforest medicinal practices are similar in nature. Healing methods and rituals are still orally passed from shaman to apprentice; herbs are learned by heart. This book focuses on the traditions of the Amazon tribes whose culture extends back to the respected Mayan *curendero* or healers.

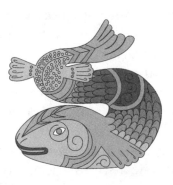

Rainforest healers never have to venture far to collect herbs for their pharmacopia. The rainforest is so rich and diverse in medicinal plants that thousands of herbal remedies lie almost literally within arm's reach. A blur to the average eye, especially to an untrained eye, each plant is easily recognizable, as a member of one's family, to the rainforest healer.

Even though the rainforest healing tradition is oral, European explorer's writings tell us that the people of the rainforests were extremely healthy (largely because of their diet of grains, fruits, vegetables and limited meats). The extent of their medicines for the few illnesses the people did have was impressive. The Europeans, who were disease-ridden in comparison, were astonished at the number of remedies available. One of the saddest commentaries of the Spanish conquest was the decimation of huge portions of the rainforest populations despite their extensive pharmacopias. (In the short time their civilizations were being destroyed or absorbed, there was no time to develop resistance or remedies for the new diseases.)

Even though it was less successful, European medicine superseded herbal knowledge,

because the Spanish used inquisition tactics to force Christianity upon the rainforest people, and Catholicism conflicted with the spiritual aspects of native healing. Only in remote rainforest areas did the traditional healing practices remain strong. Thankfully, we are beginning to rediscover them today.

Because he is the link between the earthly and spiritual worlds, the shaman, a spiritual healer, is the most powerful medicine man. Disease is seen as stemming from both physical origins and spiritual problems brought by bad spirits that inflict illness. Contact with a bad spirit, or someone who wishes another harm and uses a person of power to conjure ill will, can poison the body just as any other pathogen or pollutant. Prayers are integral to the healing response against the spiritual or emotional origins of a disease. Fortifying physical rituals are also assigned to the afflicted person to strengthen the power of the medicine. But there are many levels of healers in the rainforest tradition. Other "people of power," like the Mayan curendero, with their vast knowledge of plants, are sought to help with various aspects of a problem. Medicinal plants themselves are considered to possess a spiritual life force beyond their physical existence that may be accessed for healing. Healing spirits are often consulted through an amulet, or "sastun," about which plants to use. The healing spirit of the herbs is acknowledged through ritual or prayer, and thanked for its contribution to the restorative process.

Detoxification is also both a spiritual and a physical process. Today, detoxification is receiving a lot of attention, as even remote rainforest areas are increasingly inundated with the "western" junk food diet. The rainforest culture is being introduced to unnatural food sources and the burden that comes with them. Meanwhile, oral healing traditions are dying as young apprentices no longer want to spend years learning the thousands of herbs and their uses. Allopathic medicine is an easier option and it "comes with the territory" in the cities to which the rainforest people are migrating. With the demise of the old herbal ways goes the recognition of thousands of plants and their thousands of uses gathered over thousands of years.

Modern rainforest curenderos recognize that present day foods "are ruining people's diets, and that junk or "cuchinada" (pig food) is at the root of most patients' ailments, and getting worse. Foods full of chemicals and preservatives have made a people who had almost no instance of civilization diseases, more vulnerable to high blood pressure, heart disease, arthritis, diabetes, and cancer.

We can only hope that we learn from the Spanish conquest of centuries ago, that ancient wisdom will prevail. Unfortunately, we know the "chemical food equals disease" scenario all too well. It has happened over the last 50 years in China, Japan and Southeast Asia, where western food products have brought more disease to more people than all the wars fought there.

Detoxification and cleansing methods are largely plant based. Herbs are used for both their physical healing properties and for their purifying power. The herbs chosen are tailored to the individual and condition being treated. For example, to cleanse the body of "modern food disease," Balsam bark tea is used to detoxify the kidney and the liver.

Here is a small sampling of detox remedies currently in use:

—Purgative herbs to correct digestive problems abound throughout the rainforest tradition. Chewing gum is a favorite method of delivery.

—A yearly parasite cleanse is commonly followed in almost every rainforest healing system, sometimes with oje *(ficus insipida)*.

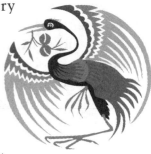

—Liver cleansing is common, with teas like aguacate *(persea gratissima)*, assacurana *(erythrina glauca)* or the bark of the Brazil nut tree *(bertholletia excelsa)*. Trumpet tree may be combined with papaya as a liver or kidney tonic during a cleanse.

—Stinking toe *(senna grandis)*, and China root *(smilax lanceolata)* are used to rid the blood and tissues of toxins and to help the body recover from toxicity resulting in fatigue and anemia.

—Blood purifying rituals use gumbolimbo *(bursera simaruba)*, jack-ass bitters *(neurolaena lobata)*, or purslane *(portulaca oleracea)*, to flush the kidneys, and to fight infections. The fresh juice from jack-ass bitters is used on the skin to heal sores and fungal infections.

Heat therapy herbal steam baths, are a respected detox practice in the rainforest to sweat out toxins. Green stick *(eupatorium morifolium)* leaves are used as a healing steam for skin conditions, flus and fevers. Steamed herbs like trumpet tree *(cecropia peltata)* or pheasant tail *(anthurium schlechtendalii)* are applied for relief from arthritic conditions and sprains.

Massage and palpation are widely used during cleansing. A skilled therapist can even move a misplaced organ to its correct setting through massage therapy. I have witnessed this phenomenon myself during a session with a Guatemalan healer.

The Native American Tradition

Native American religious and philosophical beliefs centered, as with all early human civilizations, on the idea that mankind was a part of the cosmic balance of all living things. Balance meant universal harmony and health; disruption of the balance meant illness, drought, famine, death. Respect for all life was very important— permission was even asked of plants before picking them. Indians believe that what is needed is provided. Taking too much, or more than one needed, was considered to deplete the Earth, disrupt the balance, and create bad energy.

Health in the Native American view signifies harmony and balance between the human and the supernatural world, a natural human condition given to each individual at birth. Disease was, and is today, believed due to spiritual disharmony.

Native American healing practices are often similar to rainforest medicine traditions. Healing ideas are related to spiritual beliefs. Native Americans also include bad spirits as pathogens inducing illness. As with the rainforest cultures, modern circumstances have made it difficult for Native American healing practices to flourish. Unlike rainforest cultures, Native Americans divide diseases into white man categories and Indian categories, believing that their cleansing and healing methods work only for their own people and their own health conditions. Diseases they deem as originating from the white man and the white American way of life are treated by allopathic medicine.

Still, although it's not publicized in the "white world," Native American medicine is experiencing a renaissance, especially in healing through body purification. Healing methods once again reflect the philosophy that everything is all one with both mind and spirit stimulating the healing process and cleansing actions. Purity of mind and soul are once again considered the way to good health. Purification rituals as always address all of life. Body detoxification for instance, clears out both bad influences and spirits as well as toxins. In the well-known sweat lodges, both spiritual cleansing and body cleansing take place. While the high heat helps the body kill bacteria and viruses, sweating helps the skin release toxins. Aromatherapy from the burning of cleansing herbs like cedar and sage stimulates body functions, and prayers carry the purifying herbal smoke to the creator.

Sweat lodges were first famous as cleansing places for purification prior to religious rituals, hunting, or war. It was felt that men's and women's cleansing needs were different, and they had separate sweat lodges. As social norms changed, the purpose of the sweat lodge changed to cleaning out impurities and toxins for physical as well as spiritual health. The act of sweating became the ritual instead of a precursor. Men and women used the same lodge.

Herbs were the primary cleanser and healers used in the sweat lodges. Body parts were often wrapped with an herb, then held over hot coals to allow the herb and heat combination to act upon the disease. Sage was the favorite herb in the sweat lodge, both as a sacred plant to drive out bad spirits, and as a body cleansing herb. It was spread on the floor of the lodge, made into cleansing poultices and rubbed on the body, and burned in spaces thought to be contaminated by communicable diseases.

Smudging — slowly burning bundles of fresh sage, sweetgrass, cedar or other herbs that draw in good influences, is a Native American cleansing ritual popular everywhere today. The herbal smoke is gathered in the hands, inhaled, rubbed on the body, then carried throughout a house or other space to cleanse it. Chanting or prayers are spoken or sung along with the smudging.

An interesting form of cleansing, practiced throughout Native American healing, is a shamanic extraction — the cleansing of a foreign object (like a rock, stick or bone piece) left

by a bad spirit or supernatural force. The objects are felt to be the cause of major illnesses, and must be found and removed to heal the afflicted person. Extraction takes place after a shaman journeys into the soul of the ill person either through trance or in dreams, and sees the disease. Then through a process of sucking, either with the mouth directly on the spot of the illness, or by using a hollow stick, or laying on of hands, or a sacred feather to sweep it away, the offending object is removed and destroyed. Herbs are sometimes applied to aid the extraction process. While to white Americans, this type of spiritual cleansing may seem to be based on the powers of suggestion alone, to the Native American it is as real and effective as a massage for stiff muscles.

Native Americans considered medicinal herbs as primary healing foods to restore body balance in order to restore normal health. The spring body cleanse popular in America today has its roots in Native American cleanses that celebrate the spirit of new growth and the rhythm of life with spring herbal elixirs. Slowly, the powerful effective healing ways of our Native American culture are becoming known and available to everyone who wishes to seek them out and incorporate them into an alternative medicinal approach for good health.

European Detox Techniques

Since the early middle ages, the power of the Catholic Church and its controlling influence has been extreme in Europe. Through the Church, Christian beliefs connected illness to evil, and often dealt with it through exorcisms. The idea that an illness could be the result of a natural antigen was considered blasphemy and repressed through fear. As a result, medicines and detoxification treatments for illness were slower than in other healing traditions.

The first inklings about the physical nature of illness did not develop until well into the Renaissance when man began to understand Nature as science. Thus, assigning meaning to the mystery of disease took a scientific rather than a spiritual turn.

Still, detoxification techniques had long been known. The Roman penchant for cleansing baths had been established throughout Europe. Many of the best spa locations today have been in use since Roman times. The hot springs connected to health in Scandinavian countries led to discoveries about the benefits of mineral waters, mud baths, and overheating therapy as body cleansers.

During medieval times, hot, sulphurous-smelling water boiling from the hot springs was thought to come from the devil. Yet, at the same time, there was the search for the Fountain of Youth, (an offshoot of the quest for the Holy Grail), where waters bubbled forth from the earth that could reverse the aging process or offer immortality. Eventually this idea lead to the development of therapeutic spas where special treatments were aimed at detoxifying, rejuvenating organs and overall health.

Over the last 200 years spas have developed more precise treatments. A German clergyman, Sebastian Kneipp who believed that mind, body, and spirit were all integral to health, refined many of the spa techniques used today. His therapies focused on the cause of illness, enhancing the body's natural defenses and establishing patterns for disease prevention. Kniepp suffered from tuberculosis declared incurable by allopathic medicine, yet he treated himself successfully using hot and cold hydrotherapy to improve his circulation and stimulate his immune system.

Today, spas treat psychosomatic exhaustion, recuperation from illness or postoperative conditions (with follow-up rehabilitation treatment), and support treatments for cardiovascular diseases, rheumatic disorders, metabolic imbalances, digestive tract afflictions, respiratory diseases, neurological illness, male and female hormone disturbances, childhood diseases, allergies and hypersensitive reactions.

Their programs incorporate herbal remedies, hot and cold hydrotherapy, massage, aromatherapy, special cleansing diets and exercise. Mineral mud baths and ionized hydro-treatments are popular. Herbal packs and wraps are especially used for detoxifying and cleansing effects and for long-term immune stimulation.

In fact, today, in some European countries, a "spa tune-up" is considered preventive health care, part of the general health care program. In German and Austrian Kur spas (derived from the Latin *cura* meaning care), where I worked in the early sixties there were specific spas for specific ailments, even spas to detoxify specific body parts, like the liver.

Nutrition is a focus at the spas. I worked in the spa kitchens part of my time there, and knew well the saying that "If the father of a disease is unknown, its mother will always be false nutrition." Customized therapeutic nutrition counseling, juice fasting and vegetarian diets are provided to guests for diet balance and correction based on individual needs.

Bodywork as part of the cleansing process ranges from massage therapies to tailored exercise programs like yoga, stretching and hydro-exercises to improve circulation, oxygen uptake, structural support and psychological well being. Hiking, walking, and cross-country skiing in the winter months, are encouraged.

Emotional harmony is treated as the glue binding the detoxification therapies together. Relaxation techniques, like yoga, breathing exercises, creativity exercises, autogenic training and psychological counseling are used to focus and unburden the mind so the soul and body can harmonize.

Many European spas are located in mountain settings where the clear air, aromatherapy from plants and springs, and the serenity offered by abundant trees promote better rest. (Strict noise restriction laws halt auto traffic near the spas in the afternoons and at night to improve sleep.)

Detoxing is lifestyle therapy.

Bodywork is a big part of
body cleansing.
Let your body help you detox!

This chapter has step-by-step
instructions for over thirty
different exercises, bodywork
procedures and relaxation
techniques you can use to
accelerate your detox.

Bodywork For Detoxification

Exercise has significant influence on detoxification.

—Exercise speeds up removal of toxins through perspiration. Sweating helps expel toxins through the skin, your body's largest organ of elimination. Exercising to the point of perspiration offers overheating therapy benefits, too. Tests show that when athletes sweat, for example, they excrete potential cancer causing elements, like heavy metals and pesticide PCBs from their bodies through perspiration.

—Exercise stimulates removal of toxins through deep breathing. Low impact aerobics help build a stronger diaphragm and elasticize your lungs.

—Exercise stimulates metabolism, especially before you eat, to aid in weight loss. Exercise uses up stored body fat. Calories are burned at a greater pace for several hours after you exercise.

—Exercise stimulates 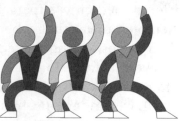 **the circulatory system,** lowering blood pressure and pre- venting heart disease by in- creasing blood flow. New heart endurance tests show exercise strengthens your circulatory system right down to your cap- illaries.... even forming new ones!

—Exercise stimulates the lymphatic systems. Blood is pumped through your body by your heart, but **lymphatic fluid depends solely on exercise for circulation.** Lymph function is critical to your body's ability to cleanse itself.

—Exercise reduces stress by increasing body oxygen levels. It improves your mood while you purify. Endorphins, the body's "feel good" hormones, are released into the brain by vigorous exercise, explaining the "high" people often experience after exercise.

—Exercise prevents disease. We know disease often results from an underactive body. Almost any kind of exercise transports oxygen and nutrients to your cells while it carries away toxins and wastes to your elimination organs.

Here are my exercise recommendations for your cleanse:

1) During initial, heavy cleansing — simple, body-balancing, stretching exercises.

2) During the rest of your cleanse — low-impact, aerobic exercise, like a walk or an easy swim for better circulation and lymph activity.

3) For your maintenance program, strengthening exercise (like a daily walk, swim or equipment workout). A moderate exercise program that raises your heart rate for a period of 20 to 30 minutes offers the most benefits.

31

Overheating therapy is an ancient cleansing technique.

Overheating therapy, or hyperthermia as a healing technique, has been known throughout history, from ancient Greek physicians (who raised body temperature as an immune defense against infection), to the elaborate bath complexes of the Romans, to the sweat lodges of the American Indians and the steam baths of the Scandinavians.

Today, high heat procedures, like overheating baths, saunas and steam rooms are experiencing new popularity as people realize their enormous benefits for health. Slightly raising body temperature speeds up metabolism, inhibits the growth of harmful viruses or bacteria, and literally burns out invading organisms. Overheating your body stimulates a slight fever. Fever is a traditional powerful healing tool against disease — a natural defense and healing force created by the immune system to rid the body of harmful pathogens.

Ancient herbalists used heat-producing herbs as protective healing measures against colds and simple infections, even against serious degenerative diseases like cancers. Today, artificially induced fevers are used in many bio-holistic clinics for treating acute infectious diseases, arthritic conditions, skin disorders and leukemia. The newest research indicates that AIDS and other virus syndromes respond to blood heating.

Despite skepticism by conventional medicine, supergerms like the HIV virus, that have no effective counteractive drug therapies, mean that other methods must be tried. In 1997, CNN Health News reported on a blood-overheating procedure for AIDS in treating Kaposi's sarcoma, a cancer that produces severe skin lesions in HIV-infected patients. The sores vanished in about four months after the therapy, along with other symptoms. Since then, many AIDS sufferers with sarcoma have undergone hypothermia with success. In some cases, the blood has even tested negative for the HIV virus! (Researchers warn that even if the blood tests free of HIV, the virus may still be in the bone and resurface.)

Here's how overheating therapy works as a detoxification mechanism:
When exposed to heat, blood vessels in the skin dilate to allow more blood to flow to the surface, activating the sweat glands, which then pour the water onto the skin's surface. As the water evaporates from the skin, it draws both heat and toxins from the body, becoming a natural detoxification treatment as well as a cooling system.

Modern health care professionals are finding that a non-life-threatening fever can do exceptional healing work. Simple overheating therapy can even be effectively practiced in your home, via either a dry sauna or an overheating bath. Both are able to stimulate the body's immune mechanism without the stress of fever-inducing drugs.

Here's how to take an overheating bath:
1) Do not eat for two hours before treatment. Empty your bladder and colon if possible.
2) Get a good thermometer so that your water temperature can be correctly measured. I recommend monitoring bath temperature at all times.
3) Use a large tub if possible. Plug the emergency outlet to raise the water to the top of the tub. You must be totally immersed for therapeutic results - with only nose, eyes and mouth left

uncovered. Start slowly running water at skin temperature. After 15 minutes raise temperature to 100°F, then in 15 minutes to 103°F. Even though the water temperature is not high, heat cannot escape from your body when you are totally covered, so body temperature will rise to match that of the water, creating a slight healing fever.

4) A therapeutic bath should be about 45 minutes. If you experience any discomfort, sit up in the tub for 5 minutes.

5) Gentle massaging with a skin brush during the bath stimulates circulation, brings cleansing blood to the surface of the skin, and relieves the heart from undue pressure.

A sauna is another way to use overheating therapy principles. Sauna therapy was developed in Finland, but today it is used all over the world by alternative physicians and clinics to help people release environmental toxins like pesticides and heavy metals. A 30 to 40 minute sauna induces a healing, cleansing fever, and also causes profuse therapeutic sweating. A good sweat uses the skin as a "third kidney" to eliminate body wastes through perspiration. Finish each sauna with a cool shower and a brisk rubdown to remove toxins that have been eliminated through the skin.

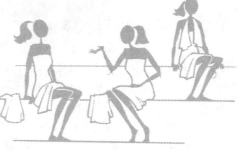

Like an overheating therapy bath, a sauna speeds up metabolism, and inhibits the replication of pathogenic organisms. It stimulates vital organs and glands to increased activity. It dramatically increases by profuse sweating the detoxifying and cleansing capacity of the skin. (For optimum skin cleansing and restoration, take a sauna once or twice a week.) Immune response is enhanced and its healing functions are accelerated.

Here's a quick overview of the cleansing benefits of a dry sauna:
- It creates a fever that inhibits the replication of pathogenic bacteria and viruses.
- It increases the number of leukocytes in the blood to strengthen the immune system.
- It provides a prolonged, therapeutic sweat that flushes out toxins and heavy metals.
- It accelerates cardiovascular activity and reduces high blood pressure.
- It stimulates vasodilation of peripheral blood vessels to relieve pain and speed healing of sprains, bursitis, arthritis and muscle pain.
- It promotes relaxation and a feeling of well-being.

Steam baths go back to prehistoric steaming hot springs of our first ancestors. Early man, like primates today in both Japan and Russia, used hot springs to clean and warm themselves, and to remove parasites.

Just as with dry heat saunas, ancient Greeks and Romans used them to sweat for health. But the benefits for a steam bath are different than for a sauna. Hot steam particularly helps respiratory diseases and rheumatic pain. The humid heat of a steam bath is ideal for skin tone and texture.

A steam bath works quicker than a sauna, cleansing the body in about 15 minutes compared to 30 to 40 minutes in a sauna. The powerful detoxification, healing process of hyperthermia does not take place until the body reaches 101-103° F. In a dry heat sauna,

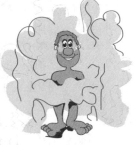

your body's cooling mechanism retards hyperthermia by natural evaporation. In a steam bath, evaporation is not possible so there is no loss of body heat. In fact, steam condensation actually becomes the heat transfer mechanism on the body.

Note: Overheating is one of the most effective treatments in natural healing. Inducing a "fever" is a natural, constructive means the body also uses to heal itself. Yet, heat methods are powerful and should be used with care. If you are under medical supervision for heart disease or high blood pressure, a heart and general vitality check is advisable. If you are ill, or have been recently, supervision is necessary during an overheating bath and reactions must be monitored closely. The pulse should not go over 130 or 140. In addition, some people who are seriously ill lose the ability to perspire; this should be known before using overheating therapy. Check with your physician to determine if overheating therapy from a sauna or a seaweed bath is all right for you.

A detox bath is pleasant, easy and stress free.

Holistic healing clinics and spas are famous all over the world for their therapeutic baths. They use mineral clays, aromatherapy oils, seaweeds and enzyme herbs to draw toxins out of the body through the skin, and to put restorative, healing nutrients into the body through the skin.

During a detox program, I recommend a therapy bath at least twice daily to remove toxins coming out on the skin. The procedure for taking an effective healing bath is important. In essence, you soak in an herbal tea, where the skin takes in the healing nutrients instead of the mouth and digestive system.

There are two good ways to take a therapeutic bath:
1) Draw very hot bath water. Put the herbs, seaweeds, or mineral crystals into a large teaball or muslin bath bag. Add mineral salts directly to the water. Steep until water cools and is aromatic. Rub the body with the solids in the muslin bag during the bath.
OR
2) Make a strong tea infusion in a large teapot, strain and add to hot bath water. Soak as long as possible to give the body time to absorb the healing properties.

Note: Food grade 35% H_2O_2 may be used as a detoxifying bath to increase tissue oxygen via the skin. Use $1\frac{1}{2}$ cups to a tub of water; or, add $\frac{1}{2}$ cup H_2O_2, $\frac{1}{2}$ cup sea salt, and $\frac{1}{2}$ cup baking soda to bath, and soak for $\frac{1}{2}$ hour.

• Before a therapeutic bath, dry brush your body all over for 5 minutes with a natural bristle, dry skin brush to remove toxins from the skin and open pores for nutrients.

• After a bath, use a mineral salt rub, such as Crystal Star LEMON BODY GLOW™, a traditional spa "finishing" technique to make your skin feel healthy for hours.

Thalassotherapy uses the sea for cleansing and health.

Thalassotherapy is another ageless, cleansing, health-restorative technique. *Thalassa* is the ancient Greek word for sea. The Greeks indeed used the sea for their well-being. I myself have seen 2500 year-old healing sites on the Greek islands of Rhodes and Corfu, and the ancient Greek healing center at Pergamum in what is now Turkey. Even judging by the therapeutic centers still known to us, much of the population of the ancient Greek and Roman world soaked in sea water hot tubs and heated seaweed baths, drank and inhaled sea water for health, got sea water massages, had seaweed facials and body wraps and used sea water pools for hydrotherapy and detoxification. Today, we are learning once again, about the ability of the sea to reduce tension and de-stress our bodies, detoxify the skin and improve circulation, relieve allergies, sinus and chest congestion, and ease arthritis symptoms.

Seaweed baths are Nature's perfect body/psyche balancer. Remember how good you feel after an ocean walk? Seaweeds purify and balance the ocean — they can do the same for your body. A hot seaweed bath is like a wet-steam sauna, only better, because the sea greens balance body chemistry instead of dehydrating it. The electromagnetic action of the seaweed releases excess body fluids from congested cells, and dissolves fatty wastes through the skin, replacing them with depleted minerals, especially potassium and iodine. Iodine boosts thyroid activity, so food fuels are used before they can turn into fatty deposits. Vitamin K in seaweeds boosts adrenal activity, meaning that a seaweed bath can help maintain hormone balance for a more youthful body.

Taking a seaweed bath even once a week stimulates lymphatic drainage and fat burning so you can keep off excess weight, reduce cellulite and rid your body of toxins.

Here is how to take a hot seaweed bath:

If you live near the ocean, gather kelp and seaweeds from the water, (not the shoreline) in clean buckets or trash cans, and carry them home to your tub. If you don't live near the ocean, dried seaweeds are available in most health food stores. Crystal Star Herbal Nutrition (ph. 800-736-6015) packages dried seaweeds, gathered from the pristine waters around the San Juan islands, in a made-to-order Hot Seaweed Bath™.

Whichever form you choose, run very hot water over the seaweed in a tub, filling it to the point that you will be covered when you recline. The leaves (whether dried or fresh) will turn a beautiful bright green. The water will turn

rich brown as the plants release their minerals. Add an aromatherapy bath oil if desired, to help hold the heat in and boost your cleansing program. Let the bath cool enough to get in. As you soak, the gel from the seaweed will transfer onto your skin. This coating increases perspiration to release system toxins, and replaces them with minerals by osmosis. Rub your skin with the seaweed during the bath to stimulate circulation, smooth the body, and remove wastes coming out on the skin surface. When the sea greens have done their work, the gel coating dissolves and floats off the skin, and the seaweeds shrivel - a sign that the bath is over. Each bath varies with the individual, the seaweeds used, and water temperature, but the gel coating release is a natural timekeeper for the bath. Forty-five minutes is usually long enough to balance body pH, encourage liver activity and fat metabolism. Skin tone, color, and circulatory improvement are almost immediately noticeable. After the bath, take a capsule of cayenne and ginger to assimilate the seaweed minerals.

Don't have time for a bath? Seaweed facials are great tonics for your skin.

The ancient Greeks said that Aphrodite, the goddess of love, rising out of the foaming sea, owed her supple skin, shiny hair, and sparkling eyes to the plants of the sea. In fact, human body makeup is a lot like that of the ocean, so taking in things from the sea can help replace nutrients we may have lost. Seaweed contains huge quantities of minerals that stress and pollution deplete from your skin. The structure of seaweed cells allows your skin to easily absorb and assimilate those minerals.

If your skin has poor tone, a seaweed facial or mask can stimulate lymphatic drainage and dilate capillaries to tone your skin. Seaweed also has mineral salts that help your skin hold its moisture better. When your skin retains moisture it plumps up, smoothing out those fine lines and wrinkles. Some seaweeds also have molecules similar to collagen that make the skin more supple and elastic, and add amazing luster. Most people report better skin texture after a seaweed treatment.

Thalassotherapy seaweed wraps are premier restorative body conditioners.

Top European and American spas use seaweed wraps to rapidly cleanse the body of toxins, and to elasticize and tone the skin. As with all sea treatments, the sea herb and mineral solution easily penetrates through the millions of pores of your skin to break down and shrink unwanted fatty cells and cellulite deposits stored in the fluids between cells. Wraps are most successful when used along with a short detox program that includes 8 glasses of water a day to flush out the loosened fats and wastes.

I have seen almost miraculous benefits from thalassotherapy wraps during my work in the European spas and with sea herbs. The results were so amazing I even formulated two wraps for health food stores to sell for home use — Crystal Star (ph. 800-736-6015), a TIGHTENING & TONING™ wrap to improve muscle, vein and skin tone, and an ALKALIZING ENZYME™ wrap to replace important minerals, enhance metabolism and balance system pH.

Water therapy helps your cleanse in almost every way.

Hot and cold hydrotherapy helps open and stimulate the body's vital healing energies. Alternating hot and cold showers, are effective for improving circulation, relieving throbbing and cramping, toning muscles, relaxing bowel and bladder tightness, and boosting energy. The form of hydrotherapy below is easy and convenient for home use.

• Begin with a comfortably hot shower for three minutes. Follow with a sudden change to cold water for 2 minutes. Repeat this cycle three times, ending with cold. Follow with a full or partial massage, or a brisk towel rub and mild stretching exercises for best results.

What are ozone pools? How do they help your body purify? Ozone, or "activated oxygen" (O_3) is the fresh, clean scent you smell in the air after a thunderstorm. Ozone is the most powerful natural oxidizer available and one of the fastest, safest and most thorough methods of purification known. Professional spas use ozone pools in their detox treatments today to destroy water and airborne viruses, cysts, bacteria and fungi on contact.

Ozone pool baths are actually the next generation of oxygen baths that you can use in your own home detox plan. They noticeably increase energy and tissue oxygen uptake.

Take an oxygen bath once a day each day of your cleanse. Here's how:
Start with a food grade 35% hydrogen peroxide. Pour in about 1 cup per bath. Oxygen baths are stimulating rather than relaxing. Most people notice a significant energy increase within 3 days. Other therapeutic benefits include body balance and detoxification, reduction of skin cancers and tumors, clearing of asthma and lung congestion, and arthritis and rheumatism relief.

If you like herbal therapy, certain herbs used in a bath can supply oxygen through the skin. Rosemary is one of the best and most popular; peppermint and mullein are also effective. Just pack a small muslin bath or tea bag with the herb, drop it into the tub or spa, and soak for 15 to 20 minutes. Use the bag as a skin scrub during the bath for skin smoothing and tone.

A baking soda alkalizing bath is a simple but remarkable therapeutic treatment for detoxification. It is especially helpful if you suffer from too little sleep, high stress, too much alcohol, caffeine or nicotine, chronic colds or flu, or over-medication. Baking soda balances an over-acid system leaving you refreshed and invigorated, with extra soft skin.

Here's how to take a baking soda bath:
Fill the bath with enough pleasantly hot water to cover you when you recline. Add 8-oz. baking soda and swirl to dissolve. Soak for 20 to 30 minutes. When you emerge, wrap up in a big thick towel or a blanket and lie down for 15 minutes to help overcome any feelings of weakness or dizziness that might occur from the heat and rapid toxin release. Zia Wesley-Hosford of Z-Line Natural Cosmetics recommends this rest time for a face mask, since the hot water will have opened up the pores for maximum benefits.

An arthritis elimination sweating bath can release a surprising amount of toxic material that aggravate your joints. Epsom salts or Dead Sea salts, and herbs with a diaphoretic action, can play a big part in the success of the bath.

Here's how to take the arthritis bath:

Make a tea of elder flowers, peppermint and yarrow. Drink as hot as possible before the bath. Then pour about 3 pounds of Epsom salts or enough Dead Sea salts for 1 bath into very hot bath water. Rub arthritic joints with a stiff brush in the water for 5 to 10 minutes; try to stay in the bath for 15 to 25 minutes. On emerging, do not dry yourself. Wrap up immediately in a clean sheet and go straight to bed, covering yourself with several blankets. The osmotic pressure of the Epsom salt solution absorbed by the sheet will draw off heavy perspiration. Your mattress should be protected with a sheet of plastic. The following morning the sheet will be stained with wastes excreted through your skin - sometimes the color of egg yolk. (This is a strong detox procedure and it happens relatively quickly. Take care if you have a weak heart or high blood pressure.)

Improvement after an arthritic sweat bath experience is notable. Repeat the bath once every two weeks until the sheet is no longer stained, a sign that the body is well cleansed. Drink pure water throughout the procedure to prevent dehydration and loss of body salts.

A sitz bath puts herbal help where you need it most.

A sitz bath is a healing technique for increasing circulation in the pelvic and urethral area It's a good way to relieve anal and vaginal irritations, and improve the pelvic muscle tone of those suffering with incontinence (a fast growing group of people in America). The best sitz baths combine herbs known for their astringent, antiseptic, emollient, and hemostatic properties that will assist the natural healing process. Sitz baths help women recover from hemorrhoids and vaginal infections. They can help men strengthen the prostate/urinary and anal area.

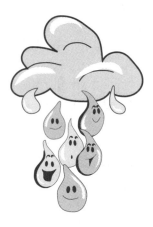

Here's how to take a sitz bath:

For a cold sitz bath, use cold water at temperatures ranging from 40° to 85°F. Make a strong, strained tea with your choice of herbs; a good combination includes herbs like goldenseal root, marshmallow root, plantain, juniper berry, saw palmetto berry, slippery elm and witch hazel leaf. Add the tea to 3" of water in a tub. Soak in the bath for 5 minutes with enough water to reach your navel, once a day for 5 minutes until healed. Use the strained herbs as a compress on the affected area.

OR

For a hot sitz bath, start with water about 100° and increase the heat by letting hot water drip continuously into the tub until the temperature reaches about 112°. The water should cover your hips when seated. Place your feet at the faucet end of the tub so that they are soaking in slightly hotter water as the water drips in. Cover your upper body with a towel, and your forehead with a cool, wet washcloth. After 20 or 30 minutes, take a quick, cool rinse in the shower, or splash the body with cool water before drying off to further stimulate circulation. Add Epsom salts, Breh or Batherapy bath salts, ginger powder, comfrey or chamomile to the bath water for therapeutic results.

Enemas use water flushing to cleanse your insides.

Enemas are an important part of a congestion cleansing detox. They release old, encrusted colon waste, discharge parasites, freshen the G.I. tract and make the cleansing process easier and more thorough. Enemas accelerate any cleanse for optimum results. They are especially helpful during a healing crisis, after a serious illness to speed healing, or to remove drug residues. Migraines and skin problems like psoriasis are relieved with enemas.

Adding herbs to the enema water serves to immediately alkalize the bowel area, control irritation and inflammation, and provide healing action to ulcerated or distended tissue.

Herbs for specific enemas. Use two cups strong brewed tea to 1-qt. water per enema.

—Garlic helps kill parasites, harmful bacteria, and cleanses mucous congestion. Blend 6 garlic cloves in 2 cups water and strain. For small children, use 1 clove garlic to 1 pint water.

—Catnip is effective for stomach and digestive conditions, and for childhood diseases. Use 2 cups of very strong brewed tea to 1-qt. of water.

—Pau d'arco normalizes body pH, especially against immune deficient diseases like chronic yeast and fungal infections. Use 2 cups of very strong brewed tea to 1-qt. of water.

—Spirulina helps detoxify both blood and bowels. Use 2 TBS. powder to 1-qt. water.

—Lobelia counteracts food poisoning, especially if vomiting prevents antidote herbs being taken by mouth.

—Aloe vera heals tissues in cases of hemorrhoids, irritable bowel and diverticulitis.

—Lemon juice rapidly neutralizes an acid system, cleanses the colon and bowel.

—Acidophilus relieves gas, yeast infections and candidiasis. Mix 4-oz. powder in 1-qt. water.

—Coffee enemas detoxify the liver, stimulating both liver and gallbladder to remove toxins, open bile ducts, increase peristaltic action, and produce enzyme activity for healthy red blood cell formation and oxygen uptake. Use 1 cup of regular strong brewed coffee to 1-qt. water. Also often effective for migraine headaches.

Here's the procedure for an effective detox enema:

Place warm enema solution in an enema bag. Hang the bag about 18 inches higher than the body. Attach the colon tube, and lubricate its attachment with vaseline or vitamin E oil. Expel a little water to let out air bubbles. Lying on your left side, slowly insert the attachment about 3 inches into the rectum. Never use force. Rotate attachment gently to ease insertion. Remove kinks in the tubing so liquid will flow freely. Massage abdomen, or flex and contract stomach muscles to relieve any cramping. When all solution has entered the colon, slowly remove the tube and remain on the left side for 5 minutes. Then move to a knee-chest position with your body weight on your knees and one hand. Use the other hand to massage the lower left side of the abdomen for several minutes.

Massage loosens old fecal matter. Roll onto your back for 5 minutes, massaging up the descending colon, over the transverse colon to the right side and down the ascending colon. Then move onto your right side for 5 minutes, in order to reach each part of the colon. Get up and quickly expel into the toilet. Sticky grey/brown mucous, small dark crusty chunks or tough ribbony pieces are usually loosened and expelled during an enema. These poisonous looking things are obstacles and toxins interfering with normal body functions. An enema removes them from you. You may have to take several enemas until there is no more evidence of these substances.

Fresh wheatgrass juice enemas stimulate the liver to cleanse. Wheatgrass enema nutrients are absorbed by the hemorrhoidal vein, just inside the anal sphincter, then circulate to the liver where they increase peristaltic action of the colon, and attract waste and old fecal matter like a magnet to be eliminated from the body. Wheatgrass juice tones the colon and is absorbed into the blood, adding oxygen and energy to the body.

—Use pure water for an initial enema rinse of the colon.

—Then use about a cup of water to 4 ounces of fresh wheatgrass juice.

—Hold the juice for ten minutes while massaging colon area. Then, expel.

Herbal implants are concentrated enema solutions for more serious health problems, like colitis, arthritis or prostate inflammation. Prepare for an implant by taking a small enema to clear out the lower bowel. You'll be able to hold the implant longer.

Mix 2 TBS. herbal powder like spirulina, or wheat grass in $\frac{1}{2}$ cup water. Lubricate the tip of a syringe with vaseline or vitamin E oil, get down on your hands and knees and insert the nozzle into the rectum. Squeeze the bulb to insert the mixture, but do not release pressure on the bulb before withdrawing, so the mixture stays in the lower bowel. Hold 15 minutes before expelling.

A colonic irrigation is a "super enema."

I have used both colonics and enemas in detox programs. Benefits are matter of degree but they're dramatically different, both in terms of waste removed and body improvement.

Your colon is over five feet long. If you want to cleanse all of it you need a colonic irrigation. Here's how a colonic works. A colonic irrigation uses special equipment and gravity (or oxygen for more control) to give your colon an internal bath. The person receiving the colonic lies on a special colema-board which is about three feet below the temperature-controlled water flow. A sterilized speculum is gently inserted in the rectum. Under the control of the practitioner, a steady flow of water gently flows from a small water tube. There is no discomfort, no internal pressure, just a steady gentle water flow in and then out of the colon through the evacuation tube, carrying with it impacted feces and mucous. Unlike an enema, a colonic irrigation does not involve the retention of water. As the water flows out of the colon the practitioner gently massages the abdomen to help the colon release its contents, recover its natural shape, tone, and normalize peristaltic wave action. A view tube is available for observation and all colonic matter is contained in the equipment. You do nothing but lie back and relax while the entire colon is cleansed.

A colonic irrigation uses about 40 gallons of water and takes about forty-five minutes. The colonic procedure is not offensive, nor painful. The first things most people feel after a colonic irrigation is a sense of lightness, energy and an improved sense of well-being. Skin condition, digestion and immune response improve. Body odor and bad breath essentially disappear, as does belly distension.

Colonics are best done in the evening so that you can relax and retire for healing rest. For a best results take a green drink before and after the colonic.

Bentonite Clay Colonic Cleanse:

Bentonite clay is a mineral substance with powerful absorption qualities; it can pull out suspended impurities in the body. It helps prevent proliferation of pathogenic organisms and parasites, and sets up an environment for rebuilding healthy tissue. It is effective for lymph congestion, cellulitic fatty tissue, blood cleansing and reducing toxicity from environmental pollutants. It may be used orally, anally, or vaginally. It works like an internal poultice, drawing out toxic materials, then draining and eliminating them through evacuation. *Note:* Bentonite clay packs are also effective applied topically to varicose veins and arthritic areas.

1.   To take bentonite as an enema, mix $\frac{1}{2}$ cup clay to an enema bag of water. Use 5 to 6 bags for each enema set to replace a colonic. Follow normal enema procedure, or the directions with your enema apparatus.

2. Massage across the abdomen while expelling toxic waste into the toilet.

Muscle kinesiology is a Traditional Chinese Medicine technique being rediscovered in America.

The word kinesiology means the study of motion, especially how muscles act to move the body. In the natural health field, kinesiology uses principles from Chinese medicine, acupressure and massage to bring the body into balance and release pain and tension.

Applied kinesiology is based on the premise that muscle, glands, and organs are linked by meridians, or energy pathways in the body. Muscle testing is the way most Americans are familiar with applied kinesiology today. Muscle testing is an effective and versatile method for detecting and correcting various energy movements and imbalances in the body.

Muscle testing identifies weak muscles. Weak muscles indicate an energy flow blockage in a body meridian. A kinesiologist uses stress release techniques to unblock the meridians. The muscles are then retested after visualization, massage techniques and movement exercises; if the muscles have regained strength, the restoration of the energy flow of the meridians is confirmed. Kinesiology does not heal, but rather restores balanced energy flow.

You can use personal muscle testing to determine your own individual response to a food or substance. It's a good technique to use before buying a healing remedy, because it lets you estimate the product's effectiveness for your own body before you buy. You will need a partner for the procedure.

Here's how to use muscle testing:

1. Hold your arm out straight from your side, parallel to the ground. Have a partner place one hand just below your shoulder and one hand on your forearm. Your partner then tries to force your arm down towards your side, while you exert all your strength to hold it level. Unless you are in ill health, you should easily be able to withstand this pressure and keep your arm level.

2. Then, simply hold the item that you desire to test against your diaphragm (under the breastbone) or thyroid (the point where the collarbone comes together below the neck). The

item may be in or out of normal packaging, or in its raw state, like a fresh food.

3. Holding the item as above, put your arm out straight from your side as before and have your partner try to press it down again. If the test item is beneficial for you, your arm will retain its strength, and your partner will be unable to force it down. If the item is not beneficial, or would worsen your condition, your arm can be easily pushed down by your partner.

Your skin is a key organ for detoxification.

Here are some cleansing methods you can use on your skin to draw out wastes and poisons:

Herbal compresses used during a cleanse, draw out waste and waste residues, such as cysts or abscesses, through the skin and release them into the body's elimination channels. Use alternating hot and cold compresses for best results. Apply the herbs to the hot compress, and leave the ice or cold compress plain. I regularly use cayenne, ginger and lobelia effectively for the hot compresses.

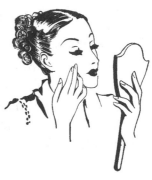

Here are some effective compresses I use:
—Add 1 teasp. powdered herbs to a bowl of very hot water. Soak a washcloth and apply until the cloth cools. Then apply a cloth dipped in ice water until it reaches body temperature. Repeat several times daily.
—Green clay compresses are effective toxin-drawing agents for growths. Apply to gauze, placed on the area, cover and leave all day. Change as you would any dressing when you bathe.

Dry skin brushing helps remove toxins during a detox and opens pores for better assimilation of nutrients. Dry skin brushing removes the top layer of old skin, helping to eliminate uric acid crystals and mucous residues. Dry skin brushing also stimulates circulation, cleans the lymph system and increases cell renewal. Dry brushing your skin every 24 hours rejuvenates your skin during detoxifcation. After your detox, dry brushing before a shower once a week will keep your skin beautiful and keep cellulitic build-up down.

Your technique for skin brushing can make all the difference to its success:
1) Use a natural bristle brush, not synthetic - it scratches skin surface.
2) Do not wet your skin. It stretches the skin and will not have the same effect.
3) All brush strokes should go towards the heart.
4) Especially brush the bottoms of your feet, nerve endings here affect the whole body.
5) Do circular, counter-clockwise strokes on the abdomen.
6) Brush lighter strokes over and around the breasts. Do not brush nipples.
7) Dry brushing is best when done before you bathe in the mornings. If done before bed, it
        can cause too much stimulation and may interrupt sleep.
8) Brush the whole body, for best results.
9) Wash your brush every few weeks in water and let it dry.

Massage therapy has been removing wastes and healing people for thousands of years.

The ancient Romans and Greeks used massage regularly as a healing treatment. Today's massage therapy has joined the alternative medicine techniques of chiropractic and reflexology as a viable health discipline. It's a wonderful detox technique, promoting mucous and fluid drainage from the lungs and increasing peristaltic action in the intestines to promote fecal elimination. I recommend at least one massage treatment during a 3 to 7 day cleanse to stimulate the body's immune response and natural restorative powers.

In the past decade, overwhelming scientific evidence has accumulated in support of massage therapy. Here are some of the research findings:

• Massage therapy is particularly helpful for pain control, stimulating the production of endorphins, the body's natural pain relievers. It is especially effective for back and shoulder pain and spinal/nerve problems.

• Massage therapy is an effective adjunct treatment for cardiovascular disorders, neurological and gynecological problems such as PMS. It is often more helpful than drugs for these problems. Massage actually helps prevent future heart disease.

• Massage therapy helps chronic fatigue syndrome, candida albicans, gastrointestinal conditions, epilepsy and psoriasis.

• Massage therapy helps correct poor posture from spinal curvatures and whiplash.

• Massage therapy helps headaches, temporo-mandibular joint syndrome (TMJ)

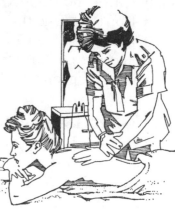

• Massage therapy helps respiratory disorders like bronchial asthma, and emphysema.

• Massage therapy promotes recovery from fatigue, muscle spasms and pain after exercise.

• Massage therapy helps break up scar tissue and adhesions.

• Massage therapy effectively treats chronic inflammatory conditions by increasing limbic circulation, especially swelling from fractures or injuries.

• Massage therapy improves blood circulation throughout the entire circulatory system.

Three types of massage therapy specifically help the body cleansing process:

Swedish massage uses kneading, stroking, friction, tapping and sometimes body shaking to stimulate and cleanse. These techniques also help cleanse muscle acids, joints, nerves and the endocrine system, by stimulating the body's circulation.

Deep tissue massage removes waste in the muscles. Deep tissue therapy uses more direct deep finger pressure across the grain of the muscles to release chronic patterns of tension, and stress accumulation. It also increases circulation to facilitate the movement of waste products out of the muscle tissue. Recent evidence shows that deep tissue massage can break up scar tissue and eliminate it.

Lymphatic drainage is a large surface, highly specialized kneading technique, a unique method that uses precise, complex hand movements to encourage the draining of lymph fluids. In comparison, normal massage techniques are much too forceful to allow drainage in the tissues and may hinder transport.

I call the lymphatic system the body's natural antibiotic. When it is flushed and clean, lymph removes body toxins as part of the auto-immune response to disease. Using slow, gentle strokes with a rhythmic pumping action, the massage technician follows the lymph pathways throughout the body to move the flow of lymph and accelerate detoxification.

There are four primary effects lymphatic massage can have on the body:

1) It balances the sympathetic and parasympathetic nervous systems.

2) It activates inhibitory reflex cells which decrease or even eliminate pain sensations.

3) It increases lymph flow for a decongestant effect on connective tissue, stimulates blood capillary flow and increases resorptive capacity of the blood capillaries.

4) It boosts immune response by increasing the lymph flow and stimulating antibodies.

Note: As wonderful as massage therapy is, there are some health conditions where massage is not a good idea.

• Don't massage a person with high fever, cancer, tuberculosis or other infections or malignant conditions which might be further spread throughout the body.

• Don't massage the abdomen of a person with high blood pressure or ulcers.

• Don't massage legs with varicose veins, diabetes, phlebitis or blood vessel problems.

• Massage no closer than six inches near bruises, cysts, skin breaks or broken bones.

• Massage people with swollen limbs gently, only above the swelling, towards the heart.

Polarity therapy is a blend of art and science.

Today's technology graphically shows that the human body consists of many electro-magnetic patterns. We can see that energy both surrounds the body and courses through it in a continual flow of positive and negative charges. Expressed in ancient times as an aura, this magnetic field makes up our physical, mental, and emotional characteristics, directs body systems and maintains energy balance. Popular in holistic spas and detox centers today, a polarity practitioner accesses the magnetic current to release energy blocks.

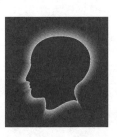

Polarity Therapy believes that balancing the flow of energy in the body is the underlying foundation of health. Rooted in Ayurveda, polarity therapy uses diet and exercise for cleansing tissues, balancing energy, improving breath and circulation and preventing illness. Polarity therapy is also helpful in treating migraines, low back pain and other stress disorders.

Gentle touch induces a relaxed, meditative state to accelerate energy flow throughout the body, inviting a return to health. There are three types of touch the therapist may use: *rajasic* is gentle and stimulating, *sattvic* is a light, balancing touch, *tamasic* touch goes deeper into the muscles and tissues. Frequently, the touch is so light that one doesn't feel anything at all.

Magnet therapy works on a balance of negative/positive magnetic energy.

Science has known since the 50's that a magnetic field is critical to normal body function and coordination. (In fact, chronic fatigue syndrome, fibromyalgia and chronic immune deficiency syndrome were first identified as magnetic field deficiency syndromes.)

The positive, acid-producing field, can create conditions like arthritis, mental confusion, fatigue, pain and insomnia- and encourage fat storage. Culprits producing this field are processed foods, caffeine, nicotine, and toxic chemicals in cosmetics, agriculture, auto exhaust, and over-the-counter and prescription drugs.

The negative, alkaline-producing field, increases oxygen, encourages deep sleep, reduces inflammation and fluid retention, relieves pain, and promotes mental acuity. A negative field can act like an antibiotic in helping to destroy bacterial, fungal and viral infections because it lowers body acidity.

In healing, magnets increase blood flow to specific areas of the body, which carries more oxygen to the region (blood is composed of positively and negatively charged particles).

Reflexology works with the body's energy zones through the hands and feet.

Reflexology is an ancient natural science based on the belief that each part of the body is interconnected through the nerve system to specific points on the feet and hands. A history of foot massage spans time and place from the Physician's Tomb in Egypt of 2300 B.C. to the Physicians Temple in Nara, Japan of 700 A.D. The ancient Egyptians are believed to have actually developed hand and foot reflexology.

Reflexology is often known as zone therapy, and it's an important part of massage therapy treatment. In reflexology, the nervous system is understood as an electrical system; contact can be made through the feet and hands with each of the electro-mechanical zones in the body to the nerve endings. The nerve endings are called reflex points (referring to the fact that these points are reflexive, like a knee-jerk reaction.) Ten reflexology zone meridians have been extensively mapped connecting all the organs and glands, and culminating in points in the hands and feet. The points are manipulated to open blocked energy pathways. Since the feet serve as reflexes for the entire body, foot reflexology is most often used.

Stress is involved in over 80% of all illness. The first step in healing is relaxation. Reflexology helps the body to heal itself through relaxation. Its goal is to clear the pathways of energy flow throughout the body, to return body balance, and increase immune response. It does this by stimulating the lymphatic system to eliminate wastes adequately, and the blood to circulate easily to poorly functioning areas.

Reflexologists look at the feet as a mini-map of the entire body, with the big toes serving as the head, the balls of the feet representing the shoulders, and the narrowing the waist area. Any illness, injury or tension in the body produces tenderness in the corresponding foot zone. Reflexologists rely on an inchworm-like massage motion of the thumb to produce light or deep pressure on each zone, concentrating on the tender spots, which often feel like little grains of salt under the skin.

For your own individual use, picture your hands and feet as your body's control panels. Get a good reflexology chart - available in health food stores. Then use your fingers or a rounded-end to locate the reflex points. Some points take practice to pinpoint. The best rule for knowing when you have reached the right spot is that it will probably be very tender, denoting crystalline deposits or congestion in the corresponding organ. However, there is often an immediate feeling of relief in the area as waste deposits break up for removal by the body.

Fifteen pounds of applied force on any reflex point can send a surge of energy to the corresponding body area, removing obstructive crystals, restoring circulation, and clearing congestion. The nerve reflex point on the foot for any afflicted area will be tender or sore indicating crystalline deposits brought about by poor capillary circulation of fluids. The amount of soreness on the foot point can also indicate the size of the crystalline deposit, and the amount of time it has been accumulating.

For effective reflexology, press on the reflex point 3 times for 10 seconds each time. The pressure treatment may be used for twenty to thirty minute sessions at a time, about twice a week. Sessions more often than this will not give nature the chance to use the stimulation or do its necessary repair work. Most people notice frequent and easy bowel movements in the first twenty-four hours after reflexology as the body throws off released wastes.

Here are some easy reflexology techniques you can use:

Finger-walking: your thumb acts as a brace as the fingers move, bending at the first joint and applying steady pressure.

•Finger walk across each toe. Cover nails and base of toe.

•Separate the big toe and second toe, exposing trough. Place finger at base of toe. Finger walk down side of trough to inside of foot. Switch hands to work outside of foot.

•Grasp the foot. Rest thumb of working hand on inside edge of the foot for leverage. Place finger on outside edge of the foot. Finger-walk around outside edge of foot.

Thumb-walking: the fingers grasp, while thumb tip exerts pressure. The thumb bends only at the first joint.

•Place thumb on the bottom of the foot, with fingers resting on top of the foot. Thumb-walk to work webbing between toes, as far into trough as padding on ball of foot allows. Don't work into soft skin between toes.

Multiple finger grip: the palm acts as a brace while the four finger tips make contact.

•Place finger in the trough between first and second toes on top of foot. Use multiple-finger grip on inside of trough. Reposition and work another part of the trough. Work on each trough. Switch hands. Use multiple-finger grip on trough toward outside of foot.

•Place tips of fingers on the ledge formed across base of toes. Grasp foot, and wrap fingers around to provide leverage. Use multiple-finger grip, with fingers downward.

Today, reflexology treatments are used for pain relief, and for faster recovery from injuries or illness without surgery or heavy medication.

Ear Coning for Ear Cleansing

Ear coning or candling is a comfortable way to clean out excess wax and other accumulations. It's an ancient healing process used by virtually every healing tradition. Chinese Traditional Medicine, Native American and Mayan societies, even the ancient Egyptians all used ear candling to gently remove ear wax, fungus, and yeast from ear canals. Some of these cultures even considered ear coning a spiritual practice that also cleared the mind and senses. Ear candling was believed to detoxify the physical body through the sinus, lymphatic and other systems to realign the flow of cranial fluids.

Ear candles are made from strips of 100% cotton muslin which are dipped into a mixture of wax and herbs with natural antibiotic, decongestant and balancing activity like *sage, Swedish bitters, cedar, spearmint, echinacea, goldenseal and rosemary.* The waxed muslin is then formed into a tapered cone.

In the coning process, the narrow end of the candle is gently placed at the ear canal, while the opposite end is lit. The spiral design of the cone creates a vacuum which draws the soothing smoke into the ear canal. The smoke goes through the Eustachian tube into the lymphatic system, then by osmosis, it draws accumulations out into the cone. The process is soothing, and takes only about 45 minutes.

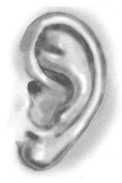

Here are the benefits of ear coning:
—helps to stimulate and detoxify the lymphatic system.
—helps remove excessive wax and allows better hearing, usually immediately.
—helps clear "swimmers ear," where ear wax stops water clearing from the ear and allows harmful bacteria to grow and fester.
—relieves pain and pressure from mucous blown into the ear from the Eustachian tube.
—helps clear itching mold caused by candida yeast allergy.
—helps remove parasites growing in the ear.

Give your body a detoxifying ascorbic acid flush.

Vitamin C (ascorbic acid) accelerates detoxification, changing body chemistry to neutralize allergens, fight infections, promote more rapid healing and protect against illness.

Here's how:
1. Use a non-acidic vitamin C or Ester C powder with bioflavonoids for best results.
2. Take $\frac{1}{2}$ teasp. every 20 minutes until a soupy stool results. (Use $\frac{1}{4}$ teasp. every hour for a very young child; $\frac{1}{2}$ teasp. every hour for a child six to ten years old.)
3. Then, slightly reduce amount taken so that the bowel produces a mealy, loose stool, but not diarrhea. The body will still continue to cleanse. You will be taking about 8-10,000mg of vitamin C daily depending on body weight and make-up. Continue for one to two days for a thorough flush.

An herbal "vag pac" can detox the vaginal/urethral area.

A cleansing herbal combination may be used as a vaginal pack by placing it against the cervix, or as a bolus inserted in the vagina. The pack acts as an internal poultice to draw out toxic wastes from the vagina, rectum or urethral areas. A "vag pac" is effective for cysts, benign tumors, polyps and uterine growths, and cervical dysplasia. It takes 6 weeks to 6 months for complete healing, depending on the problem and severity.

Here's how to make a pack:
Formula #1: Mix 1 part each with cocoa butter to form a suppository: squaw vine, marshmallow root, slippery elm, goldenseal root, pau d'arco, comfrey root, mullein, yellow dock root, chickweed, acidophilus powder.

Formula #2: Mix 1 part each with cocoa butter to form a suppository: cranesbill powder, goldenseal root, red raspberry leaf, white oak bark, echinacea root, myrrh gum powder.

1) Mix the combined, powdered herbs with warmed cocoa butter to form finger-sized suppositories. Place on waxed paper in the refrigerator to chill and harden slightly.
2) Smear a suppository on the end of a cotton tampon and insert; or insert as is, and use a sanitary napkin to catch drainage. Use suppositories at night and rinse out in the morning with white oak bark tea, or yellow dock root tea to rebalance vaginal pH.
3) Repeat for 6 days. Rest for one week. Resume and repeat.

Chelation Therapy cleans out your arteries.

Chelation therapy was developed in Germany in the early 1930's and introduced into the United States in 1948 as a method of preventing or reversing heart and artery pathology (hardening of the arteries) from diminished blood circulation. Today chelation is used by medical authorities around the world as a cleansing treatment for heavy metal and radiation toxicity, digitalis intoxication, lead and snake venom poisoning and heart arrhythmias.

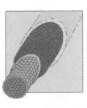

A chelating protein called EDTA, a synthetic amino acid, ethylene-diamine-tetracetic acid, is used, because it has the unique property of binding with divalent metals that are clogging arteries. When EDTA is injected, it flushes the cells of ionic minerals, especially calcium, and travels with them out of the body through the kidneys.

Oral chelation refers to specific foods and nutritional supplements that help cleanse the blood vessels of accumulated detritus (waste) and improve blood flow. While experience among chelating physicians indicates that oral chelates take about eight times longer to show health benefits than do IV chelates, oral chelation is successful in improving circulation, reversing heart disease, stroke and sexual impotency due to poor circulation. I use oral chelation as a protective against atherosclerosis and many degenerative diseases.

Detoxification can be a key
to managing the stress
in your life.

On the other hand, stress
reduction techniques like
aromatherapy, guided imagery,
magnet and polarity therapy
and biofeedback are a big part
of a successful detox.

Stress & Detoxification

Stress is a fact of everybody's life today. Maybe it's always been part of the human condition, but today, we know that it affects every cell and tissue in our bodies, it robs us of important vitamins, minerals and antioxidants, breaks down our major organs and lowers our immune response. Over time, unrelieved stress causes severe acid build-up that hinders our digestion of nutrients and stops up our elimination tracts. It interferes with our body's cleansing processes, and actually contributes to toxic buildup. Reducing stress is critical to your health. You can eat a perfect diet, cleanse your body inside and out, and exercise regularly, but if you're in a constant state of mental stress, your physical problems won't go away. **Consider stress management as a key to your detox program.**

Can your thoughts and feelings make your body toxic?

Today we have undeniable proof that they do.

Positive thoughts and emotions contribute to vitality. Negative thoughts and emotions are powerful self-poisoners that contribute to ill health. Most of us are working on a better diet, trying for a more active lifestyle and avoiding environmental toxins when we can. But a negative mental and emotional infrastructure for your lifestyle can be even more damaging, because it's subconscious and it festers. Negative thoughts and feelings are corrosive. They literally "eat away at you." Positive, optimistic thoughts are nurturing. They literally feed you by boosting digestion.

Recent proof positive of this phenomenon comes from the Institute of HeartMath™ (IHM), a nonprofit organization specializing in stress reduction and physiology improvement research. IHM has pioneered bio-medical studies on the relationship between feelings, emotional balance, cardiovascular function, and hormone and immune system health. HeartMath's projects, FREEZE-FRAME™ and CUT-THRU™, are exercise techniques that dissolve repetitive negative thought patterns to cleanse your body and pave the way for health.

What happens when your mind and emotions "get toxic?"

Our mental and emotional attitude triggers a cascade of responses for every situation we perceive. 1) the response causes electrical changes in the heart, nervous system and brain 2) the electrical changes directly affect your heart rate, blood pressure, hormone and immune responses 3) which, in turn, influence your state of health and well-being.

Our perceptions and emotional reactions are transmitted between the heart and brain via the nervous systems and can be seen in the patterns of our heart rhythms.

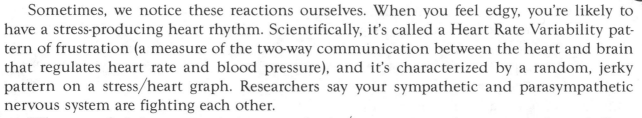

Sometimes, we notice these reactions ourselves. When you feel edgy, you're likely to have a stress-producing heart rhythm. Scientifically, it's called a Heart Rate Variability pattern of frustration (a measure of the two-way communication between the heart and brain that regulates heart rate and blood pressure), and it's characterized by a random, jerky pattern on a stress/heart graph. Researchers say your sympathetic and parasympathetic nervous system are fighting each other.

When you feel deep appreciation, your brain/heart patterns have a smooth, even flow. Researchers say your sympathetic and parasympathetic nervous system are working together efficiently.

Electrocardiogram (ECG) tests also show the effects of hostility and severe depression. Newer ECG spectral analysis shows even more subtle "negative" emotions, like frustration, worry and anxiety; as well as subtle "positive" emotions like love, compassion and appreciation. Your ECG spectra graphs have a jagged appearance (an "incoherent spectrum") on days when your life seems to be falling apart. On days that you're feeling on top of the world, your ECG spectra have a harmonious pattern (a "coherent spectrum"). Because the heart generates the most powerful electromagnetic field in the body, its electrical energy is radiated throughout your body. Every cell receives the heart's message. That's where the synthesis of your thoughts and emotions affect your physical state. (The ancient Egyptians, who saw the heart, rather than the brain, as the seat of the soul, may have had it right after all.)

And there's more......

Scientists are proving that repeated episodes of anger and frustration cause nervous system imbalances that are detrimental not only to the heart, but to the brain and the hormonal and immune systems. When your body is under stress, your nervous system increases sympathetic activity, creating reactions like nervous restlessness, hyperactivity, anxiety, muscle tension, heart arrhythmias and stomach cramps. If the stress is prolonged, your adrenal and pituitary glands produce stress-fighting hormones for emergency relief. But the relief process comes at a price because it produces chemical waste, which degenerates nerve cells and causes free radical damage in the body.

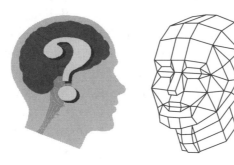

Stress also creates measureable hormonal imbalances, some of which can damage brain cells (as in new Alzheimer's studies). Other research, especially on cancer and virus-infected cells, show that feelings of happiness and joy boost white blood cell counts up to amounts needed for healing and defense against invading pathogens.

The message is becoming clear — a program of detoxification and rejuvenation is incomplete unless we understand that our thoughts and emotions have an impact on our body's internal pharmacy. We can choose angry or loving heartbeats. The challenge is managing our thoughts and emotions so that they serve us instead of harming us.

While some situations seem intrinsically "stressful," it is the way an individual perceives and reacts to the event that determines whether a stress response is activated. The HeartMath stress management techniques target the source of human emotional arousal and psychological well-being. This in turn, leads to improvements in autonomic function and balance and facilitates the healing process. Many patients report significant changes in their symptomatology after practicing the HeartMath interventions for even short periods of time.

HeartMath's "FREEZE-FRAME" is a simple, powerful technique for mental and emotional poise. It focuses on pausing to take a deeper look before making a decision, giving you a better chance to act from a point of balance.

FREEZE-FRAME takes the alpha-wave procedures of the 70's and the biofeedback technology of the eighties one step further. It's a physical exercise that produces visible chemical and electrical changes in the body. FREEZE-FRAME lets a person see a stress reaction, measure the reaction, then control the reaction to change mood and attitude.

Here's a typical comment, "I watched the pattern of my angry heartbeats rise and fall across a computer screen in jagged spikes. As I began FREEZE-FRAME, I recalled being loved, my heart responded by vibrating at a different energy frequency, and my heartbeat rhythm settled into a smoother, even pattern, that looked like ripples in a pond. It continued this way as long as I practiced FREEZE-FRAME."

FREEZE FRAME monitors show that positive feelings are instantly picked up by the brain, which responds by sending messages via neurotransmitter pathways to the body's endocrine system to generate hormones in doses that foster health. You experience a heightened state of well-being marked by greater energy, a higher pain threshold, and greater tolerance for things that would normally be frustrating.

The "CUT-THRU" technique at HeartMath documents the effects of stress-busting exercises. One impressive study tracks levels of the hormones DHEA in people practicing CUT-THRU. Low DHEA levels are linked to fatigue, exhaustion, muscle weakness, immune disorders, PMS, obesity, diabetes and Alzheimer's disease. In one study, low DHEA levels rose over 100 percent in *every* person who practiced the CUT-THRU procedure for one month. Some subjects tripled or quadrupled their DHEA levels even though no other lifestyle changes were made.

A second CUT-THRU study measured cortisol (a stress hormone) levels. Emotions of guilt, anxiety, anger, or frustration cause high cortisol levels. Chronically high levels of cortisol can damage brain cells and accelerate aging. Cortisol levels of people in the study dropped an average of 23 percent after practicing the CUT-THRU technique for one month.

Business leaders, scientists, medical doctors, and educators from around the world are beginning to see that stress reduction techniques reduce burn-out, access energy, boost the immune health and increase personal effectiveness. Today, HeartMath's techniques are used successfully in hospitals, schools, by thousands of individuals, and are being formally applied in corporations to increase productivity and reduce stress.

FYI: Institute of HeartMath, P.O. Box 1463, 14700 West Park Ave., Boulder Creek, CA 95006, 800-450-9111, www.heartmath.org

Detoxing With Aromatherapy

Volatile liquids distilled from plants are the heart of aromatherapy. They are the plant's essential oils, and they act in plants much like hormones do in humans. Aromatherapy oils, 75 to 100 times more concentrated than dried herbs and flowers, are some of the most potent herbal medicines. They are the regenerating, oxygenating immune defense of plants. The molecules of essential aromatherapy oils carry healing nutrients to your body's cells.

Did you know that plants have an electrical frequency? Aromatherapy actually heals through its bio-electrical frequency. Essential plant oils carry a bio-electrical frequency, expressed as hertz. Many of us today understand megahertz rates from our computers and electronic equipment. Plant foods have a frequency from 0 to 15Hz.; dry herbs have a frequency from 15 to 22Hz.; fresh herbs have a frequency 20 to 27Hz.; essential oils start at 52Hz and go to 320Hz.

Your body has an electrical hertz frequency, too. A healthy body has a frequency between 62 to 78Hz. Disease frequency rates begin at 58Hz. We know that a higher frequency rate destroys an entity of lower frequency. Based on this knowledge, it's easy to see that certain high frequency essential oils can create an environment in which disease, bacteria, viruses and fungus cannot live. In fact, a majority of essential oils can affect pathogenic organisms that are resistant to chemical antibiotics. They may be a good choice for overcoming today's super germs that are becoming so virulent.

Essential oils affect people first through the sense of smell. Smell is the most rapid of all the senses because its information is directly relayed to the hypothalamus. Motivation, moods, emotions and creativity all begin in the hypothalamus, so odors affect these processes immediately. (Some scents enhance your emotional equilibrium merely by inhaling them.) Essential oil molecules work through hormone-like chemicals to produce their sensations. So scents influence the glands responsible for hormone levels, metabolism, insulin levels, stress levels, sex drive, body temperature and appetite.

Scents are also intimately intertwined with thought and memory. Studies on brain-waves show that scents like lavender increase alpha brain waves associated to relaxation; scents like jasmine boost beta waves linked to alertness.

Essential oils are not oily. They are non-oily, concentrated fluids. They are highly active, and may be taken in by inhalation, steams and infusers, or applied topically to the skin. The therapeutic effects of essential oils are due both to their pharmacological properties and to their small molecule size, which allows easy penetration through the skin, the walls of the blood vessels, the lymph system and body tissues — pathways that impact the body's organ, hormonal, nervous and immune systems.

Essential oils have many therapeutic applications. In this section, we will focus on their value for detoxification, where they are quite powerful. When an oil with detoxification properties is applied, certain toxins appear to be cleared from the body. Toxins such as free radicals, heavy metals, fungi, bacteria, viruses and cell debris become attached to the essential oils which are then excreted from the body via the skin, kidneys, urine, etc.

Here are some of the ways essential oils assist detoxification:
• They stimulate immune response, partly by invigorating the production of white blood cells, and partly by increasing the activity of T-cells, NK-cells, alveolar macrophages and serum antibodies. A new study finds that all essential oils stimulate phagocytosis, the ability of white blood cells to devour harmful invading microbes.

• The aromatic molecules of essential oils have an electromagnetic charge that influences the charge on our cell magnetic fields, which studies find effective in healing.

• They are natural antioxidants which destroy free radicals.

• They boost the body's resistance to harmful bacteria, viruses, fungi and parasites. All essential oils have antibacterial properties, but each oil is effective against different pathogens. Laboratory tests show thyme oil, with a component called *thymol*, is a powerful antibiotic agent against the type of pathogens in candida and thrush infections.

• They stimulate sluggish circulation, aiding detoxification by accelerating the disposal of carbon dioxide and other waste products, by bringing oxygen and nutrients to the tissues, and by decreasing blood viscosity.

• They act as blood purifiers and normalizers. For example, rose oil helps counteract the toxic blood effects of alcohol. Rose oil and yarrow can help normalize a system invaded by allergens, such as pollens and spores.

• They improve the efficiency of the lymph system, especially the body's drainage ducts, for better elimination of metabolic residues and toxins. For example, juniper oil enhances the filtration action of the kidneys.

• Oils like eucalyptus, fennel, frankincense, ginger, peppermint and pine, are expectorants which stimulate the removal of heavy mucous in the lungs and bronchial tubes.

Essential oils high chemical groupings associated with cleansing the body, (terpenes, sesquiterpenols, phenols and diterpenols), are best delivered through the skin (in a massage or bath oil). For best results, mix them into a carrier oil, about 15 drops to 4-oz. of an oil like almond, sunflower, jojoba or a favorite massage oil.

Citrus oils like lemon, orange or grapefruit help fluid retention. Rose oil and rosemary help normalize body chemistry, particularly against allergens. Thyme oil is an anti-fungal; marjoram promotes blood flow; cedarwood promotes lymph activity. Vetiver and cypress stimulate circulation. Juniper, sandlewood and cypress release fluid retention and cellulite.

Special blends that are helpful during your detoxification process include:
• For wellness (lemon, peppermint, rosemary, thyme).
• For energy (orange, juniper berry, basil, cinnamon leaf).
• For body tone (grapefruit, lavender, cypress, basil, juniper berry).
FYI: The above oils are by Wyndmere Naturals, 153 Ashley Road, Hopkins, MN 55343, 800-207-8538.

Biofeedback Detox Therapy

Biofeedback is perhaps the most accepted alternative healing technique by the mainstream medical community - probably because it uses expensive, high-tech equipment. Before the advent of the biofeedback machine, conventional medicine held that an individual had no control over heart rate, body temperature, brain activity, or blood pressure. When biofeedback experiments proved in the 1960's, that people could voluntarily affect these functions, research began into how it might be employed for human health.

Today, biofeedback is used by health professionals in all disciplines as a tool for controlling problems like asthma, chronic fatigue, epilepsy, drug addiction and chronic pain. It is a successful specific in the treatment of migraines, poor circulation, and psoriasis, a skin disease that has a psychological foundation.

Biofeedback is used as relaxation therapy for insomnia and anxiety. Hyperactive behavior in children, bladder incontinence, back pain, TMJ syndrome, even loss of nerve-muscle control due to brain or nerve damage respond to biofeedback techniques. Biofeedback also helps heart malfunction, stress-related intestinal disorders like ulcers and irritable bowel syndrome, hiatal hernia, ringing in the ears (Meniere's syndrome), facial tics and cerebral palsy.

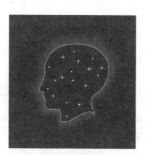

Here's how biofeedback works. First, the patient is wired with sensors. Then, by giving auditory and/or visual signals to his body he learns to control normally subconscious responses, like circulation, muscle tension, or heartbeat rate. Biofeedback computers analyze the patient's target activities. Biofeedback practitioners interpret the computer readings. Gradually, the patient learns to stabilize erratic or unhealthy biological functions. A healthy reading includes warm skin, low sweat gland activity, and a slow, even heart rate.

The effects of biofeedback can be measured by:
1) monitoring skin temperature influenced by blood flow beneath the skin;
2) monitoring galvanic skin response, the electrical conductivity of the skin;
3) monitoring muscle tension with an electro-myogram;
4) monitoring heart rate with an electro-cardiogram;
5) monitoring brain wave activity with an electroencephalogram.

One of the most popular vital signs monitored by biofeedback is muscle tension, because it can be used to treat tension headaches, muscle pain, incontinence and partial paralysis. Another is skin temperature, which can be used to treat Reynaud's syndrome, migraines, hypertension and anxiety. Other signs are perspiration, used to treat body odor and anxiety; pulse rate, used to treat hypertension, stress and heart arrhythmia; and breathing rate, used to treat asthma, hyperventilation and anxiety.

Biofeedback is seldom used by itself, but rather is combined with other relaxation techniques and therapies. Biofeedback doesn't work for everyone. Its success stories come from people who are willing to make lifestyle improvements.

Guided Imagery Connects Mind & Body

Guided imagery uses the mind/body connection to give you more control over your health. It is a communication technique for accessing the network between mind and body as a source of power in the healing process. Imagery helps clarify attitudes, emotions and lifestyle patterns that produce illness. Imagery can also help the mental and emotional part of illness recovery. By directly accessing the mind, imagery can help someone understand the healing needs that an illness represents so they can develop ways to choose wellness.

Imagery is the normal way our nervous system finds, stores, and processes information. It is a flow of thoughts that we can see, hear, feel, smell, or taste in our imagination. It has its roots in the ancient Greek understanding of how the mind influences the subconscious, and has been employed under many different names, throughout the history of medicine to speed healing by reducing stress and calming the mind.

Today, imagery is used in the sports' world to encourage athletes to better performance, to minimize discomfort from injuries like sprains, strains, and broken bones. In healing, it is successful in overcoming chronic pain, spastic colon and back pain, and for persistent problems like allergies, asthma and stress-related gastrointestinal pain. Even serious, degenerative illness such as cancer has responded to guided imagery, with patients showing heightened immune activity and shrinking tumor growths as they imagine cancer cells being gobbled up by immune antibodies.

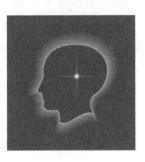

Imagery is used successfully for problems from a simple tension headache to a life-threatening disease. It can help both physical and psychological disorders, high blood pressure, acne, diabetes, heart arrhythmias and addictions. It is effective for reproductive irregularities like PMS, urinary infections, even excessive uterine bleeding. It is a proven method for helping people tolerate medical treatments, for reducing side effects, and for a less painful, faster recuperation. People using imagery for everyday health problems can accelerate healing from common colds, flus, and infections.

We know that stress is an emotional response to life's situations, and that an emotional reaction to a stressful situation shows itself in physical health. If a person responds to a loss with a prolonged state of depression, the body, too, will fall into a prolonged state of depression, manifested as illness. However, if the person is able to integrate the loss into a broader meaning of life, the feelings of loss, grief and depression will be relatively temporary. We experience a more wholesome view of life when we feel ourselves in control - as participants in life rather than as victims of undesirable circumstances.

The school of imagery believes that learning to relax is fundamental to self-healing, because if stress levels are high, immune response is reduced. Today, guided imagery in one form or another is a part of most stress-reduction techniques. Imagery is the easiest way to learn to relax, and its active nature makes it satisfying in terms of step-by-step insight.

Scientifically, imagery works like a computer to program directions that a patient wants for his body into the hypothalamus. This happens almost instantaneously, traveling from the brain through the nervous system, to the glands through the hypothalamus-pituitary-adrenal axis, and then through the vagus nerve for psychological and physical accord.

Everything that registers in our minds registers in our bodies. Messages sent through imagery, for example, are immediately translated through the parasympathetic nervous system into neurotransmitters, which direct the immune system to work better against abnormal cells, or the hormone system to rebalance and stop creating abnormal cells.

There are two types of guided imagery techniques - receptive imagery and active imagery:

• Receptive imagery involves entering a relaxed state, then visualizing an embodiment of the illness (like a sly demon) and asking why it is causing your body trouble. An answer from your unconscious can provide a great deal of information about what your body needs to heal.

• Active imagery involves envisioning an illness being cured. This may mean anything from imagining your immune system forces attacking and killing a tumor, to picturing the pain in your arm as a ball that rolls down your arm and out of your body.

Guided imagery therapists use a near-trance condition, induced through suggestion, to affect healing. Patients are asked to envision themselves in a tranquil place like a quiet woods or a mountain lake, then are directed to describe what they see, hear, smell, or feel, in order to reach a deeper state of relaxation. When a relaxation state is reached, patients are asked to visualize their immune system as an energy force battling for their health. Their immune responses are analyzed in great detail. They are then asked to join forces with the immune system, by mentally envisioning the illness and then imagining their antibodies and white cells overcoming it.

Not everyone is capable of working with guided imagery treatment. An active imagination is a must, because the vividness of the image is a key to the treatment's effectiveness. Successful subjects are those who can understand its value in relation to their problems, and who do not mentally fight it.

Deep breathing helps you detoxify.

Expanding your breathing capacity is a key to health. Body cleansing and your body's ability to heal are directly linked to the delivery of oxygen and removal of carbon dioxide. Most of us know that several deep breaths before a hard task clears our mind for the job. But deep breathing does more.... it enhances every body function. For detoxification, breathing affects lymph circulation. So when breathing is restricted, body fluid and waste products from cellular metabolism build up in the lymph.

Breathing is controlled by two sets of nerves, the involuntary (autonomic) nervous system, and the voluntary nervous system. Imbalance of the autonomic nervous system contributes to ill health. Expanding breathing capacity actually improves autonomic ner-

vous system functions. For example, studies show that people suffering from environmental illness have unhealthy, hyperventilating breathing patterns. Hyperventilation contributes to histamine release, chronic cerebral, lactic acidosis and altered immune response. Learning to breath deeply can speed the recovery of environmentally sensitive people.

Take a deep breath. Another deep breath. And another deep breath. See... how... it... feels.

Flower Essence Therapy & Detoxification

Civilization has removed us from the closeness we once had with Nature. Can people today still benefit from a flower healing therapy that is so subtle and so tuned into Nature?

Flower essence healing and homeopathy are two non-scientific therapeutic methods from times past that have been re-validated in alternative healing today. Flower essences are part of an emerging field of life-enhancing subtle therapies, like homeopathy and acupuncture, that work vibrationally through human energy fields. Vibrational essences increase disease resistance by creating internal harmony and manifesting higher energy systems.

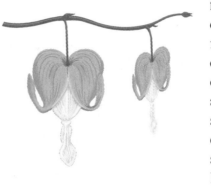

The precise application of emotions and attitudes was an English physician and homeopath in the 1930's. Bach's research showed that flowers biomagnetic energies, that power through emotional balance the mind and body is most tions. He also recognized the emotions such as depression, flower essences for specific developed by Dr. Edward Bach, discharge identified patterns of could be harnessed for healing ance. Bach's work on the relationship of stress to disease showed that the link between evident during stressful situations significance of destructive hate and fear.

Bach was one of the first modern healers to realize that true healing means the materialization of one's higher spiritual force. He saw that emotional balance strengthened the body's ability to resist disease. In the last decade, modern medicine is also beginning to see the connection between negative emotions and lower disease resistance. Deepak Chopra M.D., a well-known expert in the new field of psycho-neuro-immunology (mind-body connection), says that "the mind is in every cell of the body. Every thought we think releases neuropeptides that are transmitted to all the cells." Emotional stress disrupts nerve functions, hormone levels and immune response. Loving thoughts release interleukin and interferon, body healers. Anxious thoughts release cortisone and adrenaline which suppress the immune system. Peaceful thoughts release body chemicals similar to valium, which relax.

Flower essences can be a healing tool to assist us in emotional, mental and spiritual balance. Flower essence case studies show that people taking the remedies often experience physical and spiritual cleansing as well as emotional purification.

Bach was able to document scientifically the clinical criteria that is still used today in flower essence research. His compound, **Rescue Remedy,** is the most widely used flower essence — a gentle, effective remedy which restores the system's emotional balance during stress or anxiety. It can also be used in emergency situations or at any time of upset, shock or trauma, like impending events which produce anxiety (before giving a speech, or going to the dentist) or for working in an atmosphere of unrelenting stress.

The vitality of a plant's life force increases around the area of the flower bloom. Flower essences are captured at the plant's highest moment, the unfolding into blossom. Then, like highly dilute homeopathic remedies, their essences are potentized by vibrations. DEVA FLOWER REMEDIES are effective flower compounds that are widely available in the U.S. They are subtle liquid extracts, usually taken orally. Essences are prepared from a sun infusion of blossoms in a bowl of water, which is further diluted and potentized, then preserved with brandy. The following selection are flower essences that assist detoxification:

• **Cleansing Remedy:** A general mind, emotional and body cleanser. Relieves the feelings of toxicity. *(California poppy, chaparral, crab apple, ocotillo and star jasmine flowers with lycopodium moss extract).*

• **Radiation/Pollution:** Helps clear electromagnetic and environmental pollution effects; activates the immune system. To purify a glass of tap water, add 7 drops. *(Agrimony, crab apple, eucalyptus, French rose, mimulus, rock rose and white oleander flowers with seawater).*

• **Immunity:** Stimulates and strengthens the immune system and aligns body meridians. *(Chaparral, French rose, hawthorn, Indian corn, lotus, morning glory and pine flowers).*

• **Addictions:** Helps overcome addictive habits like drug addiction, alcoholism, smoking and overeating. *(Agrimony, California and red poppy, morning glory, self-heal, scullcap, walnut, wild mountain iris).*

• **Fatigue/Exhaustion:** For people who are tired, burned out, burdened by life, facing excessive performance pressure, low vitality and strength, or a physical or mental breakdown. *(Bindweed, bottlebrush, elm, hornbeam, olive, petunia and wild mountain iris).*

• **Stress/Tension:** Clears mental strain and headaches, relaxes tension, calms the nerves. *(Aspen, dandelion, impatiens, lotus, vervain, chamomile, sweet and white chestnut flowers).*

FYI: DEVA FLOWER REMEDIES by Natural Labs, P.O. Box 20037, Sedona, AZ 86341-0037, 800-233-0810.

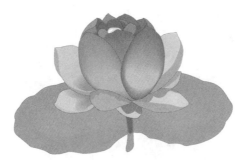

Good water is critical to your detox program.

But much of our drinking water today isn't good, and some is even dangerous.

Find out what you need to know about your water and how to use it for body cleansing in this chapter.

Water & Detoxification

Good water is essential to body cleansing. It's obvious. It sounds like a truism. Of course. Water is the basis of life. It makes up three-quarters of our bodies. Water is second only to oxygen in importance for health. It's vital to every cell. Not one of the processes in our bodies could take place without water. **Water is something that we take for granted.** But how many of us really understand how essential water is or what happens to our body if it doesn't receive pure water every day, free of chemicals and pollutants?

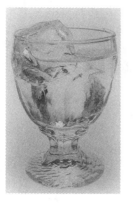

- Water is the adhesive that bonds your cell architecture. So every single body function is regulated, monitored and dependent on water.
  - Water regulates your body temperature and maintains your equilibrium.
  - Water carries every nutrient, mineral, vitamin, protein, hormone and chemical messenger in your body to its destination.
  - Proteins and enzymes, the basis for your body's healing capacity, function efficiently only when you have enough water.
  - Your daily energy depends on water, because your body's chemical reactions are water-dependent. Just like a hydro-electric system, the energy generated by your body's water is used by your two vital cell battery systems, ATP and GTP.
  - Your brain tissue is 85% water. Messages from your brain to everywhere else in your body are transported on "waterways."

And water is essential to the cleansing processes of your body.
—It lubricates and flushes wastes and toxins from all cells.
—It cleanses the internal organs.
—It helps eliminate toxins from the bloodstream.

We've all heard since we were kids that you have to drink plenty of water so your body will work at its peak. Yet, dehydration is as common here as it is in desert regions of the world, probably because Americans are not very conscious of water as part of health. Even when their fluid intake is normal, many Americans are deficient in essential fatty acids (EFAs). Severe EFA deficiency in the body opens the door to dehydration, because fatty acids act as cellular glue to prevent excessive fluid loss, particularly from the skin.

How much is enough? Your body needs about three quarts of replacement water every day under normal conditions. Strenuous activity, summer temperatures, or a diet that's high in salt increase this requirement. Your foods provide up to $1\frac{1}{2}$ quarts of water per day. (Fruits and vegetables are more than 90% water. Even dry foods like bread are about 35% water.) Water for metabolism is produced as part of the food digestion process, yielding as much as a pint per day.

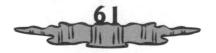

What if you just drink when you're thirsty?

That's a problem because thirst is not a reliable signal that your body needs water. Thirst is an evolutionary development that indicates severe dehydration. The sense of thirst (like sleep, appetite, satiety, and sexual responses) is controlled by the hypothalamus in the brain. You can easily lose a quart or more of water during activity before thirst is even recognized. Your thirst signal also shuts off before you have had enough for well-being.

Thinking that tea, coffee, milk or sodas are desirable substitutes is also a common mistake. These beverages contain water, but also dehydrating agents, that not only get rid of the water they bring with them but they also take away from body water reserves. Alcohol and caffeine-containing drinks are counter-productive because of their diuretic activity. Drinks loaded with dissolved sugars or milk increase water needs instead of satisfying them. Commercial sodas leach several minerals from the body.

Plain or carbonated cool water is the best way to replace lost body fluid, but if you want to vary your water intake, healthy liquids like unsweetened fruit or vegetable juices and herb teas count as replenishment. If you are physically active or working under hot weather conditions, replace lost electrolytes with electrolyte drinks like Alacer EMERGEN-C, or supplements, like Bragg's LIQUID AMINOS in water.

It is possible to consume too much water.

The general rule is 8 to 10 8-oz. glasses per day. Some enthusiastic people may feel that if ten glasses is good, twenty glasses, or even gallons, is better - every day. But drinking this much makes the body become "waterlogged," severely depressing electrolyte count. Purified water from distilled or reverse osmosis techniques compound the problem.

Poor water quality, even dangerous water, is a growing problem in most of the U.S. Today, tap water is chlorinated, fluoridated, and treated to the point where it can be an irritating, disagreeable fluid instead of a healthy drink. City tap water may contain as many as 500 different disease-causing bacteria, viruses and parasites. Chemicals and heavy metals used by industry and agriculture find their way into our ground water, adding more pollutants. Some tap water is now so bad, that without the enormous effort our bodies use to dispose of these chemicals, we would have ingested enough of them to turn us to stone by the time we were thirty! These concerns keep many individuals from drinking tap water. I recommend keeping plenty of good bottled water on hand. Tap water purifiers or a purifier for your fridge water are easy solutions for making your water consumable.

Chemicalized water contributes to the toxic overload your body must struggle with. Here are some of the "additives" you may be drinking every day:
• Fluoride • Chlorine • Pesticides • Industrial waste pollution • Home and garden chemicals • Leaching of chemicals from garbage dumps • Bacteria contamination

Americans also need to know the truth about fluoride.

Fluoride is present in commercial toothpastes used daily by both kids and adults, and it's mandatory as an additive to over 60% of U.S. public drinking water. But, it is one of the

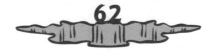

most toxic substances we know of. No other agent which is deliberately added to food or water poses the degree of health risk that fluoride does. The consequences of continual consumption are serious.

Fluoride occurs naturally in some water as calcium fluoride, but most drinking water that contains naturally-occurring fluoride has 0.1 to 0.3 ppm fluoride. The amount usually put into the drinking water is 1.0 ppm. The *type* of fluoride added to water is a hazardous waste product *(hydrofluosilicic acid)* of the phosphate fertilizer industries. It is an extremely corrosive substance. Pipes which transport fluoride have to be replaced routinely.

It is very costly to dispose of hazardous wastes. Selling *hydrofluosilicic acid* (fluoride) as a product for our water makes the industry money **and** eliminates the high cost of disposing of it as a hazardous waste material — ($1.40 per gallon in the highest-rated hazardous waste dumps). Big money is behind this movement — not concern for people's teeth.

Fluoridation has been mandated by government and rejected by citizens for years. The controversy over fluoridation of water supplies has raged every decade since fluoride was first introduced into the drinking water of Grand Rapids, Michigan in 1945. Californian's have rejected fluoridation more than 70 times! Yet, the California Legislature in October 1995 (without voter approval) passed a law requiring fluoridation of the water for the entire state. Fortunately, funds have not become available, giving citizens time once again, to organize opposition measures. Led by Santa Cruz, CA., cities are stirring to action, challenging the state, to protect its waters from fluoridation.

The city of Natick, Mass., forced to fluoridate by the public health service, recently mailed water bills to all users with the following warning boldly printed: "We recommend that pregnant women, parents of children under 3 yrs. of age, and individuals with known fluoride sensitivity consult with their personal physicians before drinking this water."

The battle for pure water in California will have an impact on the forced fluoridization of all America's water. Both sides of fluoridation/safe drinking water initiative consider the result of the fluoridation assault in California crucial to the federal government's plan to fluoridate the entire United States by the year 2000! Japan and nearly all of Europe have already rejected fluoridation and are now 98% fluoridation-free. There is active opposition in Britain, Australia, and New Zealand.

Fluoridation is mass medication whether we like it or not.

I feel it's an unnecessary toxic poison added to our drinking water. The risks of fluoridating our water supply are significant and the benefits are negligible. Don't forget that our water supply affects our food supply. If you water "organic" vegetables and fruits with fluoridated water, you get fluoride in the produce.

Studies are now coming from all over about fluoride's dangers.

In 1997, a major group, NFFE, representing toxicologists, chemists, and biologists at the Environmental Protection Agency actually went on record against adding fluoride to public drinking water.

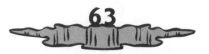

British Health, the *Journal of the American Medical Association, Lancet,* and most recently the New Jersey Dept. of Health document an enormous body of evidence from both human and animal studies showing that fluoride exposure is linked to genetic damage, nervous system dysfunction and bone disease. A new U.S. Public Health Service Review of fluoride found ample evidence that fluoride in drinking water causes an increase in cancer.

Scientists believe that interference with enzyme activity is the mechanism by which fluoride exerts its harmful impact. Effects on enzymes are some of the first detectable biological changes when an organism is exposed to a toxic agent. Enzymes mediate most of our biochemical processes, so any agent that affects a wide range of enzymes will have wide effects on an our health. Changes in certain enzyme activity are the first signs of more serious alterations that are taking place with continued exposure to fluoride.

Here are the problems:

• **Fluoridation is linked to Alzheimer's.** One study finds that fluoride increases the absorption of aluminum (a suspected Alzheimer's trigger) by over 600%! The fluoride/aluminum combination spells disaster for brain health. Researchers speculate that fluoride in water complexes with the aluminum in food, deodorants, pots and pans, enabling it to cross the blood-brain barrier.

In a 1998 study in the peer-reviewed journal *Brain Research,* low levels of fluoride in drinking water, equal to the amount in our fluoridated water today, cause damage to brain tissue similar to Alzheimer's. Both human and laboratory tests show that fluoride's link to memory impairment and diminished mental acuity can no longer be ignored.

• **Fluoride is more toxic than lead.** Even in minute doses, it accumulates in and is damaging to brain development of children. Fluoride exposure is now linked to lower than normal IQ ratings in children. Studies confirm that fluoride affects the central nervous system, and that a higher concentration of fluoride is found in embryonic brain tissue in areas where fluorosis (fluoride poisoning) is prevalent.

• **Fluoride is linked to bone damage.** Many studies clearly show that fluoride's cumulative effect on bone is devastating. The *Journal of the American Medical Association* cites chronic ingestion of fluoride as a cause of osteofluorosis, a crippling bone disease.

Hip fracture rates are much higher in people living in areas where the water is fluoridated and it occurs at even relatively low fluoride levels. Increased hip fracture has been reported in nine studies from five countries. The World Health Organization states that people consuming 2mg to 8mg of fluoride a day (2-8 litres of fluoridated water), can develop the pre-clinical arthritis-like symptoms of fluorosis. If you drink the recommended daily amount of water (8 to 10 8-oz. glasses) you are at risk, not even taking into account the potential fluoride that comes from food, juices, soft drinks, beverages, and toothpaste.

Postmenopausal women (at risk for osteoporosis), the elderly, people with nutrient deficiencies, cardiovascular and kidney problems are especially affected by fluoride's toxicity.

Isn't water fluoridation and adding fluoride to toothpastes meant to protect children and adults from tooth decay?

• The public has been misled about fluoride's health benefits for stronger teeth. A recent analysis of national survey data from the National Institute of Dental Research shows that children living in areas where the water supply is fluoridated have identical tooth decay rates of those living in non-fluoridated areas. The same is true for permanent tooth decay rates.

The Institute also admits that dental fluorosis (fluoride poisoning of the teeth) affects from 8% to 51% of children drinking fluoridated water. Its visible characteristics are discoloration or pitting of the teeth, or white flecks in the teeth. Dental fluorosis affects developing teeth but means a lifetime of damaged teeth. Incidence of dental fluorosis has steadily increased since the first introduction of fluoride to the drinking water in 1945.

Is fluoride toothpaste safe?

Believe it or not, it isn't. The poison control center receives over 11,000 calls each year because of poisoning from ingesting fluoride toothpaste (especially for small children who tend to swallow toothpaste). The problem is so bad that last year the FDA mandated a poison warning label on fluoride toothpaste.

Is there anything we can do?

You can join the fight against mandatory water fluoridation. An organization called the Citizens for Safe Drinking Water is working hard to stop water fluoridation. Dr. Kennedy heads this organization. He has practiced dentistry in San Diego for more than 20 years. He is the author of *How to Save Your Teeth*, and is an internationally recognized lecturer on toxicology and restorative dentistry. Dr. Kennedy states that increasing the fluoride intake of a patient without regard to established risk factors such as age, kidney function, weight, physical condition, water consumption, total fluoride intake, and mitigating dietary calcium is medical negligence. The court ruling which mandates fluoridation for 25 million Californians is no less negligent. **Call 888-728-3833 for more information.**

You can protect yourself and your family from the dangers of fluoride in your toothpaste. Look for one of the many non-fluoridated toothpastes at your local health food store.

Water is critical to your detoxification program.

For a healing program, several types of water are worth consideration:

• Mineral water comes from natural springs with varying mineral content and widely varying taste. The naturally occurring minerals are beneficial to digestion and regularity. In Europe, this form of bottled water has become a fine art.

• Distilled water can be from a spring or tap source; it is "de-mineralized" (only oxygen and hydrogen remain). Distilling is accomplished by reverse osmosis, filtering or boiling, then converted to steam and recondensed. It is the purest water available, ideal for healing.

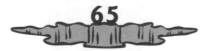

•Sparkling water comes from natural carbonation in underground springs. Most are also artificially infused with CO_2 to maintain a standard fizz. This water is an aid to digestion, and is excellent in cooking to tenderize and give lightness to a recipe.

•Artesian well water is the Cadillac of natural waters. It always comes from a deep pure source, has a slight fizz from bubbling up under rock pressure, and is tapped by a drilled well. Artesian water never comes in contact with ground contaminants.

Beyond buying bottled water, you can also take steps as an individual to conserve water and diminish pollution of ground water supplies:
— Use biodegradable soaps and detergents. Don't use water fresheners in toilet bowls.
— Don't pour wastes like paints, solvents, and petroleum based oils into drains.
— Use natural fertilizers such as manure and compost in your garden.

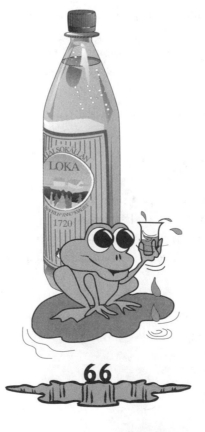

Chart Your Cleanse

There are all kinds of detox cleanses. Check out this chapter for a cleanse that suits your needs.
Then chart your cleanse. Each chart has the information you need.

• The first 2-3 pages address the reasons for each cleanse.
• The cleanse page has three columns.
  —Column 1 charts nutrition plan choices
  —Column 2 charts herb and supplement choices
  —Column 3 charts bodywork and relaxation choices

The Spring Cleanse

Cleanses come in all shapes and sizes. You can easily tailor a cleanse to your individual needs. Unless you require a specific detox for a serious illness, or recovery from a long course of drugs or chemical therapy, I recommend a short cleanse twice a year, especially in the spring, summer or early autumn when sunshine and natural vitamin D can help the process along.

A "Spring Cleaning" detox is wonderful breath of fresh air for your body after a long, closed-in winter.

A mild spring cleanse is an important, yearly vitality technique no matter how healthy you are. Even though you may exercise during the winter to keep trim, most people still feel at an energy low during the cold seasons. Our bodies still reflect the ancient seasonal need to harbor more fat for warmth and survival. In the days when people were closer to nature than we are today, the great majority farmed the land from spring to fall, and lived lives of demanding physical labor. Winter was a time of inactivity, with a natural tendency towards rest. Harvested food supplies stored in the autumn lost much of their nutrition value through the winter, so people had to eat denser foods and more of them to receive the same nutrients. Even in modern times, many days without sunshine and vitamin D mean that our bodies are less able to utilize nutrients properly.

While cold weather prompts people to consume heavier, fattier, comfort foods. Old winter "hibernation" patterns also mean that metabolism slows, sometimes by as much as 10%. So, much to the dismay of many of us, fall and winter are the most difficult times of the year to control body weight.

Winter weather illnesses like colds and flu leave us with accumulated toxins, too. Heavy winter clothing, especially thick waterproof coats, hinders normal breathing and perspiration of the skin and in this way contributes to impaired body functions. When spring finally arrives, our metabolism livens up. New, green food sources, with their metabolism-stimulating effects, abound from the first tender leafy vegetable shoots. Cleansing, antioxidant-rich herbs promote a feeling of new life and restored well-being. Nature starts chuckling in the spring. (Laughter is a good cleanser for people, too. It boosts the body's beta endorphins to induce a sense of euphoria.) Warmer weather tends to lower our appetite needs; it prompts more activity and movement, and stimulates cleansing processes. Nature has designed the perfect time for a spring cleanse.

A "spring cleaning" is actually a very light diet, focusing on digestion and the intestines to help eliminate accumulated wastes, and improve body functions. A good length for a spring or summer cleanse is 2 or 3 days or a long weekend. A weekend is enough time to fit comfortably into most people's lives, and it doesn't become too stressful on the body. The best way is to start on Friday night with a pre-cleansing salad, then follow with a cleansing diet like the one in this book, and end with a light Monday morning fruit bowl. Amplify the purifying effect with a stimulating, circulation bath or sauna and steam baths.

What are the body signs that you need a Spring Cleanse?

—Do you feel bloated, constipated and congested? (a sign that your diet has been heavier and richer than usual)

—Have you gained some unwanted pounds even though you aren't eating more food? (a sign of winter fat storage)

—Do you feel slow and low energy most of the time? (a sign of cold weather body slowdown)

—Has your digestion worsened? (a sign your body isn't using its nutrients well)

—Do your chest and lungs feel clogged and swollen? (a sign of slower, shallower breathing, and perhaps a resident colony of low-grade infective microbes)

What benefits can you expect from a Spring Cleanse?

—Your digestive tract will be "washed and brushed" of accumulated waste and putrefactive bacteria.

—Your liver, kidney and blood can be purified, impossible under ordinary eating patterns and habits.

—Your mental clarity will receive a boost, not possible under the constant overload of chemicals and food additives.

—Possible dependency on habit-forming refined sugars, caffeine, nicotine, alcohol or drugs is relieved as body chemistry normalizes.

—Bad eating habits get a break.... with a new chance for you to reform better diet patterns.

—Your stomach has a chance to reduce to normal size for weight loss and better weight control.

Nutrition Plan

• **Start with this 3 to 5 day nutrition plan.**

Your nutrition should focus on fresh plant foods. 1) high chlorophyll plants for enzymes; 2) fruits and vegetables for fiber; 3) cultured foods for probiotics; 4) eight glasses of water a day.

The evening before your spring cleanse....
—Take your choice of gentle herbal laxatives.
—Have a light salad with plenty of greens.

The next day....
—On rising: take a cleansing and flushing booster product, or 1 heaping teaspoon of a fiber drink in juice or water. Add 1000mg vitamin C with bioflavonoids 3x a day to raise body glutathione levels, an important detox compound.
—Breakfast: take your choice of fruit juices.
—Mid-morning: take a small glass of potassium broth (pg. 134), or 2 TBS. aloe juice concentrate in juice or water, or a superfood green drink (see next column); or a cup of green tea.
—Lunch: a fresh carrot juice; or raw sauerkraut or a seaweed salad (in natural or oriental food stores)
—Mid-afternoon: take a glass of fresh apple juice; or an herbal cleansing tea.
—About 5 o'clock: take another small potassium broth, a fresh carrot or vegetable juice (page 138), or a superfood green drink (see next column).
—Supper: take miso soup with 2 TBS. dried sea vegetables (dulse, nori, etc.) snipped over the top. (Note: Finish your cleanse with a small green salad with fresh sprouts on the last night.)
—Before Bed: repeat the herbal cleansers that you took on rising, and take a cup of mint tea.

Continuing Diet Notes: After the initial cleanse above, the second part of a general health system is rebuilding healthy tissue and body energy. This stage takes 1 to 2 months for best results. It emphasizes high fiber from fresh vegetables and fruits, cultured foods to replenish healthy intestinal flora, and green foods for enzyme production, and alkalizing foods to prevent irritation while healing. Avoid refined foods, saturated fats, fried foods, red meats, caffeine and pasteurized dairy foods.

Herbs & Supplements

• **Choose 2 to 3 cleansing boosters.**

Gentle herbal laxatives: HERBALTONE tablets, Crystal Star LAXATEA, AloeLife ALOE GOLD. After your initial juice detox, Zand Herbals QUICK CLEANSE KIT for the intestinal tract and the liver.

Cleansing boosters: Crystal Star DETOX™ caps with *goldenseal*; Planetary Formulas RIVER OF LIFE, clears accumulations of a long inactive winter.

Cleansing and flushing boosters: Crystal Star CLEANSING & PURIFYING™ tea; Nature's Secret SUPERCLEANSE tabs; Crystal Star FIBER & HERBS CO-LON CLEANSE™ caps.

Chlorophyll-rich plants - spring's great gift to us: Sun Wellness SUN CHLORELLA; Futurebiotics COLON GREEN caps; Green Foods GREEN ESSENCE; Crystal Star ENERGY GREEN™, NutriCology PRO-GREENS; Solgar EARTH SOURCE GREENS; Nature's Secret ULTIMATE GREEN.

Enzyme support: Transformation Enzyme RELEASEZYME to remove waste. Full spectrum enzymes: Herbal Products Development POWER-PLUS ENZYMES; Rainbow Light ADVANCED ENZYME SYSTEM.

Electrolyte boosters help detoxify cells: Nature's Path TRACE-LYTE MINERALS; Arise & Shine ALKALIZER. Probiotics replenish healthy bacteria: Prevail INNER ECOLOGY; Prof. Nutrition DOCTOR-DOPHILUS+FOS; Wakunaga KYO-DOPHILUS.

Antioxidants defeat pollutants: Country Life SUPER 10 ANTIOXIDANT; NutriCology ANTIOX FORMULA II; Biotec Food CELL GUARD; Solgar ADVANCED ANTIOXIDANT FORMULA; Rainbow Light MULTI CAROTENE COMPLEX; Enzymatic Therapy GREEN TEA ANTIOXIDANT. Fiber: All One WHOLE FIBER COMPLEX; Crystal Star CHO-LO FIBER TONE™ drink; AloeLife FIBERMATE. High-potency multiple support: Futurebiotics MAXIMUM SUPPORT MULTI; vitamin C 1,000mg daily.

Bodywork Techniques

• **Pick bodywork and relaxation techniques to accelerate and round out your cleanse.**

Irrigate: Take an enema the first, second and the last day of your spring cleansing program to help release toxins out of the body.

Exercise: take a walk for ten minutes the first day of your cleanse. Each day increase your exercise by five minutes.

Sauna: Take a hot sauna or a long warm bath with a rubdown, to stimulate circulation. Dry brush your body before your sauna to help release toxins coming out through the skin.

Massage therapy: get one good lower back and pelvis massage during your cleanse

Aromatherapy supports detoxification. Stress reducing flower remedies: STRESS/TENSION or CLEANSING REMEDY by Natural Labs; Nelson Bach RESCUE REMEDY; BODY TONER by Wyndmere Naturals.

Aromatherapy bath: add 8 to 10 drops of essential oil to a bath. Stir water briskly to disperse. Lavender and chamomile are good choices. Or try AROMATHERAPY HERBAL MINERAL BATHS by Nature's Alchemy, a blend of essential oils, herbs and ancient sea minerals.

Deep Breathing Exercise: Do this deep, relaxed breathing exercise often during your cleanse to remove stress, compose your mind, improve your mood and increase your energy: Take a deep, full breath. Exhale it slowly.... slowly. Take another deep, full breath. Release slowly. And again. Maintain a quiet rhythm, exhaling more slowly than you inhale.

Close your eyes. As you exhale, visualizes toxins dislodging and leaving your body. As you inhale, visualize pure nutrients rebuilding your vibrancy.

Can't find a recommended product? Call the 800 number listed in Product Resources.

Do you need a twenty four hour cleanse?

This cleanse is a special little jewel. It's an invaluable healing tool to put into action as soon as you realize that you are not feeling well. It can swiftly be "pulled out of your pocket" at the first signs of unexplained low energy, poor skin or congestion. It's one of the best ways I know to turn around (and get quick recovery) from a cold or flu. It's also an easy first step before making a significant diet improvement or change.

A 24 hour cleanse can be a good answer if you need a cleanse, but your busy life won't allow you to set aside even a few days. People always tell me how busy their lives are. Sometimes, even a short cleanse seems like too much time.

"Beginning" is usually the hardest part of a cleanse. You have to set apart a block of time, gather all the ingredients for a detox diet, alter your eating times and patterns; in essence change your lifestyle and that of those you live with for a while. This is very difficult to do for many people, and can delay a needed program.

A 24-hour detox is a juice and herbal tea cleanse that lets you go on with your normal activities, and "jump start" a healing program. Even though it's quick, without the depth of vegetable juices needed for a major or chronic problem, it's often enough, is definitely better than no cleanse at all, and it will make a difference in the speed of healing. Even if your program is only going to consist of lifestyle changes aimed at better health, a 24 hour cleanse can point you in the right direction.

Is your body showing signs that it needs a twenty four hour cleanse?

—Do you feel "toxic"?
—Are you tired a lot for no reason?
—Are you starting to feel congested? Do you have the first signs of a cold or flu? (Go right into this cleanse.)
—Is your skin dry or flaky? Is your skin tone sallow? Is your hair dull, dry and brittle?
—Are the soles of your feet or your palms often peeling?
—Do you frequently get mouth herpes?
—Do you get frequent yeast infections?
—Do you get frequent urinary tract infections?
—Are you getting unusual allergy reactions?

Pointers for best results from your twenty four hour cleanse:

•Drink 8 to 10 glasses of water a day to hydrate and flush wastes and toxins from all cells.
•Focus on chlorophyll-rich foods (leafy greens, sea vegetables) and juices (super green foods like chlorella, barley grass or spirulina) during this cleanse. Chlorophyll is the most powerful cleansing agent found in nature. It also has a rapid tonic effect.

Nutrition Plan

• Start your 24 hour cleanse the night before.

The evening before you begin.... have a green leafy salad to give your bowels a good sweeping. Dry brush your skin before you go to bed to open your pores for the night's cleansing eliminations.

The next day.... the next 24 hours take fresh juices, herbal drinks, water, and a long walk.

—On rising: take 2 TBS. fresh lemon or lime juice, 1 TB. maple syrup and 1 pinch cayenne in water.

—Breakfast: make a fresh fruit juice with 1 Pear, 2 Apples, 4 Oranges and 1 Grapefruit; or a glass of fresh cranberry juice from concentrate.

—Mid-morning: have a Zippy Tonic: 1 handful dandelion greens, 3 fresh pineapple rings and 3 radishes; or a cleansing, energizing tea with antioxidants like Crystal Star GREEN TEA CLEANSER™.

—Lunch: juice 4 parsley sprigs, or a handful of dandelion greens, 3 tomatoes, $^{1}/_{2}$ green bell pepper, $^{1}/_{2}$ cucumber, 1 scallion, 1 lemon wedge; or a glass of fresh apple juice with 1 packet chlorella or Green Foods GREEN MAGMA granules dissolved.

—Mid-afternoon: take a cup of Crystal Star CLEANSING & PURIFYING™ TEA or MEDITATION™ TEA.

—Dinner: take a glass of papaya/pineapple juice to enhance enzyme production; or try this high mineral broth: 7 carrots with tops, 7 celery stalks with tops, beet tops from 1 bunch, 2 potatoes, 1 onion, 4 cloves of garlic, 3 zucchini, 1 handful of parsley. Place in a large soup pot, cover with water, bring to a boil and simmer for thirty minutes. Remove and discard veggies.

—Before Bed: have a cup of mint tea, or 1 teasp. Sovex NUTRITIONAL YEAST BROTH or miso soup.

Continuing Diet Notes: The next morning: have a cup of green tea or mint tea, or Crystal Star GREEN TEA CLEANSER™. Then break your fast with a bowl of fresh fruits. Eat fresh foods during the day - have a mixed vegetable salad for lunch with a little lemon/flax oil dressing. Have another salad for dinner with a little brown rice and tamari sauce. Before bed, have a warming Miso Broth (page 150).

Herbs & Supplements

• Choose 2 to 3 cleansing boosters.

Gentle herbal laxatives: The night before your cleanse have an herbal laxative tea such as Crystal Star LAXA TEA™, M. D. Labs DAILY DETOX TEA or Traditional Medicinals SMOOTH MOVE.

Cleansing boosters: Crystal Star CLEANSING & PURIFYING™ TEA helps cleanse and detoxify the system while providing strength and nourishment or Crystal Star LIV-ALIVE™ - a cleansing formula to re-establish an alkaline environment, which is very useful at the beginning of a cleansing program.

Enzyme/nutrient support: Transformation Enzyme SUPER CELLZYME - a whole food supplement with all 45 of the vitamins and minerals required to feed the body, plus enzymes needed to allow these nutrients to do their job.

Electrolyte boosters aid in efficient removal of toxic body acids & boost energy: Nature's Path TRACE-LYTE LIQUID MINERALS; Arise & Shine ALKALIZER.

Probiotics: Have detoxifying properties, and maintain the body's vital chemical and hormone balance. Wakunaga of America KYO-DOPHILUS; Arise & Shine FLORA GROW; New Chapter ALL-FLORA.

Chlorella: Green algae are the highest sources of chlorophyll in the plant world; and of all the green algae, chlorella is the highest. Sun Wellness SUN CHLORELLA or New Chapter CHLORELLA.

Vitamin C: Take 1,000mg of vitamin C 3x per day. (complex with bioflavonoids) vitamin C raises the body's glutathione levels (an important detox compound).

Flower remedies: Flower remedies can assist the mental and emotional elements of detoxification. Natural Labs Corp. CLEANSING REMEDY.

Can't find a recommended product? Call the 800 number listed in Product Resources.

Bodywork Techniques

• Pick bodywork and relaxation techniques to accelerate and round out your cleanse.

Dry brush: The night before your cleanse, dry brush your skin before you go to bed to open your pores for the night's cleansing eliminations.

Enema: Take an enema the night before or the morning of your cleanse. After an enema there may be a heightened sense of physical well-being.

Exercise: Take a long, brisk walk during the day.

Bathe: Take a seaweed or mineral bath in the morning and one before you go to bed. (See seaweed bath, page 35.) Mineral bath: add 1 cup Dead Sea salts, 1 cup Epsom salts, $^{1}/_{2}$ cup regular sea salt and $^{1}/_{4}$ cup baking soda to a tub; swish in 3 drops lavender oil, 2 drops chamomile oil, 2 drops marjoram oil and 1 drop ylang-ylang oil.

Pamper yourself: Add some favorite beauty and skin cleansing treatments like a facial, a pedicure, or deep hair conditioning during your bath.

Rest: Get a full eight hours of rest the night before your cleanse. Add a nap during the day to allow your body's energies to focus on healing.

Essential oils Aromatherapy can support detoxification and healing, Wyndmere WELLNESS.

Visualize your detox: Close your eyes and inhale and exhale long and slowly. As you exhale, visualize toxins dislodging and leaving your body. As you inhale, visualize oxygen and nutrients renewing each cells.

Do you need an overall body stress cleanse?

You change the oil in your car because you believe it will make it run smoother and last longer. You plunge into spring cleaning, determined to make your living environment free of dirt and germs that might threaten your health. You buy air and water filters which promise to rid your environment of toxins. You sink into a hot bath, convinced that cleansing your body's exterior will keep you healthy.

How disconcerting to realize that you've left an important part of the cleansing job unattended. **Cleansing on the inside improves everything on the outside.** A whole body stress detox is the key to revitalizing your body, mind and spirit. A stress cleanse focuses on your entire body... eliminating toxins and rebuilding your tissues with cleansing juices and stress-relieving foods. Rather than targeting a specific body system or problem, this cleanse reflects broad spectrum, mild body refreshment. It clears the "junk" out of body pathways so that wholesome nutrients can get in quickly to rebuild energy and strength.

You may have been struggling with the low nutrition of a Standard American Diet (SAD) for decades. Many people do not recognize that much of the "food" in America's supermarkets doesn't really have much nutrition that the body can translate into usable nutrients. Some of the "foods" like designer fake fats may even ultimately contribute to ill health. One of the best ways to keep excess fat and sugar out of your life is to keep in mind what a really healthy diet is.

—It's fresh fruit and vegetable juices several times a week.
—It's fresh fruits and vegetables every day. At least once a day, have a fresh salad. Have steamed, stir-fried or baked veggies for at least one other meal.
—It's adding sea vegetables to a meal at least once a week for their packed, superior nutrition. (Six pieces of sushi are just fine.)
—It's cultured foods for friendly digestive flora (like raw sauerkraut, yogurt, kefir, kefir cheese or cottage cheese). Raw sauerkraut, rich in acidophilus, is especially good at deterring harmful bacteria.
—It's plenty of water - at least eight 8-oz. glasses a day.
—It's whole grains, nuts, seeds and beans for protein and essential fatty acids.
—It's healthy fats, like omega-3 oils and EFAs from cold water fish, flax and canola oil and seafood that enhance thyroid and metabolic balance; and EFAs from sea vegetables, spinach and herbs like ginger and evening primrose oil. It's just as important to include healthy fats as it is to eliminate unhealthy fats, like hydrogenated and partially hydrogenated fats.
—It's superfoods like bee pollen, royal jelly and aloe vera; or green superfoods like chlorella, spirulina or barley grass with concentrated nutrition, and they're becoming more and more popular as anti-aging factors, energy boosters, and highly supportive when dealing with a health problem, weight problem and of course detoxification.
—A healthy diet is also less meat and dairy foods. You'll feel better if you eat them in moderation. You'll feel a lot better if you avoid fried foods and chemically processed foods altogether.

Is your body showing signs that it needs an overall body stress cleanse?

- Is your immune response low? Are you catching every bug that comes down the pike?
- Are you unusually tired? Do you feel like you need a pick-me-up?
- Have you had unusual body odor or bad breath lately?
- Do you feel mentally dull?
- Have you gained weight even though your diet hasn't changed? (A cleanse is a healthy way to lose weight.)

Pointers for best results from your body stress cleanse:

- Drink eight 8-oz. glasses of bottled water each day of your cleanse (herbal teas can be part of this).
- Add 1 TB. of a superfood or green superfood mix to at least one of the juices you take per day. For the best results in energy and nourishment I like to add 1 TB. of a green superfood to all the veggie or fruit drinks.
- Alkalize the whole body. Foods which are alkalizing should be used in a ratio of at least 4:1 to foods which are acidifying. Plenty of pure water and fresh fruit or vegetable juices are especially useful. Acidifying foods tend to aggravate any health problems.

Benefits that you may notice as your body responds to a body stress cleanse:

- Your digestion will noticeably improve as your digestive tract is cleansed of accumulated waste and fermenting bacteria.
- You'll feel lighter (most people lose about 5 pounds on this cleanse) and more energized.
- You'll feel less dependent on habit-forming substances like sugar, caffeine, nicotine, alcohol and drugs as your bloodstream purifies.
- You'll feel healthier. Most people have noticeably better resistance to common colds and flu.
- You'll feel more mentally alert, less space-y, more emotionally balanced. Creativity begins to expand.
- You'll feel more energized as your body starts rebalancing. Energy levels rise physically, psychologically and sexually.

Nutrition Plan

• **Start with this 3 to 7 day nutrition plan.**

Begin with a 3 day juice/liquid diet and follow with 1 to 4 days of a diet of all fresh foods.

—On rising: take a glass of 2 fresh squeezed lemons, 1 TB. maple syrup and 8-oz. of pure water.

—Breakfast: have a nutrient-dense Kick-Off Cleansing Cocktail: juice 1 handful fresh wheat grass or parsley - extremely rich in chlorophyll and antioxidants, 4 carrots, 1 apple, 2 celery stalks with leaves, 1/2 beet with top.

—Mid-morning: have a glass of fresh carrot juice or fresh apple juice. Add 1 TB of a green superfood like Crystal Star Energy Green™ drink mix; Green Kamut Green Kamut; Vibrant Health Green Vibrance.

—Lunch: have a Salad-In-A-Glass: juice 4 parsley sprigs, 3 quartered tomatoes, 1/2 green or red pepper, 1/2 cucumber, 1 scallion, 1 lemon wedge.

—Mid-afternoon: have a cup of Crystal Star Cleansing & Purifying™ Tea, green tea or mint tea.

—Dinner: have a warm Potassium Essence Broth (page 134), for mineral electrolytes. Or try Super Soup, with antioxidants, antibiotic properties and immune boosters: 1 cup broccoli florets, 1 leek (white parts, a little green), 2 cups fresh peas, 1/2 cup sliced scallions, 4 cups chard leaves, 1/2 cup diced fennel bulb, 1/2 cup fresh parsley, 6 garlic minced cloves, 2 tsp. astragalus extract (or 1/4 cup broken pieces astragalus bark), 6 cups vegetable stock, a pinch of cayenne, 1 cup diced green cabbage, 1/4 cup snipped sea vegetables. Bring all ingredients bring to a boil, then simmer for 10 min. Let sit for 20 minutes. Strain and use broth only for a cleanse. (Use unstrained as a soup recipe when not on a cleanse.)

Herbs & Supplements

• **Choose 2 to 3 cleansing boosters.**

Use alongside the liquid juice cleanse: Crystal Star Detox™ caps with *goldenseal* stimulates the body to eliminate wastes rapidly or Crystal Star Cleansing & Purifying™ tea.

Deep cleansing: When solid food is again introduced, use Nature's Secret Ultimate Cleanse.

Cleansing support formulas: New Chapter Life Shield; Futurebiotics Oxy-Shield protects the body against oxidative damage and all-around protection against environmental assault.

Enzyme support: Prevail Detox Enzyme Formula; Transformation Excellzyme.

Antioxidants help remove toxins: Biotec Food Cell Guard; Rainbow Light Multi Carotene Complex; Jarrow Coenzyme Q_{10}.

Probiotics support detoxification in numerous ways: Professional Nutrition Doctor-Dophilus+Fos; Wakunaga Kyo-Dophilus; Prevail Inner Ecology.

Electrolytes dramatically boosts energy levels: Arise & Shine Alkalizer; Nature's Path, Trace-Lyte Liquid Minerals.

Green Superfoods: Crystal Star Energy Green™ drink mix; Green Kamut Green Kamut; Vibrant Health Green Vibrance.

Detoxing gentle flower remedies: Natural Labs Stress/Tension; Nelson Bach Rescue Remedy.

Bodywork Techniques

• **Pick bodywork and relaxation techniques to accelerate and round out your cleanse.**

Enema: Enemas can be a best friend to your cleansing program. Flushing your colon on the first, the second and the last day of your stress detox program gives your body a giant step forward in releasing toxins from your body.

Enema: Guided imagery, biofeedback and aromatherapy are especially helpful techniques for detoxing from general body stress.

Exercise: Do this body stretch daily during your cleanse. Repeat this at least 5 times.

• Stand tall — raise your hands above your head.

• Stretch your arms and fingers to reach for the sky - move your hands and fingers as if you are trying to climb up into the sky.

• As you reach, inhale deeply through your nostrils while rising on your toes.

• Exhale slowly; gradually return to your starting position, arms hanging loosely at your sides.

• Follow your stretch with a brisk walk.

Deep Breathing Exercise: Deep, relaxed breathing takes away stress, induces relaxation, composes the mind, improves mood & increases energy levels. 1. Take a deep, full breath. Exhale it, slowly. Slowly. 2. Take another deep, full breath. Release slowly. 3. And again. 4. Maintain a quiet rhythm, exhaling more slowly than you inhale.

Sauna or bath: Take a hot sauna or a long warm bath, with a rubdown to stimulate circulation. In your bath try: Aromatherapy Herbal Mineral Baths by Nature's Alchemy; or use a relaxing essential oil like lavender (10 drops in your bath water).

Massage: Have a massage therapy treatment to further remove toxins and stimulate circulation.

Continuing Diet Notes: Eat plenty of fresh vegetables and fruits for the rest of the month. Choose foods high in fiber like whole grains and beans. Especially avoid unhealthy fats, like partially hydrogenated oils. But make a point to get plenty of EFAs from sea vegetables, herbs like ginger, ginseng or evening primrose oil. Avoid refined sugars, sodas and caffeine-containing foods for the rest of the month. Don't forget to drink plenty of daily water.

Can't find a recommended product? Call the 800 number listed in Product Resources.

Do you need a mucous congestion cleanse?

Your body needs some mucous. We tend to think of body mucous as a bad thing because it obstructs our breathing during a sinus infection, asthma or a cold. But that same mucous is also a needed body lubricant, and an important body safeguard. Human beings take about 22,000 breaths a day, and along with the oxygen, we take in dirt, pollen, disease germs, smoke and other pollutants. Mucous gathers up these irritants as they enter the nose and throat, protecting the mucous membranes that line the upper respiratory system. Mucous build-up may be a sign that your body is trying to bring itself to health. The problems start when your body holds on to too much. Some of us carry around as much as 10 to 15 pounds of excess mucous!

Your body systems work together, of course. It only seems, as we address its different parts and processes, that everything isn't wholly related. But, extra pressure of disease or heavy elimination on one body part puts extra stress on another. Support for the kidneys, for example, takes part of the waste elimination load off the lungs so they can recover faster. Similarly, promoting respiratory health also helps digestive and skin cleansing problems. The lungs, though, are on the front line of toxic intake from viruses, allergies, pollutants, and mucous-forming congestives. (We can see through the need to keep our own lungs healthy the need to care for the vital lungs of the earth through rainforest preservation.)

A program to overcome any chronic respiratory problem is usually more successful when begun with a short mucous elimination diet. This allows the body to rid itself first of toxins and accumulations that cause congestion before an attempt is made to change eating habits. Foods that putrefy quickly inside your body are the same foods that spoil easily outside in the air — like meat, fish, eggs and dairy products. These same foods are the ones most likely to produce excess mucous, too, which in turn slows down transit time through your gastro-intestinal tract and colon. Mucous gathers up irritants as they enter the nose and throat, protecting the mucous membranes that line the upper respiratory system. However, excess mucus can be congestive to the respiratory system and the colon. Excess mucous may be a sign that the body is trying to bring itself to health. This is the time to do a mucous cleanse.

Is your body showing signs that it needs a mucous cleanse?

Any signs of respiratory system congestion may be thought of as sure signs of excess mucous in the body, especially in the colon and intestinal tract. The common cold and flu are usually accompanied by congestion and phlegm. A mucous cleanse helps to release excess mucous in the respiratory system and in the colon.

Pointers for best results from your mucous cleanse:

• Herbal supplements are a good choice during a mucous and congestion cleanse. They act as premier broncho-dilators and anti-spasmodics to open congested airspaces. They can soothe bronchial inflammation and cough. They have the ability to break up mucous. They are expectorants to remove mucous from the lungs and throat.

• Drink 8 to 10 glasses of water daily to thin mucous and aid elimination.

• Take 10,000mg ascorbate vitamin C crystals with bioflavonoids daily the first three days; just dissolve $1/4$ teasp. in water or juice throughout the day, until the stool turns soupy, and tissues are flushed. Take 5,000mg daily for the next four days.

76

• Take a brisk, daily walk. Breathe deep to help lungs eliminate mucous.

• Take an enema the first and last day of your fasting diet to thoroughly clean out excess mucous.

• Apply wet ginger/cayenne compresses to the chest to increase circulation and loosen mucous.

• Take a hot sauna or a long warm bath with a rubdown, to stimulate circulation.

• Drink eight to ten glasses (8-oz.) of water daily during your mucous cleanse.

• Herbal supplements are a good choice during a mucous and congestion cleanse. They act as premier broncho-dilators and anti-spasmodics to open congested airspaces. They can soothe bronchial inflammation and coughs. They have the ability to break up mucous. They are expectorants to remove mucous from the lungs and throat.

• Take 10,000mg ascorbate vitamin C crystals with bioflavonoids daily the first three days; just dissolve $^1\!/_4$ teasp. in water or juice throughout the day, until the stool turns soupy, and tissues are flushed. Take 5,000mg daily for the next four days.

Benefits that you may notice as your body responds to a mucous congestion cleanse.

• The non-mucous forming cleansing diet with supportive supplements will begin to clear any congestion in the body.

• If there is bronchial inflammation and/or cough it will give way to relief as the cleanse progresses.

• Mucous from the lungs and throat will break up and be eliminated from the body.

• Mucous from the colon may also be expelled from the body.

• Symptoms (discomfort) from colds/flu, allergies or asthma will clear faster as the cleanse speeds up recovery.

Nutrition Plan

• **Start with this 3 to 7 day nutrition plan.**

The night before your mucous cleanse....

—Mash 4 garlic cloves and a large slice of onion in a bowl. Stir in 3 TBS. honey. Cover, let macerate for 24 hours; remove garlic and onion and take only the honey/syrup infusion - 1 teasp. 3x daily. The next day....

—On rising: take 2 squeezed lemons in water with 1 TB. maple syrup.

—Breakfast: take a glass of grapefruit, pineapple, or cranberry-apple juice.

—Mid-morning: have a glass of fresh carrot juice with 1 teasp. Bragg's LIQUID AMINOS added; or a cup of congestion clearing tea, like Crystal Star X-PECT™, an expectorant to aid mucous release, or Crystal Star RESPR TEA™, an aid in oxygen uptake.

—Lunch: have a vegetable juice like V-8, or a potassium broth (page 134); or make this Mucous Cleansing Tonic by juicing: 4 carrots, 2 celery stalks, 2-3 sprigs parsley, 1 radish and 1 garlic clove.

—Mid-afternoon: have a veggie drink (page 138), or a packet of Sun Wellness SUN CHLORELLA granules in water; or a greens and sea vegetable drink like Crystal Star ENERGY GREEN™ drink.

—Dinner: apple or papaya/pineapple juice.

—Before Bed: take a hot vegetable broth (page 153), add in 1 TB. nutritional yeast. Have a small fresh salad on the last night of the cleanse.

—The next day.... begin with small simple meals. Have toasted muesli or whole grain granola for your first morning of solid food, with a little yogurt or apple juice; a small fresh salad for lunch with lemon/oil dressing; a fresh fruit smoothie during the day; a baked potato with butter and a light soup or salad for dinner.

Continuing Diet Notes: Eliminate junk foods and fried foods. Avoid pasteurized dairy foods, heavy starches and refined foods that are a breeding ground for continued congestion. Drinking eight 8-oz glasses daily helps flush body toxins and prevent the build up of excess mucous. Eat plenty of enzyme-rich foods like fresh vegetables (salads) and fruits. They form the least amount of mucous and they are the easiest to digest, passing through the body in less transit time.

Herbs & Supplements

• **Choose 2 to 3 cleansing boosters.**

Deep body cleanser for intestinal tract and lungs: Use Nature's Way 5 SYSTEM CLEANSE caps after juice fasting - along with the cleansing diet. Helps pull intestinal mucous and clear mucous congestion from the respiratory system.

Mucous cleansers: Use Crystal Star X-PECT-TEA™ as an expectorant to aid mucous release; Herbs Etc. LUNG TONIC - A mullein and horehound expectorant to loosen and remove mucous; Herbs Etc. RESPIRATONIC is an all-purpose complex which loosens mucous, clears lung congestion, and dilates the bronchioles.

Herbs to relieve mucous; *mullein* loosens and expels mucous; *slippery elm* removes excess mucous, soothes and strengthens mucous membranes; *sage* helps excessive mucous discharge; *white pine*, an antioxidant expectorant, reduces mucous.

Better oxygen uptake: Crystal Star RESPR™ TEA; NutriCology GERMANIUM.

Enzyme support: Prevail DIGESTION FORMULA; Herbal Products and Development POWER-PLUS ENZYMES; Transformation Enzyme GASTROZYME relieves bouts of mucous congestion. After congestion is relieved, use Transformation Enzyme DIGESTZYME to assist complete digestion. *Improperly digested foods putrefy and cause mucous.*

Electrolyte boosters helps digestive efficiency up to 80%: Nature's Path TRACE-LYTE LIQUID MINERALS; Arise & Shine ALKALIZER.

Probiotics help maintain proper mucous levels: Nature's Path FLORA-LYTE; Jarrow Formulas JARRO-DOPHILUS+FOS; Ethical Nutrients INTESTINAL CARE.

Can't find a recommended product? Call the 800 number listed in Product Resources.

Bodywork Techniques

• **Pick bodywork and relaxation techniques to accelerate and round out your cleanse.**

Enema: Take an enema the first, second and last day of your juice fasting to help thoroughly clean out excess mucous. Irrigate: Or, have a colonic for a more thorough colon cleanse.

Exercise: Take a brisk, daily walk on each day of your cleanse. Breathe deep to help the lungs eliminate mucous.

Massage therapy with percussion: a rubdown stimulates circulation and loosens mucous. Most people have several congestion-releasing bowel movements and expectoration incidences within 24 hours after a massage therapy treatment.

Compress: Apply wet *ginger/cayenne* chest compresses to increase circulation and loosen mucous.

Essential oil support: aromatherapy oils help clear mucous congestion in the lungs:

• *Eucalyptus* (inhale) - antiviral action works on respiratory tract to loosen mucous - treats asthma, bronchitis and sinusitis.

• *Tea tree oil* (inhale) - antiviral and antibacterial decongestant.

• *Oregano oil* (inhale) - antiviral and antibacterial properties help eradicate lung infection.

• Flower remedies: Nelson Bach RESCUE REMEDY or Natural Labs DEVA FLOWERS STRESS/TENSION.

• Visualize your detox Close your eyes —inhale and exhale long and slowly. As you exhale, visualize mucous dislodging and leaving your lungs and also from your colon. As you inhale, visualize oxygen and nutrients renewing all your cells.

Bathe & Sauna: long warm baths and saunas help loosen mucous congestion. Add to your bath 5 drops of eucalyptus, tea tree oil or oregano oil.

Do you need a brown rice cleanse?

A brown rice cleanse is a 7-day cleansing diet. I've found it's an effective option to a juice cleanse. It's especially useful for dropping a few quick pounds and a great way to transition from an unhealthy diet into a better diet. A brown rice cleanse is based on macrobiotic principles for body balance. Brown rice adds a building, warming factor to a cleanse, making your meals more satisfying, and ensuring that you get plenty of fiber and minerals. The brown rice cleanse is an option to a juice cleanse, and much easier to fit into your lifestyle.

A brown rice cleansing diet encourages an approach to eating that provides complex carbohydrates, quality protein, and energy fats by using rice as a nutrient building food, and using vegetables and vegetable juices as concentrated cleansing supplements.

Is your body showing signs that a brown rice cleanse would do you some good?

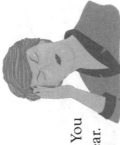

—Is your immune response low?

—Do you feel like you need to clear cobwebs from your brain?

—Do you need to lose about 10 pounds? A brown rice diet is a healthy way to lose weight!

—Are you feeling log-y and out-of-sorts?

—Are you looking for a gentle, easy transition to an improved diet? A brown rice diet is cleansing, yet filling. You don't feel like you're on a cleanse at all, yet it does the trick. It's the best cleansing diet for colder times of the year.

Pointers for best results from your brown rice cleanse:

• Drink 8 to 10 glasses of water (or herbal teas) a day to hydrate and flush wastes and toxins from all cells.

• Add 1 TB. of a green drink mix or superfood powder to each juice you take during the day.

• Use non-fat seasonings to your own taste. Use only 1 TB. of a healthy oil dressing on salads (like flax, olive or canola oil). Better yet, I like to use only sea vegetables or herbal seasoning salts on both my salads and rice during this diet.

• Follow this diet for at least seven days. You need one week to set up an ongoing body balance. Then, ease yourself into a good, ongoing diet. Include other wholesome grains like millet, amaranth, quinoa and buckwheat after you complete the brown rice cleanse.

Benefits that you may notice as your body responds to a brown rice cleanse:

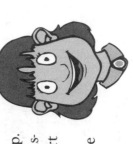

• Most people notice an improvement in vitality and energy levels right away.

• Almost everybody loses some weight during this cleanse. Most people experience about a 2 to 5 pound weight drop.

• People who have heart problems regularly notice a more stable heartbeat and better circulation. A fiber-rich cleansing diet with sea vegetables, that eliminates animal (meat and dairy) protein, almost invariably lowers the risk of heart problems, high blood pressure and diabetes risk. The diet is stimulating to the heart and circulatory system.

• Because this cleanse is so high in potassium, natural iodine, and other minerals and trace elements, most people notice improvement in their hair and skin texture and their nail growth.

Nutrition Plan

•**Start with this 7 day nutrition plan.**

The night before your brown rice cleanse.... A green leafy salad for dinner sweeps your bowels. The next day....

—On rising: take a glass of 2 fresh squeezed lemons, 1 TB. maple syrup and 8-oz. of pure water.

—Breakfast: have a drink like Pulsating Parsley Juice: 6 carrots, 1 beet, 8 spinach leaves and ¼ cup fresh parsley leaves.

—Mid-morning: take a cup of Crystal Star CLEANSING & PURIFYING™ TEA or DAILY DETOX by M.D.

—Lunch: have a veggie juice like Super V-7: 2 carrots, 2 tomatoes, handful of spinach leaves and a handful of parsley, 2 celery ribs, ½ cucumber, ½ green bell pepper. Add 1 TB. green superfood: Crystal Star ENERGY GREEN™; Body Ecology VITALITY SUPERGREEN; Ethical Nutrients FUNCTIONAL GREENS or Vibrant Health VITALITY SUPERGREEN.

—Mid-afternoon: have a glass of carrot juice.

—Dinner: have steamed brown rice and mixed steamed vegetables. Sprinkle with sea vegetables (like dulse or kelp, easily purchased in flakes or granules). (Use 1 TB. flax or olive oil, if desired, and 1 TB . Bragg's LIQUID AMINOS). Add flavor and nutrition by sprinkling with nutritional yeast.

—Before Bed: have a cup of herbal tea such as peppermint, spearmint or chamomile.

—The next 6 days: have 2 to 3 glasses of mixed vegetable juices throughout the day. Any blend of your favorite vegetables is fine. Don't eat any solid food during the day. Have steamed brown rice and mixed vegetables for an early dinner each evening. Either steamed or raw vegetable salads can be used. The enzymes in raw vegetables provide a greater cleansing quality.

Herbs & Supplements

•**Choose 2 to 3 cleansing boosters.**

Cleansing boosters: Crystal Star FIBER & HERBS COLON CLEANSE™ caps stimulate the body to eliminate waste rapidly; Nature's Secret ULTIMATE CLEANSE helps detoxify all five channels of elimination and is taken along with a cleansing diet.

Cleansing teas: Crystal Star CLEANSING & PURIFYING™ TEA helps cleanse and detoxify the system while providing strength and nourishment; DAILY DETOX by M.D. is a mild cleanser, gentle enough to take on a daily basis, yet stimulates all the major elimination organs.

Enzyme support: Transformation Enzyme DIGESTZYME.

Cleansing support formulas: Futurebiotics Oxy-SHIELD and New Chapter LIFE SHIELD protect against oxidative damage and environmental assault;

Electrolyte boosters: electrolytes play a major role in detoxifying cells, and enhance uptake of essential nutrients, macro minerals and proteins from food sources and other supplements. Nature's Path TRACE-LYTE LIQUID MINERALS; Arise & Shine ALKALIZER.

Probiotics: the number one factor in creating and maintaining health and well-being of the intestines. Premier Labs MULTI-DOPHILUS; Prevail INNER ECOLOGY; Jarrow Formulas JARRO-DOPHILUS+FOS.

Essential Fatty Acids: Evening primrose oil 1000mg.

Chlorella: Chlorophyll is the most powerful cleansing agent found in nature. Green algae are the highest sources of chlorophyll in the plant world — Sun Wellness SUN CHLORELLA or New Chapter CHLORELLA.

Bodywork Techniques

•**Pick bodywork and relaxation techniques to accelerate and round out your cleanse.**

Enema: Take an enema the night before or the morning of your cleanse. Flushing the colon is one of the best ways to jump-start any cleanse. Cleaning the colon allows more expedient release of toxins from all other body cells.

Exercise: Take a brisk walk, or workout on an exercise bicycle or a treadmill. Exercise increases oxygen uptake, and boosts blood transport to carry nutrients to cells and waste products and toxins away from the cells.

Massage therapy: It's one of my cardinal cleansing points. —Get a massage once a week for the month of your cleanse. Health experts agree that a regular massage promotes the movement of body fluids. There's also noticeable improvement in overall health because most of the body's processes rely on movement of fluids, including getting nutrients to cells, oxygenating tissues and removing wastes from all body parts.

Flower remedies: Nelson Bach RESCUE REMEDY or Natural Labs DEVA FLOWERS STRESS/TENSION.

•Essential oils: Aromatherapy supports relaxation, detoxification and healing. Wyndmere STRESS MANAGEMENT (*Lavender, Ylang Ylang, Clary Sage, Pine Needle*) or WELLNESS (*Lemon, Peppermint, Rosemary, Thyme*) are good choices for this cleanse.

•Visualize your detox: Close your eyes and inhale and exhale long and slowly. Visualize a free movement of body fluids. As you exhale, visualize toxins dislodging from cells, being carried by the bodies fluids, and leaving your body. As you inhale, visualize oxygen and nutrients flowing to and renewing all your cells.

Continuing Diet Notes: Eating whole foods is the first principle to remember as you choose the foods for your continuing diet. Eating from the sea is the second important principle. Include fish or shellfish, or sea vegetables at least three times a week. Work at eliminating (completely if possible) fried and fast foods. Reduce your consumption of meats and dairy foods. Consciously add more grains and vegetables. Eat your fruits and fruit juices in the morning or late at night.

Can't find a recommended product? Call the 800 number listed in Product Resources.

Do you need a pollutant or heavy metal cleanse?

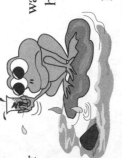

Chemical pollutants and toxic by-products affect every facet of our lives, from our workplace and our homes. Heavy metal poisoning and pollutant toxicity are now major health problems of the American culture. We have moved from fetid air to undrinkable water to severe allergy reactions to serious diseases caused by pollution. There seems to be no way to avoid toxic exposure. The main effect is reduced immune response, especially in the way that our filtering organs, the liver and kidneys, are impacted. Periodic detoxification needs to be a part of life to keep our bodies able to defend us.... against yet more pollutants. (An astounding twenty-five thousand NEW chemicals enter our society every year.) A hair analysis can help you determine which heavy metals are lodged in your body, and also nutrient deficiencies you may have that result from environmental toxin overload.

Is your body showing signs that it needs a pollution/heavy metal cleanse?

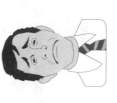

—Are you far more sensitive to odors like perfumes and strong cleansers than most people? Do you feel worse in certain stores?
—Do you have an unusually small tolerance for alcohol?
—Are there medications you can't take, some vitamins or other supplements that make you feel worse?
—Do you have small black spots along your gum line? Unusually bad breath or body odor?
—Is your reaction time when driving noticeably poorer in city traffic?
—Do you have unexplained seizures, memory failure or psychotic behavior?
—Have you become infertile or impotent?

Pointers for best results from your pollutant/heavy metal cleanse:

• Drink 8-10 glasses of bottled water each day of your cleanse.
• A heavy metal and pollutant detox is one of the most likely cleanses for a "healing crisis" to occur. You may feel head-achy, slight upset stomach or nausea as toxins are released into the bloodstream for elimination. The feelings should pass quickly, usually within 24 hours. But I don't recommend an all-liquid diet if you're trying to release heavy metals or chemicals. They may enter the bloodstream too fast and heavily for your body to handle safely. Eat solid cleansing foods instead to release the toxins more slowly and safely.
• Chlorophyll is the most powerful cleansing agent found in nature. Green veggie drinks and green superfoods are key.
• Sea vegetables are powerful in releasing environmental toxins, heavy metals and radiation from the body. They can be sprinkled on salads, steamed veggies, baked potatoes, into vegetable juices, etc.

Benefits that you may notice as your body responds to a pollution cleanse.

• Your immune response will improve as the toxins leave your body and you build up resistance.
• Providing high quality nutrients gives your body a choice and allows the natural law of selective uptake to kick in. This means your cells and tissues will naturally admit the nourishing nutrients and more easily release toxins that would otherwise lodge in them.

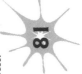

Nutrition Plan

• **Start with this 7 day nutrition plan.**

—On rising: take 2-3 TBS. cranberry concentrate in 8-oz. water with $^1/_2$ teasp. ascorbate vitamin C crystals; or Crystal Star GREEN TEA CLEANSER™, or blend half a lemon with pit, 1 tsp. honey, 1 cup water and 1 tsp. acidophilus in 8-oz. aloe vera juice.

—Breakfast: have a glass of fresh carrot juice, with 1 TB. of a green superfood like Crystal Star ENERGY GREEN™ or Green Foods GREEN MAGMA, and whole grain muffins or rice cakes w. kefir cheese or yogurt; or a cup of soy milk or plain yogurt blended with a cup of fresh fruit, walnuts, and $^1/_2$ teasp. Natren TRINITY (or acidophilus) in 8-oz. aloe vera juice.

—Mid-morning: take a cup of green tea, with $^1/_2$ teasp. ascorbate vitamin C crystals; or a fresh vegetable juice with 1 TB. green superfood such as Nutricology PRO-GREENS or Wakunaga KYO-GREEN.

—Lunch: have a leafy salad with lemon/flax oil dressing; or have an open-faced sandwich on rice cakes or a chapati, with soy cheese and fresh veggies; or a cup of miso soup with brown rice; or steamed vegetables with brown rice and tofu; and pau d'arco tea with $^1/_2$ teasp. ascorbate vitamin C and $^1/_2$ teasp. acidophilus powder.

—Mid-afternoon: have a carrot juice with 1 TB. green superfood like Crystal Star ENERGY GREEN™.

—Dinner: have a baked potato with Bragg's LIQUID AMINOS and a fresh salad w. lemon/flax dressing; or a black bean or lentil soup; or a Chinese steam/ stir fry with vegetables, shiitake mushrooms and brown rice; or a tofu and veggie casserole.

—Before Bed: take a 8-oz. glass of aloe vera juice with $^1/_2$ teasp. ascorbate vitamin C with bioflavs; and another carrot juice, or papaya juice with 1 teasp. acidophilus powder.

Herbs & Supplements

• **Choose 2 to 3 cleansing boosters.**

Deep Cleansing product: Along with the cleansing diet use a deep cleanser like Arise & Shine CLEANSE THYSELF PROGRAM or Creation Garden 14 DAY TOTAL BODY CLEANSE (can be used as a 7 day cleanse). Pollutant/Heavy Metal cleansers: Crystal Star HEAVY METAL CLEANZ™ caps.

Herbal immune protection: Crystal Star REISHI/ GINSENG™ extract; *astragalus* extract; *propolis* extract; *panax ginseng; Siberian ginseng; aloe vera and garlic.*

Liver enhancers: Crystal Star LIV-ALIVE™ caps/ tea; Crystal Star GINSENG/LICORICE ELIXIR™; MILK THISTLE SEED extract; *dandelion* extract.

Antioxidants defeat pollutants: Alpha Lipoic Acid is among the most powerful liver detoxifiers ever discovered. Jarrow Formulas ALPHA LIPOIC ACID or ALPHA-LIPOIC ACID by MRI; NutriCology ANTIOX FORMULA II; Futurebiotics OXY-SHIELD.

Chelation: Oral chelation cleanses circulatory of heavy metals. Hayestown Assoc. TRICARDIA; Golden Pride FORMULA ONE, oral chelation with EDTA.

Enzyme support: Protease binds to heavy metals, sparing metabolic enzyme destruction. Transformation Enzyme PUREZYME (high doses effective in lowering blood mercury toxins).

Probiotics help deactivate drugs: Professional Nutr. DOCTOR-DOPHILUS+FOS; Nature's Path FLORA-LYTE; Chlorella supplements: *chlorella's* high chlorophyll content and powerful detox ability are available through its unique cell wall. Sun Wellness SUN CHLORELLA or New Chapter CHLORELLA.

Sea Vegetables: Seaweeds bind with and neutralize many heavy metals and environmental toxins. Nature's Path TRACE-MIN-LYTE; Bio-Tec PACIFIC SEA PLASMA; New Chapter OCEAN HERBS caps.

Bodywork Techniques

• **Pick bodywork and relaxation techniques to accelerate and round out your cleanse.**

Enema: Enemas greatly assist removal of toxins and relieving stress on the body. Take an enema the first and second day of your cleansing program. Take additional enemas as you feel the need. See enemas in this book. Better yet - have at least one colonic irrigation during your cleanse.

Exercise: Exercise only moderately during this cleanse. Allow your body to use its energy for healing and repair. Take a walk every day, breathing deeply. Get plenty of tissue oxygen. Do deep breathing exercises on rising, and in the evening on retiring to clear the lungs and respiratory system.

Shower: Take a hot and cold hydrotherapy treatment at the end of your daily shower. Alternating hot for 1 minute, then cool for 1 minute to stimulate circulation. Use a dry skin brush before and after the shower to remove toxins coming out on the skin (quite common in a heavy metal cleanse).

Bathe: A detoxifying, relaxing mineral bath: Add 1 cup Dead Sea salts, 1 cup Epsom salts, $^1/_2$ cup regular sea salt and $^1/_4$ baking soda to a tub. If you have access to seaweed (either dried or freshly gathered), add it to the bath to help draw out toxins. If you wish to add essential oils, swish in 4 drops lavender oil, and 4 drops chamomile oil.

Flower remedies: Natural Labs STRESS/TENSION; Nelson Bach RESCUE REMEDY.

Visualization Exercise: Close your eyes and inhale and exhale long and slowly. As you exhale, visualize toxins dislodging and leaving your body. As you inhale, visualize pure, nourishing nutrients building health and vibrancy.

Continuing Diet Notes: Protection against pollutants begins with a healthful whole foods diet. Eat organically grown foods as much as possible to reduce the intake of toxins. Green drinks are a key against all kinds of contaminants. One of the easiest ways to do this is to add 1-2 TBS of a green superfood mix to juice or water at least once a day.

Can't find a recommended product? Call the 800 number listed in Product Resources.

Do you need an Excess Fat Cleanse?

Weight control today is a strategy of prevention lifestyle - an attitude of keeping weight down. Even though Americans are still looking for the "miracle magic bullet" for slimness, everyone is slowly realizing that a good diet has to be front and center for health and body tone. Long term weight control is always the result of a sound nutritious eating plan, rather than a try at the latest fad diet. One of the great advantages of achieving weight loss through improved nutrition is the extra energy you feel from the fresh juices, superfoods, herb teas and healing broths. Most weight loss diets have little nutrition to offer so they leave you feeling tired and lifeless. In the end, even if you lose weight, your body feels so deprived that it starts ravenous cravings for foods that put the weight right back on.

An excess fat cleanse is one of the best ways to jump start a new health program. Unhealthy fats, like saturated fats in meats and dairy foods, trans-fats like those in many dairy foods, hydrogenated or partially hydrogenated oils like those in margarine, shortening and many snack foods, and oxidized fats, like those in all fried foods, collect into excess body fat. Sugary foods and highly processed foods (like fast foods) are so devoid of digestive enzymes that they end up collecting as excess fat, too. Further, if you are congested, your body tries to dump its metabolic wastes to get them out of the way — one of the places that receives metabolic wastes is excess fat.

Is your body showing signs that it needs a Excess Fat Cleanse?

—Is cellulite collecting on your hips, thighs or tummy? Cellulite is a combination of fat, water and trapped wastes beneath the skin.
—Are your upper arms slightly flabby or your waistline noticeably thicker?
—Does your face look jowl-y or puffy?
—Have your wrists and ankles thickened?

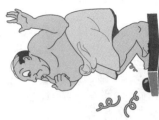

Pointers for best results from your Fat Cleanse:

• Drink plenty of water! Eight glasses of bottled water each day of your cleanse (can include herbal teas).
• Enzymes are a dieters best friend! Enzyme-rich juices and foods help you lose and maintain your ideal weight.
• Include a superfood drink once or twice a day for energy and nutrient content.
• Boost your fiber intake. Fiber is another key to weight control, especially for men.
• Watch your fats like a hawk! Unhealthy fats (see above) contribute greatly to weight gain—healthy fats assist weight loss.

Benefits that you may notice as your body responds to a fat cleanse:

• Energy levels rise almost every day as you go forward with the cleanse.
• Elimination problems which are often associated with weight problems will almost certainly lessen.
• Circulation will noticeably improve, especially in terms of cardiopulmonary performance.
• Your weight will drop as you go forward with the cleanse.
• Your digestion noticeably improves as toxins are flushed from your system and high-quality nutrients are more quickly absorbed.

Nutrition Plan

• **Start with this 3 to 7 day nutrition plan.**

Begin with a 3 day juice/liquid diet and follow with 1 to 4 days of all fresh cleansing foods. *Note:* Drink plenty of water during this cleanse. Water naturally suppresses appetite and helps maintain a high metabolic rate. In fact, water is the most important catalyst for increased fat burning. It enhances the liver's main function of detoxification and metabolism, and allows it to process more fats. Don't be concerned about fluid retention; high water intake actually decreases bloating, because it flushes out sodium and toxins. Expert dieters drink 8 glasses of water a day.

—On rising: take a glass of lemon juice and water regularly in the morning.

—Breakfast: have a Fat Melt Down Juice: juice 2 apples, 2 pears, 1 slice of fresh ginger to help reduce fat from places where it is stored in cellulite. The ginger stimulates better blood circulation.

—Mid-morning: have fresh carrot or apple juice to restore normal pH. Add 1 TB. green superfood into the juice: Arise & Shine Power Up; Rainbow Light Hawaiian Spirulina; Transitions Easy Greens.

—Lunch: have a liquid Salad Special: juice 3 broccoli flowerets, 1 garlic clove, 5 carrots or 2 tomatoes, 2 celery stalks, 1/2 red or green pepper.

—Mid-afternoon: have Crystal Star Lean & Clean™ Super Tea or a cup of green tea.

—Dinner: have an electrolyte broth: In 3 cups water, cook 2 cups fresh mixed vegetables (carrots, broccoli, dark leafy greens, celery and parsley), and 2 tsp. miso. Add in mixed sea vegetables. Seaweeds add minerals and improve sluggish metabolism.

—Before Bed: have licorice or peppermint tea with a dash of honey.

Herbs & Supplements

• **Choose 2 to 3 cleansing boosters.**

Deep liver cleanser: The liver is your body's chemical plant responsible for fat metabolism. Weight gain and energy loss are often the result of a liver which has become enlarged through overwork, alcohol exhaustion or congestion. Crystal Star Cel-Lean™ caps or Vale Enterprises Perma-Clean.

Essential fatty acids: Without essential fatty acids (EFA's), poor fat metabolism is certain. Unhealthy excess fluid retention is also controlled by EFAs. EFA deficiency increases appetite and promotes obesity.

EFAs to consider:

• Flax Oil -1 or 2 TBS. over a salad.
• Evening Primrose Oil - 1000mg daily.
• CLA - an Omega-6 fatty acid with fat-burning properties, 1800mg daily.

Capillary strengthening: you must tighten capillary walls in order to keep extra fat and cellulite from returning. Bioflavonoids are important: Ethical Nutrients Super Flavonoid; Crystal Star Bioflav. Fiber & C Support™ drink or Cel-Lean™ tea..

Herbal weight loss help: Crystal Star Appe-Tight™ is a mild, subtle herbal formula that helps you from overeating; Nature's Secret Ultimate Phen-Solution; Gaia Herbs Elim/Slim Supreme; Source Naturals Diet-Phen.

Enzyme support: Transformation Enzyme Balance-Zyme Plus for weight loss.

Electrolytes dramatically boost energy levels: Arise & Shine Alkalizer; Nature's Path Trace-Lyte Liquid Minerals.

Bodywork Techniques

• **Pick bodywork and relaxation techniques to accelerate and round out your cleanse.**

Enema: Take an enema the first and last day of your excess fat cleanse to help release toxins out of the body.

Exercise: Take a brisk walk or do 15 minutes of aerobic exercise. One pound of fat represents 3500 calories. A 3-mile walk burns up 250 calories. In about 2 weeks, you will have lost one pound of real extra fat. That means 3 pounds a month or 30 pounds a year *without changing your diet.* With your cleanse *and* diet improvements the result is obviously even greater! Exercise promotes an "afterburn" effect, raising metabolic rates for up to 24 hours afterwards. Exercise before a meal raises blood sugar levels and decreases appetite, often for several hours after the exercise.

Dry brushing: Fatty wastes can get trapped beneath the skin's surface easily (especially in women) when the liver or lymphatic systems are sluggish. Use a natural bristle brush - brush vigorously in a rotary motion and massage every part of your body in this order: feet and legs, hands and arms, back and abdomen, chest and neck. Five to fifteen minutes is the average time.

Massage: Have a massage therapy treatment at the beginning and end of your cleanse to move excess fluid wastes and unattached fats into elimination systems, and to stimulate skin circulation.

Bathe away excess fats: Crystal Star Hot Seaweed Bath; or a sea salt bath: add 1 cup Dead Sea salts, 1 cup Epsom salts, 1/2 cup regular sea salt and 1/4 cup baking soda to a tub; swish in 3 drops lavender oil, 2 geranium drops oil, 2 drops sandalwood oil and 1 drop neroli oil.

Continuing Diet Notes: Drink plenty of water for good weight maintenance. Water can help an overeater get past weight loss plateaus; decreasing water intake causes increased fat deposits. Drink all liquids before eating, to suppress appetite and maintain a high metabolic rate. Make sure at least 50 percent of your diet is composed or fresh foods and juices. Fresh food calories are relatively non-stimulating to glands and tend to stabilize weight.

Can't find a recommended product? Call the 800 number listed in Product Resources.

Chart Your Body System Cleanse

It's so easy..... each cleansing chart tailors your detox program for the body system you need to cleanse.

•The first 2-3 pages set up the diagnostics for each cleanse.

•The cleanse page has three columns:

—Column 1 charts your nutrition plan choices

—Column 2 charts your herb and supplement choices

—Column 3 charts your bodywork and relaxation choices

Do you need a colon cleanse?

A colon elimination cleanse is a cleanse most of us need. As the solid waste management organ for the entire body, mucous and rubber-like waste can easily adhere to colon walls. It's also the easiest breeding ground for putrefactive bacteria, viruses and parasites. (A nation-wide survey reveals that one in every six people has parasites living somewhere in the body.)

The latest estimates show that over 90% of disease in America is directly or indirectly attributable to an unhealthy colon. Health problems like headaches, skin blemishes, senility, bad breath, fatigue, arthritis and heart disease can be linked to a congested colon. Colon and bowel malfunctions are one of the biggest factors in accelerated aging, too. When colon health is compromised, waste backs up, becomes toxic, and releases the toxins from the bowel into the bloodstream. Other elimination organs become overburdened in their detoxification duties, and it's easy to see why health problems begin.

Cleansing your colon lightens the toxic load on every other part of your body... even your mind (mental dullness is a sign of colon congestion). In fact, hardly any healing program you have in mind will work without a colon cleanse as part of it. Real healing takes place at the deepest levels of your body, your cells. All your cells are fed by your blood. The nutrients that reach your blood get there by the way of the colon. So a clogged, dirty colon means toxins in your blood.

Is your colon toxic? Here are some questions to ask yourself:

Is your elimination time slow? Bowel transit time should be approximately twelve hours. Slow bowel transit time allows wastes to become rancid. Blood capillaries lining the colon absorb these poisons into the bloodstream, exposing the rest of your body to the toxins.

Do you eat a lot of highly processed, chemicalized food, fast foods or synthetic foods? A clean, strong system can metabolize or eliminate many pollutants, but if you are constipated, they are stored as unusable substances. As more and different chemicals enter your body they tend to inter-react with those that are already there, forming second generation chemicals more harmful than the originals. Colon cancer, now the second leading cancer in the United States today (only slightly behind lung cancer in men and breast cancer in women), is a direct result of accumulated toxic waste. Colitis, irritable bowel syndrome, diverticulosis, ileitis and Crohn's disease, are all signs of poor waste management. They're on the rise, too. Over 100,000 Americans have a colostomy every year! An incredible fact.

Is your digestion poor? The most common signal of toxic bowel overload is poor digestion. A lot of us eat way too many acid-forming foods — rich, red meats and cheeses, refined-flour bread, sugary foods, salty foods and fried foods. They rob your body of critical electrolytes and they have almost no fiber for digestion. A high fiber, whole foods diet is both cure and prevention for waste elimination problems. Fiber's significance comes from its ability to move food through the digestive system quickly and easily. A low residue diet causes a gluey state that can't be efficiently processed by the intestines. You can picture this if you remember the hard paste formed by white flour and water when you were a kid. A lot of the food we eat today is simply crammed into the colon and never fully excreted.

So much media attention has been focused on high fiber foods for so long, that everybody in America should have changed their diet to a more colon-health oriented pattern. This is simply not the case. Most diet attention has been targeted at reducing fat at all costs, often at the expense of a healthy, fiber-rich diet. Even a gentle, gradual change from low fiber, low residue foods helps almost immediately. In fact, a gradual change is better than a sudden, drastic about-face change, especially when the colon is inflamed.

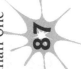

Check your fiber. The protective level of fiber in your diet is easily measured:

—The stool should be light enough to float.
—Bowel movements should be regular, daily and effortless.
—The stool should be almost odorless, signalling decreased bowel transit time.
—There should be no gas or flatulence.

Is your body showing signs that it needs a colon cleanse?

—Are you constipated most of the time? (a colon cleanse softens and removes clogging colon congestion)
—Do you feel heavy and logy? (a colon cleanse helps you lose colon congestive weight)
—Do you have gas, bloating and flatulence after you eat? (a colon cleanse helps you remove gluey materials impairing your digestion)
—Do you catch a cold, or flu every few weeks? (a colon cleanse releases excess mucous that harbors hanging-on cold and flu viruses)
—Are you tired most of the time for no real reason? (a colon cleanse boosts immune and liver response to give you more energy)
—Do you have a white-coated tongue, bad breath or body odor frequently? (a colon cleanse removes rancid foods that cause smells)
—Do you feel mentally slow and tired? (a colon cleanse lets more blood circulation get to your brain)
—Is your skin unusually sallow and dull? (a colon cleanse can remove toxic elements that are coming out through your skin)
—Do you have a degenerative disease like cancer, arthritis, M.S. or lupus? (a colon cleanse can remove disease-causing toxic settlements)
—Are your cholesterol numbers too high? (a colon cleanse increases absorption of cholesterol-lowering foods)

You can easily combine a colon cleanse with a cholesterol cleanse.

Pointers for best results from your colon cleanse:

• A colonic irrigation is a good way to start a colon/bowel cleanse. (See how to take a colonic, page 40.) Grapefruit seed extract (15 to 20 drops in a gallon of water) is effective, especially if there is colon toxicity along with constipation. Or take a catnip or diluted liquid chlorophyll enema every other night during the cleanse. Note: Enemas may be given to children. Use smaller amounts according to size and age. Allow water to enter very slowly; let them expel when they wish.
• Drink six to eight glasses of water daily during your colon cleanse.
• Take a brisk walk for an hour every day to help keep your colon elimination channels moving.
• Take several long warm baths during your cleanse. A lower back and pelvis massage and dry skin brushing will help release toxins coming out through your skin.

Note 1: Drugstore laxatives aren't really body cleansers. They offer only temporary relief, are usually habit-forming and destructive to intestinal membranes and don't even get to the cause of the problem. The bowels tend to expel debris simply because the colon becomes so irritated by the laxative that it expels whatever loose material is around.

Note 2: Bowel elimination problems are often chronic, and may require several rounds of cleansing. You can space out more than one colon cleanse by alternating it with periods of eating a healthful diet.

Nutrition Plan

• **Start with this 3 to 5 day nutrition plan.**

The 4 keys: 1) high chlorophyll plants for enzymes; 2) fruits and vegetables for fiber; 3) cultured foods for probiotics; 4) eight glasses of water a day.

The night before your colon cleanse.....

—Take your choice of gentle herbal laxatives.

—Soak dried figs, prunes and raisins in water to cover; add 1TB. molasses, cover, leave over night.

The next day....

—On rising: take a cleansing and flushing booster product, or 1 heaping teaspoon of a fiber drink in juice or water. Add 1000mg of vitamin. C with bioflavonoids 3x a day to raise body glutathione levels, an important detox compound.

—Breakfast: discard dried fruits from soaking water and take a small glass of the liquid.

—Mid-morning: take 2 TBS. aloe juice concentrate in a glass of juice or water.

—Lunch: take a small glass of potassium broth (page 134); or a glass of fresh carrot juice.

—Mid-afternoon: take a large glass of fresh apple juice; or an herbal colon cleansing tea.

—About 5 o' clock: take another small glass of potassium broth, another fresh carrot juice, or a vegetable drink (page 138).

—Supper: take a glass of apple or papaya juice. (Note: Finish your cleanse with a small raw foods salad on the last night.)

—Before Bed: repeat the herbal cleansers that you took on rising, and take a cup of mint tea.

Herbs & Supplements

• **Choose 2 to 3 cleansing boosters.**

Gentle herbal laxatives: HERBALTONE tablets, Crystal Star LAXATEA, M. D. Labs DAILY DETOX TEA.

Note: If you have a sensitive colon or irritable bowel disease (IBS), heal your colon before you cleanse. Avoid products with senna or psyllium. Use a gentle herbal cleansing formula, with peppermint oil, like Crystal Star BWL TONE I.B.S.™ to lessen inflammation and irritation of bowel mucosa which make the bowel more permeable to toxins.

Cleansing and flushing boosters: Nature's Secret SUPERCLEANSE tabs; Crystal Star FIBER & HERBS COLON CLEANSE™; *una da gato* extract drops in water.

Chlorophyll sources: Sun Wellness SUN CHLORELLA; Futurebiotics COLON GREEN; Crystal Star ENERGY GREEN™ drink.

Enzymes: Transformation Enzyme DIGEST-ZYME.

Electrolyte boosters speed up the cleanse: Nature's Path TRACE-LYTE LIQUID MINERALS; Arise & Shine ALKALIZER.

Probiotics replenish healthy bacteria: Professional Nutrition DOCTOR-DOPHILUS+FOS; Nature's Path FLORA-LYTE; Arise & Shine FLORA GROW.

Antioxidants defeat pollutants: Country Life SUPER 10 ANTIOXIDANT; NutriCology ANTIOX FORMULA II.

Fiber support: All One FIBER COMPLEX; Crystal Star CHO-LO FIBER TONE™ drink; AloeLife FIBERMATE.

Bodywork Techniques

• **Pick bodywork and relaxation techniques to accelerate and round out your cleanse.**

Irrigate: Take a colonic irrigation 2 to 3 times during your cleanse. Colonic irrigation products:

Exercise: take a brisk walk for an hour every day to help keep your elimination channels moving.

Bathe: take several long warm baths during your cleanse. Dry brush your lower back, abdomen, hips and thighs to help release colon toxins coming out through the skin. Lemon Detox Bath: add into warm bath - 5 drops lemon & 2 drops geranium essential oil.

Massage therapy: get one good lower back and pelvis massage during your cleanse

Reduce stress: Deva Flower Remedies STRESS & TENSION or CLEANSING REMEDY.

Visualize your detox: Close your eyes and inhale and exhale long and slowly. As you exhale, visualizes toxins dislodging and leaving your colon. As you inhale, visualize pure, nourishing nutrients rebuilding your vibrancy.

Continuing diet notes: After the initial cleanse above, the second part of a colon health system is rebuilding healthy tissue and body energy. This stage takes 1 to 2 months for best results. It emphasizes high fiber from fresh vegetables and fruits, cultured foods to replenish healthy intestinal flora, green foods for enzyme production, and alkalizing foods to prevent irritation while healing. Avoid refined foods, saturated fats, fried foods, red meats, caffeine and pasteurized dairy foods.

Can't find a recommended product? Call the 800 number listed in Product Resources.

Do you need a bladder/kidney cleanse?

Kidney function is vital to health. The kidneys are largely responsible for the elimination of waste products from protein breakdown (such as urea and ammonia). If the movement of salts, proteins or other bio-chemicals goes awry, a whole range of health problems arises, from mild water retention to major kidney failure, and mineral loss. Concentrated protein wastes can cause chronic inflammation of the kidney filtering tissues (nephritis), and can overload the bloodstream with toxins, causing uremia.

But your bladder and kidneys do more than just remove water wastes. Channeling pollutants and chemicals out of our systems before they build up in the tissues and contaminate our cells is obviously crucial to the body's internal hygiene. The bladder and kidneys are primary removal sites for toxic and potentially toxic chemicals in the bloodstream.

The urinary system is also part of a complex process that maintains your body's fluid stability. Urinary controls are involved with the brain, hormones, and receptors all over the body. They are smart controls that register what your body needs for fluids. Sometimes, they remove very little salt or water; at other times, they remove a lot. By the way... dehydration is the most common stress on the kidneys. Natural medicine emphasizes the importance of ample, high-quality water for kidney health.

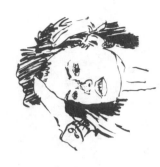

Is your body showing signs that it needs a bladder/kidney cleanse?

Do you have chronic lower back pain, irritated urination, frequent unexplained chills, fever, or nausea or unusual fluid retention? If you do, a gentle, natural, three to five day cleansing course might be just the thing to keep you from getting a full-blown, painful bladder infection.

Pointers for best results from your bladder/kidney cleanse:

—Drink 10 glasses of bottled water each day of your cleanse. Body purification systems can operate efficiently only if the volume of water flowing through them is sufficient to carry away wastes.
—Avoid dietary irritants on the kidneys, such as coffee, alcohol, and excessive protein.
—Herbal supplements provide excellent support for a kidney cleanse. Take them as liquids (drinks or teas) for best results.
—Take a liquid green supplement each day of your cleanse, such as Green Foods GREEN ESSENCE, or Sun Wellness CHLORELLA.
—Apply wet, hot compresses on the lower back to speed cleansing; or take alternating hot and cold sitz baths.

Improvement signs show that your body is responding to the cleanse.

• The flow of urine will be enhanced (increased).
• Infection of the bladder and/or irritated urination will abate.
• The kidneys will be relieved of any undo stress from their detoxification duties.

If you have been diagnosed with kidney stones or think you might have them, turn to page 92 for a kidney stone removal cleanse.

Nutrition Plan

• **Start with this 3 to 5 day nutrition plan.**

Water is the key to this cleanse. Drink 8 to 10 glasses of pure water each day.

The night before your bladder cleanse....
—Take a cup of bladder cleansing herb tea, (see next column). Add ¹/₄ tsp. non-acidic C crystals. **The next day....**
—On rising: take 1 lemon squeezed in a glass of water, with 1 teasp. acidophilus liquid; or 3 tsp. cranberry concentrate in a small glass of water, add ¹/₄ teasp. non-acidic vit. C crystals. (Cranberry juice reduces ionized calcium in the urine by over 50% to create an unfavorable environment for urinary tract infections.)
—Breakfast: have a glass of watermelon juice or cranberry juice with ¹/₄ tsp. non-acidic vit. C crystals or a glass of organic apple juice with ¹/₄ tsp. acidophilus powder.
—Mid-morning: take 1 cup watermelon seed tea. (grind seeds, steep in hot water 30 minutes, add honey); or a potassium broth (page 134) with 2 tsp. Bragg's LIQUID AMINOS; or a cleansing tea from column 2.
—Lunch: have a carrot/beet/cucumber juice. (page 138), or a chlorophyll-rich superfood drink, or a glass of carrot juice.
—Mid-afternoon: take a cup of healing herb tea, (parsley/oatstraw, plantain, watermelon seed tea or cornsilk tea); or a cleansing tea from column 2.
—Dinner: have a carrot juice, add 1 tsp. spirulina powder; or another cranberry juice, add ¹/₄ teasp. ascorbate vitamin C crystals.
—Before Bed: take a glass of papaya or apple juice with ¹/₄ tsp. acidophilus powder.

Herbs & Supplements

• **Choose 2 to 3 cleansing boosters.**

Liquid supplements are best with this cleanse.

Bladder/kidney cleansers: Crystal Star BLDR-K™ tea or extract; cornsilk tea; Jean's Greens P.P.T. tea; Nature's Apothecary DETOX FORMULA.

Anti-biotic/anti-infective/anti-inflammatory: Crystal Star ANTI-BIO™ caps or extract; marshmallow tea; vitamin C-1,000mg 3x/day; Nature's Answer BLADDEX or Nature's Plus AQUAACTIN.

Enzyme support: Transformation Enzyme EXCELLZYME (kidney antioxidant), and PUREZYME (a protease supplement that breaks apart protein-based viscid matter that cements salts into stones).

Bladder/kidney healing tonics: Crystal Star GREEN TEA CLEANSER™, Herbs Etc. KIDNEY TONIC; Gaia Herbs PLANTAIN/BUCHU SUPREME; Nature's Apothecary KIDNEY SUPPORT; dandelion tea; parsley tea.

Electrolyte mineral support: Nature's Path TRACE-LYTE LIQUID MINERALS; Arise & Shine ALKALIZER.

Probiotic support: Professional Nutrition DOCTOR-DOPHILUS + FOS; Wakunaga KYODOPHILUS.

Chlorophyll rich superfoods: Sun Wellness CHLORELLA drink or tablets; Crystal Star ENERGY GREEN™ drink or capsules; spirulina powder.

Fiber supplements reduce risk of stones: All One WHOLE FIBER COMPLEX; Nature's Secret ULTIMATE FIBER.

Bodywork Techniques

• **Pick bodywork and relaxation techniques to accelerate and round out your cleanse.**

Exercise: Take a daily brisk walk to keep kidney function flowing.

Enemas: Take a spirulina or catnip enema the first, second and the last day of your kidney cleanse to help release toxins. See enema instructions (page 39) in this book.

Heat therapy: 1) Take hot saunas to release toxins and excess fluids, and to flush acids out through the skin. 2) Apply hot compresses to the kidney area. Combine your choice — ginger and oatstraw, or cayenne and ginger, or mullein and lobelia.

Massage therapy: Have at least one massage during your cleanse to stimulate circulation.

Bladder/Kidney Baths: Add 8-10 drops of essential oils to your bath - a combination of two or three oils, like juniper, cedarwood, sandalwood, lemon, chamomile, eucalyptus or geranium. Stir the water to disperse.
Or use about 15 drops essential oil in 4-oz of jojoba oil and rub on kidney area).

Note: Avoid commercial antacids during healing. Some NSAIDS drugs have been implicated in kidney failure cases.

Continuing Diet Notes: After your cleanse, add sea foods and sea vegetables, whole grains and vegetable proteins. Continue with a morning green drink or Crystal Star GREEN TEA CLEANSER™. Kidney healing foods include garlic and onions, papayas, bananas, watermelon, sprouts, leafy greens and cucumbers. Take these frequently for the rest of the month. Avoid heavy starches, red or prepared meats, dairy foods (except yogurt or kefir), salty, fatty and fast foods. They all inhibit kidney filtering.

Can't find a recommended product? Call the 800 number listed in Product Resources.

Do you have kidney stones?

Every decade since World War II, the U.S. has seen a steady rise in kidney stone cases. Today 10% of American men and 5% of American women have a kidney stone by the time they're seventy. Kidney stones are a diet-related illness directly linked to low dietary fiber, high fat and high calcium (usually from dairy sources), and large amounts of animal protein, refined sugar, alcohol and salt. They parallel the rise of the Standard American Diet, full of fat, fried foods, rich dairy products and sugar. Excessive use of antacids and adrenal exhaustion also contribute to kidney stones.

Kidney stones form when minerals that normally float free in the kidney fluids combine into crystals. When there is an overload of inorganic mineral waste and too little fluid, the molecules can't dissolve and form sharp-edged stones. There are three types of kidney stones: those composed of calcium salts, the most common type (75-85% incidence); struvite, or non-calcium-containing crystals (10-15% incidence); and uric acid crystals, at about 5-8% occurrence. It takes from 5 to 15 hours of vigorous, urgent treatment to dissolve and pass small stones.

Kidney stones plague people who eat a rich, high fat diet. A vegetarian diet, low in proteins and starches, that emphasizes fresh fruits, vegetables and cultured foods to alkalize the system, is the key to avoiding kidney stone formation. This type of diet is high in fiber to reduce urinary calcium waste. It eliminates acid-forming foods, like caffeine-containing foods, salty, sugary and fried foods and soft drinks that inhibit kidney filtering. It avoids mucous-forming foods, like pasteurized dairy products, heavy grains, starches and fats, to relieve irritation and inhibit sediment formation.

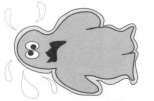

Is your body showing signs that it needs a kidney stone cleanse?

There may be no apparent symptoms at first except a dull ache in the lower back. When the stone(s) become large enough to block the urinary tract, there is excruciating, radiating pain with extremely painful urination. The abdomen becomes distended. A woman may have heavy menstrual bleeding or anemia, signs of a vitamin K deficiency, which can lead to stones. As infection sets in, there are chills, nausea, vomiting and fever.

Pointers for best results from your kidney stone cleanse:

• Dehydration which causes a reduction in urine volume and an increased rate of excretion of stone constituents is a factor relating to kidney stones. Drink 8-10 glasses of bottled water each day of your cleanse, so that waste and excess minerals are continuously flushed.

• Use fresh vegetable and fresh fruit juices during your cleanse.

After your cleanse:

—When you begin eating solid foods, make sure you are eating enough fresh fruits and vegetables. Studies have shown that even meat eaters showed a lower incidence of stones when they ate higher amounts of fresh fruits and vegetables.

—Keep salt and protein low for at least 3 weeks.

—Establish a diet with plenty of fiber.

Nutrition Plan

• **Start with this 3 to 5 day nutrition plan.**

Vitamin K is an important part of your body's natural inhibitors of kidney stone formation. Spinach and sea vegetables, high in vitamin K, help vegetarians have a lower incidence of kidney stones.

Take 2 TBS. olive oil through a straw every 4 hours to help dissolve stones.

The night before your kidney stone cleanse ..
—Take a cup of chamomile tea.
The next day....
—On rising: take cranberry juice (from concentrate) in water with 1 tsp. honey; or 2 TBS. apple cider vinegar in water with 1 tsp. honey; or Crystal Star GREEN TEA CLEANSER™; and a cup of chamomile tea.

—Breakfast: have a glass of cranberry juice, or fresh watermelon juice, or watermelon chunks.

—Mid-morning: take 1 cup watermelon seed tea. (grind seeds, steep in hot water 30 minutes, add honey); or a green drink (see column 2); or dandelion tea, or Crystal Star BLDR-K™ tea.

—Lunch: have a carrot/beet/cucumber juice. (pg. 138), and a spinach salad with cucumbers.

—Mid-afternoon: have a cup of chamomile tea; and asparagus stalks and carrot sticks with kefir cheese; or fresh apples with kefir or yogurt dip.

—Dinner: have brown rice with tofu and steamed veggies; or steamed asparagus with miso soup and snipped, dry sea veggies on top; or a baked potato with kefir cheese and a spinach salad; or baked or broiled salmon with rice and baked onions.

—Before Bed: take a glass of aloe vera juice and another cup of chamomile tea; or miso/ginger soup with sea vegetables snipped on top.

Continuing diet notes: Avoid oxalic acid-forming foods, like cooked spinach, chard or rhubarb, chocolate, black tea, coffee and grapes during your cleanse. Avoid all yeast-containing foods during a kidney stone cleanse.... no baked breads. After the cleanse follow, a low salt, low protein, vegetarian diet with 75% fresh foods for 2 weeks. Avoid all refined, fried, fatty foods, cola drinks, salty, sugary foods, and caffeine-containing foods. Eliminate dairy and reduce animal protein for 1 month.

Herbs & Supplements

• **Choose 2 to 3 cleansing boosters.**

Kidney stone cleansers: ascorbate or Ester C powder in water; $1/4$ tsp. every hour to bowel tolerance until stones pass - about 5000mg daily.

Mineral balancers to prevent stones: Flora VEGE-SIL caps 2 daily for kidney stone prevention; Solaray CALCIUM CITRATE 4 daily, with QBC to reduce inflammation.

Vitamin C 3000mg with bioflavonoids daily for a month to acidify urine and prevent stones; Futurebiotics VITAL K or vitamin K 100mcg daily.

Enzyme support: Transformation Enzyme EXCELL-ZYME (kidney antioxidant), and PUREZYME (a protease supplement that breaks apart protein-based viscid matter that cements salts into stones).

Dissolve kidney sediment wastes: Enzymatic Therapy ACID-A-CAL caps to dissolve sedimentary waste, with bromelain 500mg daily; Chamomile, rosemary, or dandelion/nettles tea - about 5 cups a day for one to 2 weeks. Jean's Greens P.P.T. tea.

Chlorophyll superfood for vitamin K to inhibit growth of stones: Crystal Star ENERGY GREEN, Transitions EASY GREENS, Aloe Falls ALOE w. GINGER, Sun Wellness CHLORELLA 2 pkts. daily.

Fiber supplements reduce risk of stones: All One WHOLE FIBER COMPLEX; Nature's Secret ULTIMATE FI-BER.

Bodywork Techniques

• **Pick bodywork and relaxation techniques to accelerate and round out your cleanse.**

Exercise: Take a daily brisk walk to keep kidney function flowing. Stagnate urine flow is a factor in kidney stone formation.

Enemas: Take an enema the first, second and the last day of your kidney cleansing program to help release toxins. Use spirulina, or catnip enemas. See enema instructions (page 39) in this book.

Heat therapy: Apply wet, hot compresses and lower back massage when there is inflammation flare up, especially lobelia or ginger fomentations. Take hot saunas when possible to release toxins and excess fluids, and to flush acids out through the skin.

Massage therapy: at least once during your cleanse to stimulate circulation and reduce pain.

Bladder/Kidney Baths: Take hot and cold, or Epsom salts sitz baths to stimulate circulation.

Aromatherapy kidney stress relief: Add a total of 8-10 drops of essential oil to your bath. Stir the water briskly to disperse evenly. Use a combination of two or three of the following essential oils: juniper, cedarwood, sandalwood, lemon, chamomile, eucalyptus or geranium.

Can't find a recommended product? Call the 800 number listed in Product Resources.

Your liver is your most important organ of detoxification. Do you need a liver cleanse?

Your life depends on your liver. To a large extent, the health of your liver determines the health of your entire body. The liver is really a wonderful chemical plant that converts everything we eat, breathe and absorb through the skin into life-sustaining substances. The liver is a major blood reservoir, forming and storing red blood cells, and filtering toxins at a rate of a quart of blood per minute. It manufactures natural antihistamines to keep immune response high.

More than any other organ, the liver enables us to benefit from the food we eat. Without the liver, digestion would be impossible and the conversion of food into living cells and energy nonexistent. It is the primary metabolic organ for proteins, fats and carbohydrates. It also synthesizes and secretes bile, a substance that not only insures good food assimilation but also is critical to the excretion of toxic material from the gastrointestinal tract. Blood flows directly from the gastrointestinal tract to the liver, so it can neutralize or alter toxic substances from our food before they are distributed to the rest of the body through the blood. Blood also keeps returning to the liver, processing toxins again and again through the lymph system until they are excreted by the bile or kidneys.

Liver congestion and exhaustion interfere with all of these vital functions. Unfortunately, since the common American diet is high in calories, fats, sugars and alcohol, with unknown amounts of toxic substances in the form of preservatives, pesticides and nitrates, almost everybody has liver malfunction to some extent. Still, a healthy liver can deal with a wide range of toxic chemicals, drugs, solvents, pesticides and food additives. Your liver also has amazing rejuvenative powers, continuing to function when as many as 80% of its cells are damaged. Even more remarkable, the liver can regenerate its own damaged tissue.

Yet, even in life-threatening situations, such as cirrhosis, hepatitis, acute gallstone attacks, mononucleosis or pernicious anemia, the liver can be rejuvenated, and major surgery or even death averted. Health problems occur after many years of abuse, when the liver is so exhausted it loses the ability to detoxify itself. We can help the liver take a "deep cleansing breath"..... something I've found you can almost feel as its miraculous powers of recovery begin to flow.

A liver detox is often the first vital step for the body to begin to heal itself.

Look at all the health problems you can improve or prevent with a liver cleanse:

Liver health normalizes other gland and organ functions, especially adrenal, pituitary, kidney, gall bladder, and spleen problems. In fact, gland function and digestion often improve right away. You will notice this in terms of fewer instances of swollen glands during cold and flu season, and less lower back fatigue (adrenal swelling). Weight and cellulite control difficulties may be solved, especially if you notice unusual stomach distension, a clear sign of a swollen liver. Both gallstone and kidney stone accretions lessen. Drug and alcohol cravings reduce. Most women notice that PMS and other menstrual difficulties like endometriosis are far less severe. Seemingly unrelated problems like breast and uterine fibroids or infertility, even osteoporosis may be corrected. Male impotence is normally improved. Inflammatory conditions like shingles flare-ups, neuritis pain, herpes outbreaks are helped. Brown skin spots and spots before the eyes (signs that the liver is congested and eliminating poisons by other body avenues) begin to fade.

Is your body showing signs that it needs a liver cleanse?

As the world becomes more prosperous, more people are suffering from liver disorders, mostly due to too many rich foods and alcoholic beverages, but also environmental, air and water pollutants. We lose energy and our sense of well-being when the liver is congested.

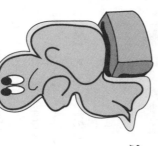

Body signals that your liver needs some TLC include:
· Unexplained fatigue, listlessness, depression or lethargy, lack of energy; numerous allergy reactions
· Unexplained weight gain and the appearance of cellulite even if you are thin
· A distended stomach even if the rest of the body is thin
· Mental confusion, spaciness
· Sluggish elimination, general constipation alternating to diarrhea
· Food and chemical sensitivities, usually accompanied by poor digestion, and sometimes unexplained nausea
· PMS, headaches and other menstrual difficulties; bags under the eyes
· A yellowish tint to the skin and/or liver spots on the skin; poor hair texture and slow hair growth; skin itching and irritation.
· Anemia and large bruise patches indicate severe liver exhaustion.

Pointers for best results from your liver cleanse:

—Relieve your liver of toxic build-up and strain by eliminating red meats, partially hydrogenated fats and oils (except for essential fatty acids), refined sugars, food preservatives and food dyes.

—Drink 8 glasses of bottled water each day of your cleanse to encourage maximum flushing of liver tissues.

—Liver regeneration needs optimum nutrition for three to four months. Have a dark green leafy vegetable salad every day.

—Get adequate rest and sleep during a liver cleanse. The liver does some of its most important work while you sleep!

I recommend a short liver detox twice a year in the spring and fall, using the extra vitamin D from the sun to help. Your liver is probably the most stressed in the spring and early summer (one of the reasons that people with skin problems get more flare-ups in the spring). As movement of energy in the spring as plant sap rises and nature springs to life are mirrored in the human body with ascending, outgoing energy that can most readily get rid of waste products accumulated during the fall and winter.

Improvement signs show that your body is responding to the cleanse.

—Many skin conditions can be traced back to digestive and liver problems, so skin conditions will show signs of clearing. If there are no skin problems, the skin will become more radiant.

— Stiff and aching muscles will receive relief as the liver is replenished.

—Warmth may come to cold hands and feet.

—Relief from recurring migraine or other headaches.

Nutrition Plan

• **Start with this 3 to 5 day nutrition plan.**

Follow with a diet of 100% fresh foods for the rest of the week. Add $1/4$ tsp. vitamin C crystals to each drink you take. It's a natural chelator of heavy metal toxins that deteriorate liver function. (Don't forget - 8 glasses of water through the day.)

The night before your liver cleanse.....
—Take a cup of miso soup with sea veggies.
The next day....
—On rising: take 1 lemon squeezed in a glass of water; or 2 TBS. lemon juice in water; or 2 TBS. cider vinegar in water with 1 teasp. honey.
—Breakfast: take a glass of potassium broth, (page 134) or carrot/beet/cucumber juice, or organic apple juice or Crystal Star SYSTEMS STRENGTH drink™. Add 1 teasp. spirulina to any drink.
—Mid-morning: take a green veggie drink (See the Green Cuisine for juicing recipes); or take a green superfood powder mixed into water or vegetable juice (Some superfood choices: Green Foods GREEN MAGMA, Crystal Star ENERGY GREEN or NutriCology PRO-GREEN).
—Lunch: have a glass of fresh carrot juice or a glass of organic apple juice.
—Mid-afternoon: have a cup of peppermint tea, pau d' arco tea, or Crystal Star LIV-ALIVE TEA™; or another green drink.
—Dinner: have another carrot juice or a mixed vegetable juice; or have a hot vegetable broth (See the Green Cuisine for recipes).
—Before Bed: take another glass of lemon juice or cider vinegar in water. Add 1 tsp. honey or royal jelly; or a pineapple/papaya juice with 1 tsp. royal jelly.

Herbs & Supplements

• Choose 2 to 3 cleansing boosters.

Bitters herbs stimulate the liver and bile flow: Crystal Star BITTERS & LEMON CLEANSER™; Floradix HERBAL BITTERS; Solaray turmeric caps; dandelion root and leaf tea.

Liver cleansers: Crystal Star LIV-ALIVE™ tea or caps, or GREEN TEA CLEANSER™ tea; Nature's Apothecary LIVER CLEANSE; Gaia Herbs SUPREME CLEANSE.

Liver tonics and vitality support: Milk thistle seed extract (accelerates liver regeneration by a factor of four); Enzymatic Therapy SUPER MILK THISTLE COMPLEX WITH ARTICHOKE; Herbs Etc. LIVER TONIC.
A liver tonic tea: 4-oz hawthorn berries, 2-oz. red sage, and 1-oz. cardamom seeds. Steep 24 hours in 2 qts. water. Add honey. Take 2 cups daily.

Enzyme support: Transformation Enzyme DIGESTZYME.

Lipotropics prevent fatty accumulation: Phos. Choline or choline 600mg, or Solaray LIPOTROPIC PLUS; sea vegetables (any kind) every day; dandelion tea; gotu kola or fennel seed tea.

Chlorophyll rich superfoods: Green Foods GREEN ESSENCE or Sun Wellness CHLORELLA.

Antioxidants for the liver: ALPHA-LIPOIC ACID by MRI. (Lipoic acid is one of the most powerful liver detoxifiers ever discovered); CoQ$_{10}$ 60mg 3x daily; Solaray CENTELLA ASIATICA or Solaray ALFA-JUICE caps; Transformation Enzyme EXCELLZYME; vitamin E 400IU with selenium 100mcg.

Bodywork Techniques

• **Pick bodywork and relaxation techniques to accelerate and round out your cleanse.**

Enema: Take a coffee enema (1 cup coffee to 1 qt. water) the first and last day of your liver cleansing program to help release toxins out of the body. See enemas in this book for instructions.

Exercise: Take a brisk, daily walk on each day of your cleanse. Breathe deep to help the liver eliminate toxins. The liver is dependent on the amount and quality of oxygen coming into the lungs. Exercise, an air filter, or time spent walking in the forest and at the ocean can be of great benefit.

Massage therapy: Have a massage to stimulate circulation.

Heat therapy: a sauna every day possible to induce sweating and faster elimination.
Early morning sunlight will boost your cleanse with natural vitamin D.

Stress & Relaxation techniques:
• Flower remedies: Natural Labs STRESS/TENSION COMBO.
• Essential oil support: To assist your liver cleanse use the essential oils of fennel, lemon & rosemary. You can use one or a combination of all three oils. Put a total of 15 drops essential oil in 1oz of a carrier oil (such as jojoba) and rub on the skin.
• Bathe: Take several long hot baths if possible during a liver cleanse for faster, easier detoxification. Add to your bath 5 drops fennel, 5 drops lemon and 5 drops of rosemary essential oils.

Continuing diet notes: Keep fat low in your nutrition plan. It's crucial to liver regeneration and vitality. Beets, artichokes, radishes and dandelions are good liver foods because they promote the flow of bile, the major pathway for chemical release from the liver. A permanent diet for liver health should be lacto-vegetarian, low in fats, rich in vegetable proteins, with plenty of vitamin C foods for good iron absorption. A complete liver renewal program can take from 3 to 6 months.

Can't find a recommended product? Call the 800 number listed in Product Resources.

Do you need a gallstone cleanse?

In the United States, high bile cholesterol levels are the main cause of gallstones, with most stones (80%) composed of cholesterol and varying amounts of bile salts, bile pigments and inorganic calcium salts. When bile in the gallbladder becomes supersaturated with cholesterol, it combines with other particulate matter present and begins to form a stone. A stone may grow for 6 to 8 years before symptoms occur. Since continued formation of the gallstone is dependent on either an increased accumulation of cholesterol or reduced levels of bile acids or lecithin, it's easy to see that anywhere along the way, diet improvement will deter, even arrest, stone development.

What else causes gallstones? Although high bile cholesterol is the main problem (bile cholesterol levels do not necessarily correlate with blood cholesterol levels), other dietary factors like high blood sugar, high calorie and saturated fat intake which leads to obesity are also involved. Gastrointestinal diseases, like Crohn's disease and diverticulitis may be involved. Drugs like oral contraceptives and some estrogen replacement drugs have been implicated. Blood cholesterol lowering drugs that contain fibric acid derivatives like clofibrate and gemfibrozil increase the level of bile cholesterol in the bile.

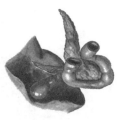

Is your body showing signs that it needs a gallstone cleanse?

Gallstones are present in 95% of people suffering from cholecystitis (gallbladder inflammation). There may be no identifiable symptoms, except for periods of nausea and intense abdominal pain that radiates to the upper back. Ultrasound provides a definitive diagnosis.

Important note:

Although I have personally seen several gallstone sufferers use the 9 day program on the following page pass gallstones without surgery, I recommend it only under the supervision of a qualified health professional. The liver and gallbladder are interconnecting, interworking organs. Problems with either affect both. Before undertaking a Gallstone Fast and Flush to pass gallstones, have an ultrasound test to determine the size of the stones. If they are too large to pass through the urethral ducts, other methods **must** be used.

Pointers for best results from your gallstone cleanse:

—Once stones have passed, concentrate your diet on strengthening the liver/gallbladder area to prevent further stone formation.
—Drink at least eight 8-oz. glasses of bottled water each day.
—Eliminate any foods that create an allergy response. Allergenic substances cause swelling of bile ducts, impairing bile flow. Common allergy-causing foods that may induce gallstone symptoms are eggs (very troublesome), pork, onions, milk, citrus, corn, beans and nuts.
—Coffee (including decaf) generates gallbladder contractions. Avoid coffee until the stones are resolved.

Improvement signs show that your body is responding to the cleanse:

• Relief from any nausea or pain in the abdomen. A healthy appetite should return if it has been lost.
• The gallbladder plays an important part in the digestion of fats. Digestion of fats and overall digestion will improve.

Nutrition Plan

• This is a 9 day gallstone flush plan.

<u>Three day Olive Oil and Lemon Juice Flush:</u>
—On rising: take 2 TBS. olive oil and juice of 1 lemon in water. Sip through a straw if desired.
—Breakfast: have a glass of organic apple juice.
—Mid-morning: have 2 cups of chamomile tea.
—Lunch: take another glass of lemon juice and olive oil in water; and a glass of fresh apple juice.
—Mid-afternoon: have 2 cups of chamomile tea.
—Dinner: have a glass of carrot/beet/cucumber juice; or a potassium juice or broth (pages 134).
—Before Bed: take another cup of chamomile tea.

<u>Follow with a 5 day Alkalizing Diet:</u>
—On rising: take 2 TBS. cider vinegar in water with 1 teasp. honey; or a glass of grapefruit juice.
—Breakfast: have a glass of carrot/beet/cucumber juice, or a potassium broth or juice.
—Mid-morning: have 2 cups of chamomile tea, and a glass of organic apple juice.
—Lunch: take a vegetable drink with Sun Wellness CHLORELLA, or Crystal Star ENERGY GREEN DRINK™, a small green salad with lemon-olive oil dressing and a cup of dandelion tea.
—Mid-afternoon: have 2 cups of chamomile tea, and another glass of apple juice.
—Dinner: have a small green salad with lemon-oil dressing; and another glass of apple juice.
—Before Bed: 1 cup chamomile or dandelion tea.

<u>End with a One Day Intensive Olive Oil Flush:</u>
At 7 p.m. on the evening of the 5th day of the alkalizing diet, mix one pint of olive oil and 10 juiced lemons; take ¼ cup every 15 minutes until it is gone. Lie on the right side for best assimilation.

Herbs & Supplements

• Choose 2 to 3 cleansing boosters.

Fiber supplements reduce risk of stones: Fiber absorbs excess cholesterol so it can be eliminated. Fiber is most important in preventing and removing gallstones. Crystal Star CHO-LO FIBER TONE™; Futurebiotics COLON GREEN; Rainbow Light EVERYDAY FIBER SYSTEM; All One WHOLE FIBER COMPLEX.

Form more bile: Low levels of lecithin in the bile help cause formation of gallstones. Increased lecithin also increases the solubility of cholesterol. Solgar PHOSPHATIDYL-CHOLINE (triple strength lecithin); Nature's Plus LECITHIN; taurine 1000mg daily. Vitamin C 2000mg per day, has been shown to positively effect bile composition and reduce cholesterol stone formation.

Lipotropics remove fat deposits: Nature's Plus LIPO-PLEX; Flax oil 3 TBS. daily; vitamin E 400 IU daily. Enzyme support: Transformation Enzyme LYPOZYME contains highest amount of lipase found in any product to help break down of gallstones.

Herbal sediment dissolvers: Crystal Star STN-EX caps (with *dandelion, gravel root, milk thistle and hydrangea*) and Planetary Formulas STONE FREE have a long successful history of dissolving gallstones.

Milk thistle extract increases solubility of the bile to help dissolve gallstones. *Hydrangea* is a stone solvent for gall and kidney stones. *Gymnema sylvestre* capsules balance blood sugar to reduce a cause of stones. *Turmeric* contains curcumin which increases the solubility of bile to keep prevent gallstones from forming and helps eliminate already formed stones, Jarrow Formulas CURCUMIN-97.

Peppermint and chamomile tea helps dissolve gallstones. Peppermint oil in an enteric-coated capsule may also be used between meals.

Bodywork Techniques

• Pick bodywork and relaxation techniques to accelerate and round out your cleanse.

Enema: Take an enema at the beginning of the cleanse to release toxins in the colon and remove undo stress on the gallbladder through backup of colonic toxins. (Enema instructions page 39).

Apply castor oil packs to the abdomen daily throughout the cleanse for 1 to 2 hours at a time.

Take a gallstone essential oil bath: Add a total of 10 drops of essential oils to your bath. Stir the water briskly to disperse evenly. Use a combination of two or three of the following essential oils: *bergamot, lemon, eucalyptus, chamomile, camphor, geranium, hyssop, lavender, or rosemary.*

Or, put a total of 15 drops of these above essential oils in 1-oz of jojoba oil and rub on gallbladder area.

Flower Essence Remedies: Bach Flower RESCUE REMEDY or Natural Labs Corp. DEVA FLOWERS STRESS/TENSION oil.

Continuing diet notes: The key to both prevention and control of gallstones is diet improvement. Increase your fresh fruit and vegetable intake for more food fiber. Vegetable proteins from foods like soy, oat bran and sea vegetables help prevent gallstone formation. Reduce your intake of animal protein, especially dairy products (casein in dairy products increases formation of gallstones). Avoid fried foods and sugary foods altogether if you are at risk for gallstones.

Can't find a recommended product? Call the 800 number listed in Product Resources.

Do you need a lung/respiratory cleanse?

Lung and respiratory diseases of all kinds have increased dramatically in just the last decade. Air, water and environmental pollutants may have finally reached an overload point on the general population where having a congestive "cold" is more common than breathing free. During high risk seasons, almost a third of Americans have a cold every two or three weeks. Cold symptoms are usually your body's attempt to cleanse itself of wastes and toxins that have built up to the point where natural immunity cannot handle or overcome them.

Your glands are always affected, (since the endocrine system is on a 6 day cycle, a cold usually runs for about a week) as the body works through all its detoxification processes.

Your lungs are on the front line of toxic intake from viruses, allergies, pollutants, and mucous-forming congestants. If you are highly sensitive to chemicals and pollutants, you will more than likely have many respiratory problems. I have found that an occasional lung cleanse is a wise way to support your respiratory system in releasing and healing from pollutant-caused infections.

But don't forget that your body works together. Extra pressure of disease or heavy elimination on one part of the body puts extra stress on another. Cleansing your kidneys, for example, takes part of the waste elimination load off your lungs so they can recover faster. Similarly, promoting respiratory health through a lung cleanse also helps digestive and skin problems.

Any program to overcome any chronic respiratory problems is usually more successful when begun with a short mucous elimination plan like a lung cleansing diet. This allows the body to rid itself first of toxic accumulations that cause congestion before an attempt is made to change eating habits that support better health.

Is your body showing signs that it needs a lung and respiratory cleanse?

Do you have a chronic phlegmy cough? Do you wheeze with asthma? Is your head stuffy with congestive allergies? Do you have bronchitis or severe sinusitis? Do you have a runny nose in any weather? Are you a cigarette smoker? These are signs that you might need a lung cleanse.

Pointers for best results from your lung and respiratory cleanse:

• Drink plenty of non-dairy fluids, like water, juices, herb teas or broth, to hydrate and flush the body. Milk congests and constipates.
• Stimulate the immune system. Maintaining a healthy immune system is a primary way to support lung/respiratory health.
• Alkalize your body during a lung cleanse. Acid-forming foods tend to aggravate or prolong colds, flus and other respiratory problems. Alkalizing foods like fresh fruits, high chlorophyll vegetables, sea veggies and non-gluten grains like brown rice or millet should be used in a ratio of about 4:1 over acid-forming foods during a lung and pulmonary detox.
• Chlorophyll-rich super green foods like chlorella, spirulina and barley grass speed up lung cleansing, increase oxygen in the body and help treat respiratory tract infection.
• Get plenty of quality sleep, fresh air and sunshine.
• Consciously steer clear of air pollution to the best of your ability. Environmental and heavy metal pollutants, like chlorofluorocarbons, tobacco smoke (even secondary smoke) contribute greatly to respiratory problems and can undo all your hard cleansing work.

Nutrition Plan

• **Start with this 4 to 7 day nutrition plan.**

Begin with a 3 day juice/liquid diet and follow with 1 to 4 days of a diet of 100% fresh foods.

The night before your lung cleanse....
—Take your choice of gentle herbal laxatives.
The next day....
—On rising: take 2 squeezed lemons in water with 1 TBS. maple syrup.
—Breakfast: have a water-diluted grapefruit juice with 1 TBS. of a green superfood, such as Transitions EASY GREENS or Nature's Secret ULTIMATE GREEN; or water-diluted pineapple juice as a natural expectorant - add in 1 TBS. of a green superfood for additional detox support.
—Mid-morning: take a carrot juice or mixed fresh vegetable juice such as Personal Best V-8 (page 138). This juice is cleansing, neutralizes acids and rebuilds the body. It provides rapid energy and system balance.
—Midafternoon: have a cup of mucous cleansing tea like Crystal Star X-PEC™ tea with *mullein, marshmallow, comfrey, pleurisy root, rose hips, calendula, boneset, ginger, peppermint and fennel seed.*
—Dinner: have a warm Potassium Essence broth (page 134), for energy and mineral electrolytes. Or try this broth, soothing to gastric mucosa, rich in zinc, vitamin A, C, potassium and magnesium electrolytes: In 2 ¹⁄₂ cups water, cook 1 ¹⁄₂ cups fresh mixed vegetables (carrots, broccoli, dark leafy greens, celery and parsley) with 1 TBS. miso. Strain and take broth. Blender blend veggies, broth and 4TBS. sunflower seeds for a hearty version.
—Before Bed: have cranberry or celery juice.

Continuing diet notes: After your initial juice cleanse, your diet for lung health should be high in vegetable proteins and whole grains, low in sugars and starches. Include cultured foods like raw sauerkraut, yogurt, and kefir for probiotics to assist friendly G.I. flora. Include lung-specific pitted fruits such as apricots, peaches and plums. Include nutritional yeast 2 tsp. daily. Take a green superfood drink at least three mornings a week for a month after your cleanse to "set" the cleanse benefits.

Herbs & Supplements

• **Choose 2 to 3 cleansing boosters.**

Deep Cleansing: Nature's Secret ULTIMATE CLEANSE. Lung cleansers: Creation's Garden LNG-1 (assists respiratory ailments settling in the lungs) and LNG-3 (clears lung congestion, bronchial inflammation).

Herbal lung support: North American Herb & Spice OIL OF OREGANO & OREGAMAX for lung conditions like cough, asthma, colds, flu, bronchitis and pneumonia; Crystal Star RESPR™ CAPS a decongestant rich in herbal antioxidants; Crystal Star X-PECT-TEA™, an expectorant to aid mucous release; Herbs Etc. LUNG TONIC supports lung cleansing.

Immune support: Immunity herbs: *panax ginseng, echinacea, ashwagandha, astragalus, Siberian ginseng, goldenseal, licorice, ligustrum, suma, codonopsis, pau d' arco, chaparral, dumontiaceae (red marine algae), garlic* and immune-enhancing mushrooms, like *reishi & shiitake.* Chlorophyll rich superfoods: Solgar EARTH SOURCE GREENS & MORE; Country Life SHIITAKE/REISHI COMPLEX.

Enzyme support: Transformation Enzyme GASTROZYME (clears mucous congestion) and PUREZYME (strengthens immune system).

Electrolyte increase oxygen uptake: Nature's Path TRACE-LYTE LIQUID MINERALS; Arise & Shine ALKALIZER.

Probiotics inhibit growth of harmful organisms: Source Naturals LIFE FLORA; Arise & Shine FLORA GROW; Nature's Path, FLORA-LYTE.

Anti-infective agents: NutriCology PROLIVE WITH ANTIOXIDANTS (olive leaf extract); North American Herb & Spice OIL OF OREGANO.

Antioxidants are linked to improved lung function: Vit. C 1,000mg 3x day raises body's glutathione levels to protect the lungs; Futurebiotics OXY•SHIELD; Source Naturals PROANTHODYN.

Bodywork Techniques

• **Pick bodywork and relaxation techniques to accelerate and round out your cleanse.**

Enema: Take an enema the first, second and the last day of your lung cleansing program to thoroughly clean out excess mucous.

Deep Breathing Exercise: Do this deep breathing exercise often during your cleanse to remove stress, compose your mind, improve your mood and increase your energy: Take a deep, full breath. Exhale it slowly... slowly. Take another deep, full breath. Release slowly. And again. Maintain a quiet rhythm, exhaling more slowly than you inhale.

Exercise: If you are cleansing your lungs and not ill with a cold, flu, or other respiratory infection, take a brisk, daily walk on each day of your cleanse. Breathe deep to help the lungs eliminate mucous.

Compress: Apply wet ginger/cayenne compresses to chest to increase circulation and loosen mucous.

Essential oil support: To assist your lung cleanse use oregano, tea tree, and eucalyptus oils (singly or in combination). Put a total of 15 drops essential oils in 1-oz of a carrier oil (such as jojoba) and rub on the chest.

Inhalant: 6 drops of the essential oils can be added to one quart hot water - inhale the steam:
• Eucalyptus has antiviral action to loosen mucous, and treat asthma, bronchitis and sinusitis.
• Tea Tree has decongestant, antiviral and antibacterial properties.
• Oregano oil has antiviral and antibacterial properties help eradicate lung infection. Also thins mucous and stops excessive mucous secretion.

Bathe/Sauna: Take a hot 20 minute bath or sauna at the onset of a cold, flu or beginning of a respiratory cleanse to stimulate your body's defenses and increase toxin elimination.

Can't find a recommended product? Call the 800 number listed in Product Resources.

Do you need a gland cleanse?

Your glands (and their hormone secretions) work at your body's deepest levels. They are involved with almost every body function and biochemical reaction, so they're a key to good health, especially as you age. The comment "you are as young as your glands" has merit. There are two types of glands in the body: **Exocrine glands**, like salivary and mammary glands, that are regulated by the hypothalamus and secrete their fluids through ducts; and **Endocrine glands**, like the pituitary, pineal or ovaries that emit their secretions (primarily hormones) directly into the bloodstream and lymph system.

In their turn, hormones are chemical messengers exerting wide-ranging effects on other glands and on virtually every body organ. Hormones also affect our moods, energy level, mental alertness, even metabolism. With this broad base in the body, you can imagine that glands and their substances like adrenaline, insulin, and thyroid hormones, are extraordinarily affected by nutritional deficiencies, environmental pollutants, chemicalized foods and synthetic hormones. Strangely enough, even though they are in our bodies, glands and hormones are affected **first** by harmful toxins and poor nutrition. A mineral deficiency, for instance, something most Americans are affected by today, undermines the health of almost every gland and organ. The chronic stress loads most Americans live under have a direct effect on hormone levels and balance. We can see this easily in low levels of steroidal hormones produced by our "stressed-out" adrenals.

Is your body showing signs that it needs a gland cleanse?

Some of the first signs to look for might be unexplained weight gain and sluggish metabolism (indicating impaired thyroid activity), and blood sugar problems (indicating unbalanced insulin levels). Poor assimilation of nutrients may mean low enzyme output from a congested pancreas, chronic fatigue may indicate adrenal exhaustion.

What body improvement signs can you look for to see if your cleanse is working?

* Your energy level should noticeably rise indicating less stressed and inflamed adrenal glands.
* Your mood should improve and be more stable, indicating better blood sugar balance from the pancreas.
* Bloating, unexplained weight gain and metabolism should improve, indicating a more active thyroid.
* Your sleep and rest should improve, indicating pineal balance and adrenal health.
* Your digestion should improve, indicating more pancreas, gallbladder and liver vitality.
* You should have noticeably less colds and flu. Glands are always affected by chronic respiratory infections.

Pointers for best results from your gland cleanse:

—The glands are affected first by dehydration. Drink 8 glasses of water a day.
—Trace minerals and protein are important for gland function. Add green superfoods to your diet.
—After long periods of stress, the whole gland system becomes depleted and exhausted. Herbal adaptogens noticeably improve the way your body handles stress. Add herbs from the ginseng family, like *panax and Siberian ginsengs, suma, gotu kola, dong quai and ashwagandha* to your healing program.

Nutrition Plan

• Start with this 4 to 7 day nutrition plan.

Begin with a 3 day juice-liquid diet and follow with 1 to 4 days of a diet of all fresh foods.

The night before your gland cleanse....

—Take your choice of gentle herbal laxatives, like Crystal Star LAXA-TEA™, M. D. Labs DAILY DETOX TEA. (See Product Resources page 254.)

The next day.... If possible, depending on the season, for the first day of your juice cleanse, go on a watermelon juice only cleanse. Drink throughout the day to rapidly flush and alkalize. If watermelon is not available, start with the following:

—On rising: take lemon juice in water with 1 tsp. honey. Add 2 tsp. brewer's yeast flakes.

—Breakfast: have a carrot juice with 1 TBS. green superfood, like Vibrant Health GREEN VIBRANCE or Country Life SHIITAKE/REISHI COMPLEX WITH CHLORELLA.

—Mid-morning: take a carrot or mixed vegetable drink. Add 1 tsp. sea veggie flakes (dulse or kelp).

—Lunch: have a bowl of miso soup. Sprinkle with dulse flakes and 1 tsp. brewer's yeast.

—Mid-afternoon: have a mixed vegetable juice like Personal Best V-8 (page 138), a high vitamin/mineral drink for body balance.

—Dinner: have a Mineral Rich Broth: Simmer 30 minutes: 3 carrots, 1 cup parsley, 1 onion, 2 potatoes, & 2 stalks celery. Strain and add 1 TBS. Bragg's LIQUID AMINOS.

—Before Bed: have an apple or pineapple/papaya juice. If desired, blend in 1 fresh fig.

Herbs & Supplements

• CHOOSE 2 to 3 cleansing boosters.

Deep gland cleanser: Gaia Herbs SUPREME CLEANSE. Herbal gland support: Use herbal compounds that contain phytohormone-rich herbs, like ginseng, licorice root, sarsaparilla, dong quai, and black cohosh. Bioflavonoid-rich herbal complexes like Crystal Star BIOFLAV., FIBER & C SUPPORT™ drink have gland balancing properties. For gland homeostasis, Crystal Star FEEL GREAT™ and ADRN™ formulas, or Planetary Formulas SCHIZANDRA ADRENAL SUPPORT; mineral compounds for the glands, Crystal Star MINERAL SPECTRUM™, Crystal Star HEAVY METAL CLEANSE™ caps if you are regularly exposed to toxic pollutants.

Essential Fatty Acids: Barlean's Organic OMEGA TWIN FLAX/BORAGE COMBO, Futurebiotics VITAL K LIQUID.

Enzyme support: Transformation Enzyme Corp. PUREZYME supports adrenal insufficiencies; Rainbow Light DOUBLE-STRENGTH ALL-ZYME.

Electrolytes expedite the cleanse: Nature's Path TRACE-LYTE LIQUID MINERALS; Arise & Shine ALKALIZER.

Probiotics assist detoxification & protection from toxins: Source Naturals LIFE FLORA; Arise & Shine FLORA GROW.

Chlorophyll rich superfoods for glands: Body Ecology VITALITY SUPERGREEN; Solgar EARTH SOURCE GREENS & MORE.

Raw glandular extracts offer biochemical nutritional support for gland-affecting stress and fatigue: Premier Labs RAW MULTIPLE GLANDULAR; Enzymatic Therapy glandulars are highly recommended - THYMUPLEX, PARA-CAL, NUCLEO-PRO M, and NUCLEO-PRO F and RAW MAMMARY for women.

Bodywork Techniques

• Pick bodywork and relaxation techniques to accelerate and round out your cleanse.

Enema: Take an enema the first, second and the last day of your gland cleansing program to help release toxins out of the body.

Or have a colonic irrigation to deep cleanse the glands.

Exercise: Take a regular 20 minute "gland health" walk every day.

Environmental concerns: Avoid air and environmental pollutants as much as possible. Your glands are the first to feel their damaging effects.

Acupressure points: Stroke the top of the foot on both feet for 5 minutes each to stimulate endocrine and hormone secretions.

Massage therapy: Have a massage therapy treatment to stimulate circulation and re-establish clear meridian pathways in the body.

Essential oil support: To assist your gland cleanse use bergamot, chamomile, eucalyptus and lavender. You can use one or more of the oils in a combination. Put a total of 15 drops essential oil in 1-oz of a carrier oil (such as jojoba) and rub on the skin.

Bathe/Sauna: Try a relaxing mineral bath. Add 1 cup Dead Sea salts, 1 cup Epsom salts, 1/2 cup regular sea salt and 1/4 baking soda to a tub; swish in 3 drops lavender oil, 2 drops chamomile oil, 2 drops marjoram oil and 1 drop ylang-ylang oil.

Continuing Diet Notes: Good gland foods: sea veggies, fresh figs and raisins, pumpkin and sesame seeds, green leafy veggies, broccoli, avocados, yams and dark fruits. Trace minerals, essential fatty acids and protein are important for glandular function. Herbal digestive tonics (especially with ginger), mineralizers (especially from dark leafy greens like spinach) and herbal adaptogens (like ginseng) are helpful when you feel your glandular system is weak.

Can't find a recommended product? Call the 800 number listed in Product Resources.

Do you need a blood purifying cleanse?

Your blood is your river of life. The health of your blood is critical. The blood must supply oxygen to the body's sixty trillion cells, transport nutrients, hormones and wastes, warm and cool the body, ward off invading microorganisms, seal off wounds and much more. It is the chief neutralizing agent for bacteria and toxic wastes. Although not immediately obvious, toxins ingested in sublethal amounts can eventually add up to disease-causing amounts. For example, slow viruses that lead to nerve diseases like M.S. can enter the cells and remain dormant for years, mutating and *feeding on toxic substances*, then reappear in a more dangerous form. While the body has its own self-purifying complex for maintaining healthy blood, the best way to protect yourself from disease is to keep those cleansing systems in good working order. A blood purifying diet may be followed for 1 to 2 months, or longer if the body is still actively cleansing, or needs further alkalizing. The diet may also be returned to when needed, to purify against relapse or additional symptoms.

Note: for persons suffering from severe blood toxicity: Most serious immune deficient diseases are the result of blood toxins and can benefit from a blood purifying diet to boost compromised immunity. However, in serious degenerative conditions like AIDS, Lupus, Chronic Fatigue Syndrome or Fibromyalgia, there are usually large amounts of toxins and pollutants in the blood. When this is the case, an all-liquid fast is *not recommended*, since it is often too harsh for an already weakened system, and in fact may dump more toxins out into the bloodstream than the body can handle. The initial diet in these severe cases, should be as pure as possible in order to be as cleansing as possible - totally vegetarian - free of all meats, dairy foods, fried, preserved and refined foods and saturated fats.

Is your body showing signs that it needs a blood cleanse?

• A simple blood-color test monitors blood improvement. Make a small, quick, sterilized razor cut on your finger. If the blood is a dark, bluish-purplish color it is not healthy. A bright red color indicates healthy blood.

- a deep, choking, chronic cough
- unexplained depression, memory loss or unusual insomnia, schizophrenic behavior, seizures, periodic black-outs
- sexual impotence or dysfunction
- black spots on the gums, bad breath/body odor, unusual, severe reactions to foods and odors
- loss of hand/eye coordination, especially in driving

Pointers for best results from your blood cleanse:

—Food should be organically grown. Avoid canned, frozen, prepackaged foods or foods with colors, preservatives and flavor enhancers.
—Avoid sodas, artificial drinks, concentrated sugars, fried foods and sweeteners.
—Mild herb teas and bottled mineral water (6 to 8 glasses) are recommended throughout each day, to hydrate, and alkalize.
—For optimum results, $1/2$ tsp. ascorbate vitamin C crystals with bioflavonoids may be added to any drink.
—Sprinkling $1/2$ tsp. lactobacillus powder over any food makes a big difference to your body chemistry improvement.

Nutrition Plan

• **Start with this 4 to 7 day nutrition plan.**

Begin with a 3 day juice/liquid diet; follow with 1 to 4 days of 100% fresh solid and liquid foods.

The night before your blood cleanse.....
—Take your choice of gentle herbal laxatives or Gaia Herbs SUPREME CLEANSE.
The next day.....
—On rising: Take 2 to 3 TBS. cranberry concentrate in 8 oz. water with $^1/_2$ teasp. ascorbate vitamin C crystals, or use a green tea blood cleansing formula, such as Crystal Star GREEN TEA CLEANSER™, or cut up a half lemon with skin and blend in the blender w. 1 teasp. honey, and 1 cup distilled water; and $^1/_2$ teasp. Natren TRINITY in 8-oz. aloe vera juice.

—Breakfast: have a glass of fresh carrot juice, with 1 TB. Bragg's LIQUID AMINOS added; or an 8-oz. aloe vera juice with $^1/_2$ teasp. Natren TRINITY.

—Mid-morning: take a potassium broth (page 134) and $^1/_2$ teasp. ascorbate vitamin C crystals; and another fresh carrot juice, or pau d'arco tea.

—Lunch: have a glass of fresh Personal Best V-8 juice (page 138) or a carrot or apple juice. Mix in 1 TB. of a green superfood such as Crystal Star ENERGY GREEN™ or NutriCology PRO-GREENS.

—Mid-afternoon: have a vegetable juice such as Blood Regenerator Juice: handful spinach, 4 romaine leaves, 4 sprigs parsley, 6 carrots, $^1/_4$ turnip. Dinner: have a cup of miso soup with 2 TBS. dried sea vegetables (dulse, nori, wakame, kombu or sea palm) snipped over the top.

—Before Bed: take a 8-oz. glass of aloe vera juice with $^1/_2$ teasp. ascorbate vitamin C with bioflavs and $^1/_2$ teasp. Natren TRINITY lactobacillus powder.

Continuing diet notes: Vegetable and fruit juices stimulate rapid, heavy waste elimination, a process that can generate mild symptoms of a "healing crisis." A slight headache, nausea, bad breath, body odor and dark urine occur as the body accelerates release of accumulated toxins. If you are detoxifying from alcohol or drug overload, 5000 to 10,000mg. of ascorbate Vitamin C is recommended daily during serious cleansing, to help keep the body alkaline and encourage oxygen uptake.

Herbs & Supplements

• **Choose 2 to 3 cleansing boosters.**

Herbal blood cleansers: Crystal Star GREEN TEA CLEANSER™ and LIV-ALIVE™ capsules; M.D. Labs DAILY DETOX II tea; Herbal Magic COL-LIV HERBAL BASE; Planetary Formulas COMPLETE PAU D'ARCO PROGRAM; Nature's Way DANDELION WITH GOLDEN SEAL.

Blood cleansing herbs: *red clover, dandelion, burdock, yellow dock, echinacea, Oregon grape root, sarsaparilla, astragalus, pau d' arco, goldenseal root, garlic and cayenne.*

Blood purifiers with immune stimulants: HEMATONIX-Nature's Answer; RIVER OF LIFE-Planetary.

Enzyme support: Transformation Enzyme PUREZYME, breaks down protein invaders in the blood supply leaving them vulnerable to destruction by the immune system. A potent blood purifier: Rainbow Light ADVANCED ENZYME SYSTEM.

Electrolytes establish healthy blood and strengthen the immune system: Arise & Shine ALKALIZER; Nature's Path TRACE-LYTE LIQUID MINERALS.

Probiotics provide nutrients for building blood: Arise & Shine FLOR GROW; Source Naturals LIFE FLORA; or Premier Labs MULTI-DOPHILUS.

Chlorophyll enhances blood cleansing: SUN CHLORELLA by Sun Wellness; New Chapter CHLORELLA.

Antioxidants strengthen white blood and T cells: Schiff PHYTOCHARGED ANTIOXIDANT; Solgar ADVANCED ANTIOXIDANT FORMULA; Jarrow Formulas COENZYME Q₁₀; Enzymatic Therapy GRAPE SEED PHYTOSOME 100;

Antioxidant blood cleansers: germanium, 100 to 150mg; Vitamin E 1000IU with selenium 200mcg; CoQ₁₀ 180mg daily; Vit. C-1,000mg w. bioflavs. 3x daily; Quercetin and bromelain 500mg 3x daily, for auto-immune reactions; shark cartilage to stimulate interferon, interleukin, lymphocytes.

Bodywork Techniques

• **Pick bodywork and relaxation techniques to accelerate and round out your cleanse.**

Enema: Take an enema the first, second and the last day of your blood cleansing program to help release toxins out of the body.

Irrigate: Take a colonic irrigation or a Nature's Secret SUPERCLEANSE once a week to remove infected feces.

Exercise: Exercise daily in the morning, if possible. Aerobic oxygen intake alone can be an important nutrient.

Massage therapy: Have a massage to stimulate blood circulation.

Essential oil support: To assist your blood cleanse use rosemary, cypress & vetiver. You can use one or a combination of all three oils. Put a total of 15 drops essential oil in 1oz of a carrier oil (such as jojoba) and rub on the skin.

Stress & Relaxation techniques:
• Flower remedies: Natural Labs Corporation STRESS/TENSION.

• Bathe/Sauna: Take several saunas or long hot baths if possible during a blood cleanse for faster, easier detoxification. Add a total of 8-10 drops of essential oil to your bath. Stir the water briskly to disperse evenly. Use a combination of two or three of the following essential oils: rosemary, cypress & vetiver.

Can't find a recommended product? Call the 800 number listed in Product Resources.

Do you need a lymph cleanse?

The lymphatic system includes lymphatic vessels and nodes, thymus gland, tonsils and spleen. It's really a network of tubing that drains waste products from tissues, produces disease-fighting white blood cells (lymphocytes) and antibodies and carries the bulk of the body's waste from the cells to the final elimination organs. Experts call the lymphatic system **a secondary circulatory system**, because it assists the bloodstream with millions of tiny vessels and ducts throughout the body to collect tissue fluid not needed by the capillaries or skin and return it to the heart for recirculation. Special filtering lymph nodes in groups along the lymph ducts remove infective organisms. So your lymph system is also a key to your body's immune defenses and a major player in your health.

The liver produces the majority of lymph in the body. It's a major route for nutrients from the liver and intestines, so it's rich in fat-soluble nutrients produced in the liver, especially protein. The integrity of the lymph system is dependent on special immune cells in the liver that filter out harmful bacteria and destructive yeasts. Liver health is a key to lymphatic health.

The spleen is the largest mass of lymphatic tissue. It destroys worn-out red blood cells, and serves as a healthy blood reservoir for fresh red blood. During times of demand, such as hemorrhage, the spleen can release its stored blood and prevent shock from occurring.

Here's an even more amazing fact: The valves of the lymph system move the waste-filled fluids to be flushed and filtered. But since there is no pump as there is with the heart, lymph circulation depends solely upon breathing and muscle movement. **This is why physical exercise and diaphragmatic deep breathing are so critical to lymph cleansing program and to healthy immune response.**

Is your body showing signs that it needs a lymph cleanse?

If you are under chronic stress; if you are constantly tired (indicating liver exhaustion); if your skin is very pale; if you are extremely thin; if your memory is noticeably failing; if you have low immune response with frequent colds, a revitalizing lymph cleanse can make a difference. If your body looks uncharacteristically soft and pudgy or has newly noticeable cellulite (indicating too many saturated fats and sugary foods), you probably need a lymph-draining cleanse.

Pointers for best results from your lymph cleanse:

• Drink 8-10 glasses of bottled water each day of your cleanse.
• Include potassium-rich foods regularly — sea vegetables, broccoli, bananas and seafood.
• Avoid caffeine, sugar, dairy products and alcoholic drinks for the duration of your cleanse. They contribute to lymphatic stagnation.
• Spicy foods like natural salsas, cayenne pepper, horseradish and ginger boost a sluggish lymph system and cut mucous congestion.

Improvement signs show that your body is responding to the cleanse:

• Most people notice an energy increase in their daily activity.
• Most people notice they no longer catch every cold that comes their way, and the illnesses they do get don't last as long.
• Most people notice far fewer stress reactions as body chemistry normalizes.
• Most people notice better weight control (especially if they were overweight) and less cellulite formation as congestion lessens.

Nutrition Plan

• **Start with this 4 to 7 day nutrition plan.**

• Start your lymph cleanse:

Begin with a 3 day juice-liquid diet and follow with 1 to 4 days of a diet of 100% fresh foods.

Note: Nutrient deficiency is the most frequent cause of a sluggish lymph system. Immune-boosting vegetables for juicing: cabbage, kale, carrot, bell pepper, collards and garlic. Lymph-enhancing juice fruits: apple, pineapple, blueberry and grape.

—On rising: take a glass of lemon juice and water regularly in the morning for lymph revitalization.

—Breakfast: have a fresh mixed vegetable lymph juice builder: handful parsley, 1 garlic clove, 5 carrots, and 3 celery stalks. Add 2 TBS. of a green superfood like Solgar EARTH SOURCE GREENS & MORE or Wakunaga of America KYO-GREEN.

—Mid-morning: have two cups of Crystal Star LIV-ALIVE™ tea for liver and lymph cleansing, or a lymph tea blend of *white sage, astragalus, echinacea root, Oregon grape root and dandelion root.*

—Lunch: have a vitamin A/carotene/vitamin C rich drink: 3 broccoli flowerets, 5 carrots, 1 garlic clove, 2 celery stalks and ¹⁄₂ green pepper. Add 2 TBS. of a green superfood like Vibrant Health GREEN VIBRANCE or Arise & Shine POWER UP.

—Mid-afternoon: a glass of apple or grape juice.

—Dinner: have a potassium essence broth (page 134), for mineral electrolytes. Or try a broth rich in zinc, vitamin A and C, potassium and magnesium electrolytes: In 2 ¹⁄₂ cups water, cook 1 ¹⁄₂ cups fresh veggies (carrots, broccoli, dark leafy greens, celery and parsley) and 1 tsp. miso. Strain and use broth. Hearty version: blend warm broth and vegetables. Add 4 TBS. sunflower seeds.

—Before Bed: have a glass of papaya juice.

Herbs & Supplements

• **Choose 2 to 3 cleansing boosters.**

Deep lymph cleanser: Gaia Herbs SUPREME CLEANSE; *echinacea* extract and *astragalus* extract are highly successful deep lymph cleansing single herbs.

Lymphatic cleansers: Crystal Star ANTI-BIO™ caps for white blood cell formation, a lymph purifier with immune-stimulant properties. Herbs Etc. LYMPHATONIC, with *echinacea*, (reduces lymphatic swelling and congestion), *red root* (powerful lymphatic cleanser, synergistic with echinacea), and *ocotillo* (flushes lymph congestion); Nature's Apothecary LYMPH CLEANSE; Enzymatic Therapy LYMPHO-CLEAR; Gaia Herbs ECHINACEA RED ROOT SUPREME a lymphatic and liver cleanser.

Immune Support: Silica decisively affects the functions of the lymphatic nodes and system, increasing the phagocytes to strengthen the immune response. Eidon SILICA MINERAL SUPPLEMENT; Flora VEGE-SIL.

Supporting lymph nutrients: Vitamins A, C, E, B-complex, carotenes, iron, zinc and selenium.

Herbal lymph immune support: Crystal Star REISHI/GINSENG™ extract.

Enzyme support: Protease is a powerful lymph immune booster. Transformation Enzyme PUREZYME; shark cartilage, about 1400mg for leucocyte production.

Electrolyte boosters: Mineral electrolytes play a major role in detoxifying the lymph glands, helping to remove acid crystals. Nature's Path TRACE-LYTE LIQUID MINERALS.

Deficiencies to watch for: Protein and B₁₂ deficiency also effect efficiency of the lymphatic system.

Bodywork Techniques

• **Pick bodywork and relaxation techniques to accelerate and round out your cleanse.**

Colonic irrigation: take a colonic irrigation or a Sonné BENTONITE CLAY CLEANSE once a week to remove lymph congestion and infected feces from the intestinal tract.

Exercise: exercise is critical to lymphatic flow. To stimulate lymph flow activate muscles with regular exercise and stretching. Start every exercise period with deep, diaphragmatic breathing. Mini-trampoline exercise clears clogged lymph nodes.

Massage therapy: elevate feet and legs for 5 minutes every day, massaging lymph node areas.

Lymph supporting therapies: acupuncture and acupressure have both been successful.

Essential oil support: to assist your lymph cleanse use geranium, juniper and black pepper. Use one or a combination of all three oils. Put a total of 15 drops essential oil in 1-oz of a carrier oil (such as jojoba) and rub on the skin.

Shower: Take an alternating hot and cold hydro-therapy treatment at the end of your daily shower to stimulate lymph circulation.

Stress relaxation techniques: the mind and emotions have a great effect on immune response. The following techniques are important:

Bathe: —A relaxing mineral bath. Add 1 cup Dead Sea salts, 1 cup Epsom salts, ¹⁄₂ cup regular sea salt and ¹⁄₄ baking soda to a tub; swish in 3 drops lavender oil, 2 drops chamomile oil, 2 drops marjoram oil and 1 drop ylang ylang oil.

—Lymph support essential oil bath mixture. Add a total of 8-10 drops of essential oils (see above) to your bath. Stir the water briskly to disperse evenly.

Eliminate aluminum: cookware, food additives, and alum-containing foods and deodorants.

Continuing Diet Notes: Poor nutrition profoundly impairs the immune system. Excessive dietary sugars and alcohol over consumption especially inhibit white blood cell activity. Be sure to eliminate or limit their use. Adequate protein intake is critical to immune health and the ability to heal. The best sources for immune response are those with plenty of EFAs: salmon and fresh tuna, sea vegetables, green superfoods like spirulina and barley grass and sprouts.

Can't find a recommended product? Call the 800 number listed in Product Resources.

Do you need a skin cleanse?

Your skin is the surest mirror of your lifestyle. Almost everything that's going on inside you shows on your skin. Your skin is your body's largest organ of elimination and detoxification. The skin acts as a backup for the other elimination organs. When the colon becomes overloaded and stagnant with toxins, or the liver cannot efficiently filter the impurities coming from the digestive tract, the skin will try to compensate in every way it can to release toxins from your body. It sweats them out, or throws them off through rashes or abscesses. Fortunately, our skin is the essence of renewable nature... it sloughs off old, dying cells every day, and gives a the body a clean, new start.

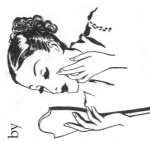

Your skin is also your body's largest organ of absorption and ingestion — both for nutrients and toxins. Good dietary care and habits show quickly. By the same token, chemicalized food toxins and nutritional deficiencies from a poor diet show up first on your skin. Toxins eliminated through the oil glands in the skin, for example, show up as acne and boils. The skin mirrors our emotional state and our hormone balance, too. So stress reactions and hormone disruption show up as poor skin tone and texture, or spots and blemishes. Luckily, immune response elements speed to help the skin's protective acid mantle when it's assaulted by disease-causing bacteria.

Is your body showing signs that it needs a skin cleanse?

Do you have sallow skin? Poor skin coloring may indicate waste build-up from liver malfunction or drug residues.

Do you have age spots? Brown mottled spots on the hands, neck or face may reflect waste accumulation in the liver.

Do you have adult acne, or uneven skin texture? Waste build-up from environmental pollutants, poor diet, liver exhaustion and stress allow increased free radical formation which attack skin cell membranes.

Do you have wrinkles, or sagging skin contours? Free radical activity also affects skin collagen and elastin proteins, resulting in wrinkling and dry skin.

Do you have puffy or swollen eyes, dark circles under your eyes, or crusty, mucous formations in your eyes? If your breath is also bad, it's a pretty solid sign your body has an overload of fluid wastes.

Do you have a skin disorder? Psoriasis, dermatitis and seborrhea all indicate its time for a skin cleanse.

Do you have skin sores or rashes that aren't healing? or hard bumps on the skin? They may be your body's way of saying it's overloaded with wastes that you're not eliminating.

Do you have unusually oily skin? or scaly, itchy skin? or chronically chapped and red skin? A skin cleanse will probably help.

Note: Poor circulation (cold hands and feet, swollen ankles), poor digestion and chronic constipation are also signs that your body lacks tissue oxygen uptake. Poor skin tone is a sign of antioxidant deficiency.

Pointers for best results from your skin cleanse:

• Drink 8-10 glasses of bottled water each day of your cleanse (herbal "skin" teas are fine, too). Water keeps the system flushed, so waste and body toxins will not be dumped out through the skin as blemishes or rashes. Bottled water is best. Fluoridated water may leach Vitamin E out of your body.

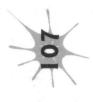

• Your diet is the quickest way to change your looks. You can make effective improvements easily. Skin tissues need a rich, high oxygen, high blood supply, and plenty of mineral building blocks. Silica, sulphur, calcium and magnesium are specific minerals for your skin. Plants are the most absorbable way for your body to get them.

So, soft smooth skin depends on a diet rich in fresh fruits and vegetables. Beautiful skin tone needs vitamin A, vitamin C, mineral-rich foods, and high vegetable protein foods, for collagen and interstitial tissue health. Eliminate or limit sugary foods, fried foods and trans-fats, like those in milk and dairy products, margarine, shortening and hydrogenated oils. Avoid red meats and refined foods of all kinds.

• Include a green superfood drink daily during your skin cleanse. Superfood powders can be mixed into any juice or water.

• Don't forget good bodywork for your skin: 1) The healthiest skin needs some fresh air and sunlight every day. Early morning sunlight on the body for natural vitamin D is a key. 2) Daily mild exercise keeps your skin's circulation free and flowing. 3) Dry brush your skin once a week to increase circulation and slough dead cells.

Benefits you may notice as your body responds to skin cleansing:

Most people experience noticeable appearance improvement in about 3 weeks.
—Your face will look rested, rejuvenated and revitalized.
—Your skin's natural glow will return as capillary circulation and lymphatic drainage improve.
—Skin blemishes, blotches and spots diminish or disappear.
—The whites of your eyes will become whiter; dark circles will disappear.
—Your skin texture will appear smoother and softer; fine lines will appear less noticeable.

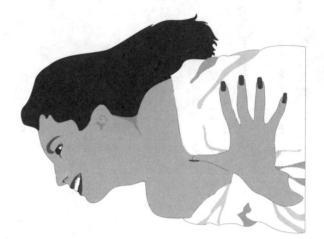

Nutrition Plan

• **Start with this 3 to 5 day nutrition plan.**

Begin with a 3-day liquid elimination diet and follow with 1 to 4 days of a diet of fresh foods.

—On rising: take a glass of lemon juice and water; add New Moon GINGER WONDER syrup if desired.

—Breakfast: make a Complexion Booster: juice 2 slices of pineapple and 2 apples. Add 1 TBS. Crystal Star BIOFLAV, FIBER & C SUPPORT™, 1 teasp. brewer's yeast and 1 teasp. wheat germ oil.

—Mid-morning: have watermelon juice when available (rich in natural silica), or a skin tonic drink: juice 1 cucumber, 1 handful fresh parsley, 1 4-oz. tub fresh sprouts and sprigs of fresh mint. Or have a superfood green drink, such as Crystal Star ENERGY GREEN™ or Transformation EASY GREENS.

—Lunch: have a fresh carrot juice; or a Skin Nutrient drink: juice 5 carrots, 2 apples and add 15 drops GINGER EXTRACT.

—Mid-afternoon: have a carrot/beet/cucumber juice (once a week for the next month) to keep the liver clean and support the skin's health.

—Dinner: have a warm potassium essence broth (page 134) for mineral electrolytes. Or make this high luster skin broth: In 2 1/2 cups water cook 2 cups chopped fresh mixed vegetables, add 1 tsp. miso and 2 TBS. chopped dried sea vegetables (you can snip some wakame into pieces). Hearty version: Blender blend luster skin broth above; then add 4 TBS. sunflower seeds for a protein boost. Vegetable protein aids faster healing for damaged skin.

—Before Bed: have Crystal Star BEAUTIFUL SKIN™ TEA or Japanese green tea for skin support; or a pineapple/papaya, papaya or apple juice; or VEGEX yeast broth for high B complex vitamins.

Continuing Diet Notes: Follow a whole foods diet. Eat mineral-rich foods such as leafy greens, bell peppers, broccoli, sesame and sunflower seeds, fish and sea vegetables. Include 4 to 5 servings of vegetables a day—if possible eat half raw—as salads. Eat fruits 1 to 3 times per day. Increase fiber to help keep your colon clean. Besides the fiber of vegetables and fruits include: flax seed meal, whole grains (like oats and rice), and beans (pinto and black beans).

Herbs & Supplements

• **Choose 2 to 3 cleansing boosters.**

Deep skin blood cleansing: Creations Garden TOTAL BODY CLEANSE, Crystal Star SKIN THERAPY #1™ CAPS; *sage or burdock root tea.*

Smoothing/hydrating herbs for skin: Crystal Star SKIN THERAPY #2™ CAPS; chamomile tea or CamoCare FACIAL THERAPY; lavender aromatherapy oil to reduce puffiness.

Skin vitamins and minerals: Diamond HERPANACINE superior skin support; Futurebiotics HAIR, SKIN & NAILS - results in just 2 weeks; Crystal Star MINERAL SPECTRUM™ caps.

Skin herbal support: Crystal Star BEAUTIFUL SKIN™ CAPS - for blemishes and skin maintenance; Nature's Apothecary SKIN SUPPORT - blood purifiers and mineralizers; Herbs Etc. DERMATONIC - stimulates waste elimination; *burdock root* normalizes production of the skin's beneficial oils.

Antioxidants are important for skin health: Beta carotene protects against the effects of the sun's free radicals; Vitamin E protects against the lipid peroxidation caused by UV rays; Bioflavonoids improve vascularization of the skin.

Essential fatty acids: deficiency reflected by skin dehydration and wrinkling: Crystal Star EVENING PRIMROSE; Spectrum ORGANIC ESSENTIAL MAX EFA OIL.

Enzyme support: Protease heals skin disorders; Transformation Enzyme PUREZYME.

Electrolyte boosters: Nature's Path TRACE-LYTE.

Silica, a mineral for collagen support, reduces dry, wrinkled skin: Eidon SILICA MINERAL SUPPLEMENT; Flora VEGESIL; Crystal Star SILICA SOURCE™.

MSM (Methyl Sulfonyl Methante):MSM enhances tissue pliability and helps repair damaged or scarred skin: Nature's Path MSM-LYTE.

Bodywork Techniques

• **Pick bodywork and relaxation techniques to accelerate and round out your cleanse.**

Enema: Take an enema the first, second and the last day of your skin cleansing program to help release toxins out of the body and help clear the skin. Or have a colonic for a more thorough cleanse.

Dry brushing: Use a natural bristle brush. Start with the soles of your feet - brush vigorously making rotary motions and massage every part of your body - starting at the feet and work up to the neck. Massage: Skin circulation for better tone.

Healing, beautifying skin application treatments:
—Crystal Star BEAUTIFUL SKIN™ GEL - a cleansing, restorative phytotherapy gel.
—Skin Beauty Face tea: steep chamomile, calendula, rosehips, juice of 1 lemon and 2 teasp. rose water. Strain; apply with cotton balls to the face.
—Herbal Answers HERBAL ALOE FORCE GEL boosts circulation and stimulates new cell growth.
—AloeLife ALOE SKIN GEL with antioxidant herbs.
—Nature's Path SKIN-LYTE a liquid electrolyte spray.
—Fruit acid treatment: Rub face with the insides of papaya and cucumber skins. They alkalize wastes that come out on the skin.

Essential oil support: Essential oils assist a skin cleanse: lavender, geranium, sandalwood and neroli. Use one or a combination of all three oils. Put a total of 15 drops essential oil in 2-oz of a carrier oil (such as jojoba) and rub on the skin.

Bathe: High mineral bath. Add 1 cup Dead Sea salts, 1 cup Epsom salts, 1/2 cup regular sea salt and 4 TBS. baking soda to a tub; swish in 3 drops lavender, 2 drops geranium, 2 drops sandalwood and 1 drop neroli oil.

Flower remedies: Natural Labs STRESS/TENSION; Nelson Bach RESCUE REMEDY.

Can't find a recommended product? Call the 800 number listed in Product Resources.

Chart Your Cleanse

Some health problems are a direct result of body toxicity... so they respond rapidly to body detoxification.

The ailments considered in the following charts have shown great improvement in my experience from cleansing techniques.

Each of the cleanses discussed may be used for a three to seven day period. If you need more detoxification, simply wait a week or two and repeat your program.

Chart Your Cleanse

It's so easy..... each cleansing chart has all the information you need to make it work.

• The first 2-3 pages set up the diagnostics for each cleanse.

• The cleanse page has three columns:

—Column 1 charts your nutrition plan choices

—Column 2 charts your herb and supplement choices

—Column 3 charts your bodywork and relaxation choices

A modified macrobiotic detox for cancer:

Detoxification followed by diet improvement is a major weapon against cancer. Dietary factors are undeniably involved with the largest number of cancers. Improving your diet directly improves your defenses against cancer. Massive new research is validating what naturopaths have known for decades. The more fruits and vegetables you eat, the less your cancer risk from colon and stomach cancer to breast and even lung cancer. For many cancers, people who eat plenty of fruits and vegetables have half the risk of people who eat few fruits and vegetables. Most studies show that even small to moderate amounts of fruits and vegetables make a big difference.

Do we know what causes cancer? Even though there are many types of cancer, diet is always the first place to look. The latest estimates list nutritional factors as accounting for 60% of women's cancers and 40% of men's. Extrapolating from that number means that good food choices could have helped prevent 385,000 to 700,000 new cancer cases, and between 170,000 to 325,000 cancer deaths in 1994 in the United States alone.

Hormone-driven cancers like ovarian, breast, uterine, kidney, bladder, prostate and colon cancers are closely related to the kind of protein and fat we eat, especially protein and fat from meats, and oxidized fats from junk foods and fried foods. Dietary factors are also directly linked to cancer of the rectum, stomach, intestines, mouth, throat, esophagus, pancreas, liver and thyroid.

Yet, there is encouraging evidence that certain dietary factors also act as anti-carcinogens, preventing tumor development and growth, inhibiting tumor metastasis of cancerous growths, and helping to normalize cancer cells. Nutritional therapy for cancer relies on re-establishing metabolic balance. Whole food nutrition allows the body to use its built-in restorative and repair abilities.

A cancer-fighting diet can intervene in the cancer process at many stages, from its conception to its growth and spread. Even if your genetics and lifestyle are against you, your diet may still make a tremendous difference in your cancer odds.

For example, we know that certain body chemicals must be "activated" before they can initiate cancer. Certain foods can block the activation process. Antioxidant foods can snuff out carcinogens, nip free radical cascades in the bud, and even repair some cellular damage. Some food compounds in cells can determine whether a cancer-causing virus or a cancer promoter (like too much estrogen) will turn tissue cancerous. Even after cells have massed into benign structures that may grow into tumors, food compounds can intervene to stop further growth. Some actually shrink the patches of precancerous cells.

Other foods accelerate body detoxification, and prevent the genetic ruin of cells, a prelude to cancer. It's one of the reasons I emphasize a detoxification diet as part of a cancer control program.

Although far less powerful at later stages, diet can still influence the spread of cancer. Wandering cancer cells need the right conditions in which to attach and grow. Food agents can foster a hostile or a favorable environment. So even after cancer is diagnosed, the right foods may help prolong your life.

Two fruits and three vegetable servings a day show amazing anticancer results. Eating fruit twice a day, instead of twice a week, can cut the risk of lung cancer by 75% even in smokers. One National Cancer Institute spokesman said it is almost mind-boggling, that ordinary fruits and vegetables could be so effective against such a potent carcinogen as cigarette smoke. The evidence is so overwhelming that some researchers are beginning to view fruits and vegetables as powerful preventive drugs that could even wipe out the scourge of cancer. What an about-face this has been for cancer study!

Here are the foods that provide prime nutrition with cancer-fighting and immune-enhancing properties:

—Fruits and vegetables, rich in vitamin C, for immune support and antioxidant protection: citrus fruits, tomatoes, peppers and broccoli.

—Active culture yogurt, to help neutralize carcinogens, and deactivate enzymes that allow body substances to turn into cancer.

—Antioxidant foods: wheat germ, soy foods, yellow, orange and green vegetables, green tea, citrus fruits, and olive oil help normalize precancerous cells, and neutralize cancer-causing free radicals. Normal cells multiply with oxygen, and cancer cells multiple without oxygen (anaerobic cell activity).

—Eating plenty of enzyme-rich fresh fruits and vegetables and using supplemental enzymes offer potent defense in fighting cancer. (See enzyme therapy below.)

—Fiber-rich foods: whole grains, fruits and vegetables to absorb excess bile and improve healthy intestinal bacteria.

—Phytochemical food elements, especially those found in cruciferous vegetables, break down carcinogens and remove them from the body. These same vegetable substances also break down excess estrogens responsible for some breast cancers, and inhibit tumor growth.

—Folic acid foods: whole wheat and wheat germ, leafy vegetables, beets, asparagus, fish, sunflower seeds, and citrus fruits are critical to normal DNA synthesis so healthy cells do not mutate and turn cancerous.

A modified macrobiotic diet switches the reliance on animal proteins and fats over to vegetable proteins like grains, beans, sprouts and sea vegetables. Essential Fatty Acids replace the unhealthy fats, such as saturated fats (typically from animal sources), or "hydrogenated" oils, such as found in margarine. The process of hydrogenating an oil is what transforms unsaturated fat into an unhealthy "trans fat." Healthy fat choices include olive oil, flaxseed oil and evening primrose oil. This modified macrobiotic diet also switches the reliance on highly processed foods over to the benefits of enzyme rich and phytochemical/antioxidant rich foods such as fresh, raw vegetables & fruits. Red meat and other animal proteins have not only the undesirable baggage of unhealthy saturated fats, but and are laden with pesticides, hormones, and various body-polluting substances. Also the super high protein diets have given way to the more commonly accepted view (approximately 50 to 80 grams of protein per day) by many current researchers. The traditional macrobiotic diet consists of 50 to 60% grains, 20 to 30% vegetables; fruit and eggs is a tiny percent.

A macrobiotic diet's greatest benefit is that it is cleansing and strengthening at the same time. Those who advocate macrobiotics for serious diseases like cancer also believe that the high percent of enzyme-rich vegetables and fruits in the modified macrobiotic diet are the most potent cancer fighters. Cancer cells grow because there is an absence of enzymes to fight them off. The fiber (fibrin) around a cancer cell is made of protein. Proteolytic enzymes digest this protein coating which allows the body's white blood cells to attack and destroy the cancer cell. At the same time, the enzymes also reduce the stickiness of the cancer cell, the mechanism the cell uses to attach itself and form tumors. The more cancer cells—the more enzymes the body needs. Protease is a proteolytic enzyme available in supplement form.

Enzyme therapy has earned a special position as an ethical, rational and highly promising preventive measure for cancer, especially in preventing the formation of cancer cells. Even though this is not always possible, European scientists, who have been in the vanguard of enzyme therapy, feel the goal should be to combat new cancer cells from being formed when the cancer is still at the single-group stage, or has made only small metastases with small numbers of cells into the blood or lymph vessels. Enzyme therapy has been effective prophylaxis

for metastatic spread. Enzyme therapy is also recommended before and after cancer surgery in order to help compensate for the weakening of the immune system which accompanies surgical intervention. A significant number of European oncologists now use enzymes for their cancer patients in hospitals.

European physicians also use enzyme therapy as an adjunct to traditional treatments. Recent radiotherapy studies show that when enzymes are administered along with radiation, lower radiation doses can produce the same effect. The enzymes also protect against radiation sickness and radiation therapy side effects. Patients regain their morale, their appetite, and feel more alive, both physically and mentally.

Please note: If you wish to use enzymes beyond the scope of a dietary supplement for "enzyme therapy," consult a health practitioner familiar with enzyme therapy. A resource which may be helpful in locating doctors using this approach is: Third Opinion - An International Directory to Alternative Therapy Centers for the Treatment and Prevention of Cancer", by John M. Fink. (Third Edition, 1997).

Is your body showing signs that it needs a modified cancer cleanse?

—Immune strength is a key to protection against cancer. Do you have recurrent or chronic infections? Do you catch colds easily? Even mild colds are signs of weak immune response.

—Do you get frequent cold sores or have genital herpes?

—Do you have swollen, sore lymph glands?

—Do you have chronic indigestion? Do you take large amounts of antacids on a regular basis?

Pointers for best results from your modified cancer cleanse:

•Drink 8-10 glasses of bottled water each day of your cleanse, including herbal teas. Water lubricates and flushes wastes and toxins from all cells, accelerating the cleansing program.

•Use green superfoods like chlorella, spirulina and barley grass. They are rich in every known cancer-fighting nutrient—chlorophyll, phytochemicals, antioxidants, vitamins, minerals, enzymes, and more. Superfoods are also powerful immune builders.

•Cancers are opportunistic, attacking when immune defenses and bloodstream health are low. Promote an environment where cancer and degenerative disease can't live - where **inherent immunity** can remain effective. These diseases do not seem to grow or take hold where oxygen and nutrients are high in the vital fluids. The cleansing and quality nutrients of this cleanse boost the immune system and create an unfavorable environment for cancer cells. Persist with your efforts to change unhealthy eating habits and incorporate healthy ones.

Benefits that you may notice as your body responds to the modified cancer cleanse:

•Most people notice an increased sense of well-being.

•Since this diet is non-mucous forming, low in fat foods and high in vegetable fiber, most body congestion will begin to clear.

•Circulation improves due to the stimulating effect on the heart and circulatory system from foods like miso, green tea, and shiitake mushrooms.

•Your stronger immune response system will begin to protect you from all the colds, flus and chronic infections.

Nutrition Plan

• Start with this 3 to 7 day nutrition plan.

The night before your cancer cleanse....

—Have a green leafy salad for dinner to give your bowels a good sweeping.

Before each meal (wait 20 minutes before eating), and before bed: take 2-oz. Herbal Answers HERBAL ALOE FORCE in water.

The next day....

—On rising: take 2 fresh squeezed lemons, 1 TBS. maple syrup and 8-oz. of water; or a ginseng restorative tea like Crystal Star GINSENG SIX™.

—Breakfast: have Pulsating Parsley Juice: 6 carrots, 1 beet, 8 spinach leaves and ¼ cup fresh parsley; or have a mixed fresh fruit salad.

—Mid-morning: take a cup of Crystal Star CLEANSING & PURIFYING™ TEA or DAILY DETOX by M.D.

—Lunch: have a Super V-7 veggie juice: 2 carrots, 2 tomatoes, handful each of spinach and parsley, 2 celery ribs, ½ cucumber, ½ green bell pepper. Add 1 TBS. of a green superfood: Crystal Star ENERGY GREEN™, NutriCology PRO-GREENS; Ethical Nutrients FUNCTIONAL GREENS; Vibrant Health VITALITY SUPERGREEN. Or have steamed broccoli or cauliflower with brown rice; or have a big fresh green salad.

—Mid-afternoon: have a fresh carrot juice; or a recovery broth like Crystal Star SYSTEMS STRENGTH™.

—Dinner: have brown rice and steamed vegetables with maitake or shiitake mushrooms. Maitake's unique natural killer cells are powerful against tumors and boost interleukin, an immune protein that fights cancer. Snip on dry sea vegetables, 1 TBS. flax or olive oil, and nutritional yeast.

—Before Bed: have green tea or Crystal Star GREEN TEA CLEANSER™. Green tea exhibits anticancer and cancer chemoprotective effects.

Continuing Diet Notes: The best chance for cancer isn't drugs or surgery - it's diet and lifestyle choices you make yourself. Cancers live and grow in unreleased fatty waste and mucous deposits. Fat intake is the key dietary risk factor linked to cancer. Avoid unhealthy fats - add essential fatty acids. Organic fruits and vegetables are essential to a successful cancer program. Refined sugars and junk foods have a direct effect on cancer growth. Have at least one daily drink of a green superfood.

Herbs & Supplements

• Choose 2 to 3 cleansing boosters.

Cleansing support formulas: Arise & Shine CLEANSE THYSELF PROGRAM - a specific for cancer patients, with many reports of success.

Antioxidants fight cancer/elevate T-cell levels: Biotec CELL GUARD; NutriCology ANTIOX FORMULA II; Crystal Star ANTI-OXIDANT extract; Jarrow GINKGO BILOBA + GRAPE SEED; Country Life SUPER 10 ANTIOXIDANT; Schiff PHYTOCHARGED ANTIOXIDANT; Source Naturals COENZYME Q₁₀ ULTRA POTENCY.

Enzyme support: Transformation Enzyme PUREZYME between meals dissolves the fibrin coating on cancer cells allowing immune defenses to work. Helps shrink tumors by stimulating removal of abnormal tissue. Purifies the blood by breaking down protein invaders. Use DIGESTZYME with meals.

Immune support: Herbs: *panax ginseng, echinacea, ashwaganda, Siberian ginseng, goldenseal, licorice, astragalus, ligustrum, suma, dandelion and cayenne.* Supplements: Allergy Research THIODOX (lipoic glutathione); NutriCology LAKTOFERRIN and TOTAL IMMUNE; Flora VEGESIL; Eidon SILICA MINERAL SUPPLEMENT.

Oxygen support: *"The prime cause of cancer is the replacement of normal oxygen respiration body cells by anaerobic cell respiration." - Otto Warburg, 2x Nobel Laureate.* NutriCology ORG. GERMANIUM and MODIFIED CITRUS PECTIN inhibit tumor metastasis.

Green Superfoods: Crystal Star ENERGY GREEN™; NutriCology PRO-GREENS; Vibrant Health GREEN VIBRANCE; Sun Wellness SUN CHLORELLA; Country Life SHIITAKE/REISHI COMPLEX WITH CHLORELLA.

Cancer Fighters: Herbal Answers HERBAL ALOE FORCE - proteolytic enzymes help remove tumors growths; NutriCology CAR-T-CELL or Kal BOVINE TRACHEAL CARTILAGE.

Bodywork Techniques

• Pick bodywork and relaxation techniques to accelerate and round out your cleanse.

Enema: Enemas are a specific for cancer detoxification: Take an enema the first, second and the last day of your cleansing program to help release toxins out of the body. Irrigate: Or have a colonic once a week for more thorough elimination.

Exercise: Regular exercise is almost a "cancer defense" in itself. Exercise acts as an antioxidant to enhance body oxygen use and boost immune response; it accelerates waste passage out of the body. Exercise alters body chemistry to control fat retention, a key involvement with cancer.

Rest: Immune power builds the most during sleep—essential to long-term recovery from cancer.

Overheating therapy: highly effective against cancer. See page 32 for an in-home method.

Guided imagery: effective in helping the immune system to work better, and the hormone system to stop producing abnormal cells.

Deep Breathing Exercise: Deep, relaxed breathing removes stress, composes the mind, improves mood and increases energy levels. It's the simplest form of concentration - a basic principle of yoga meditation. 1. Shift your focus away from your racing mind or stressful emotions to focus attention on your breath. 2. Consciously take slow, deep, regular breaths, the mind will become calm. 3. Recall a pleasant past experience. 4. Physically feel thankfulness or love about the good things and people you have in your life. 5. Sincerely question your inner intuition to help find your health solution, one that will minimize future stress.

Can't find a recommended product? Call the 800 number listed in Product Resources.

Do you need a cleanse from drug or alcohol addiction?

Americans have an expensive river of chemicals coursing through our national veins. We take some $19 billion worth of prescription drugs each year. At a cost to taxpayers of *276 billion dollars a year*, some believe that it's the nation's number one health problem. The use of "hard" or "pleasure" drugs in today's society is also prevalent. Still, experts believe that the most serious addictions are those to pharmaceutical drugs. More than one million people a year (3 to 5 percent of admissions) end up in hospitals as a result of negative reactions to prescription drugs.

Clearly, modern drugs play lifesaving roles in emergency situations and they can help numerous health problems, especially short term, but most people begin taking drugs to alleviate boredom and fatigue, or to relieve physical or psychological pain. A detox program helps enormously to release drugs and alcohol from your system, but withdrawing after long time use can produce harsh effects (see following page). I highly recommend the supervision of a qualified health professional for an addictions cleanse, especially if the dependency has been long term and highly addictive. Sometimes, the best way is to wean yourself gradually from the addictive substance while you do your addiction cleanse.

The symptoms that drugs or excessive alcohol address are merely the warning signs of deeper internal imbalances. Alcohol abuse especially may be brought on and marked by stress and depression. Drugs and alcohol can even aggravate an original health problem and add to the poisons in your body. Drug detoxification is a process of releasing the stored substances while at the same time changing lifestyle habits so that you are no longer dependent on them. It is critical to fortify your body enough to give it the power to resist returning to the addictive substance. I have found that only a well-nourished body can offer both your body and mind enough of a sense of well being and strength to melt the relapse urges and desires.

Is your body showing signs that it needs an addiction cleanse?

—Do you only feel happy and relaxed after having a drink or taking an antidepressant or mood elevating drug?
—Do you find that you can't relieve stress, or escape daily problems without alcohol or drugs?
—Do you have liver problems? Does your stomach protrude but you are thin everywhere else? It's a sign of liver enlargement and inflammation.
—Do you have esophagus impairment, high blood pressure, or pancreatitis? Are your stools pale?
—Are the whites of your eyes dingy? Is the eye lower lid yellow? Is your skin slightly jaundiced? Do you sweat a lot?
—Have you lost your appetite? Have you gotten noticeably, or unusually thin? Do you have a marked intolerance for fatty foods?
—Is your digestion always bad? Do you have a metallic taste in your mouth? Are you drowsy after meals? In the overwhelming number of cases, habitual drug and alcohol users suffer from chronic subclinical malnutrition, and from multiple depletions of critical nutrients. Vitamins, minerals, amino acids, fatty acids and enzymes are all depleted, some by 50 to 60 percent.
—Are you often foggy mentally? Do you have a lot of food allergies or chemical sensitivities? Do you crave sweets? Is your blood sugar usually low? These signs indicate rampant hypoglycemia from alcohol or drug overload.
—Do you feel shaky and sweaty? Do you often get a "wired," nervous feeling, sometimes with heart palpitations? Central nervous system overload is a sign of addiction.

—Do you have frequent memory loss? Short term memory loss is one of the first signs of alcohol abuse; damage to the brain is another.

—Are you unusually anxious, even paranoid? Do you lose your temper or get in a bad mood easily? Do you feel depressed and cry a lot? Do you ever get dizzy or black out? These are typically late symptoms of alcohol abuse.

—Is there pain on your right side or under your right shoulder blade? Do you get stomach or muscle cramps frequently?

—Do you get frequent frontal headaches that feel like a continual hangover?

—Are you continually tired? Extreme fatigue usually results from poor liver health, adrenal exhaustion or thyroid malfunction

—Is your immune response low? Do you seem to have a cold or flu all the time? All drugs weaken the immune system over time

Pointers for best results from your addiction cleanse:

• Drink 8 glasses of water each day of your cleanse (can include herb teas). Water flushes alcohol and drugs from every corner of your body.

• Natural mood enhancers, such as *St. John's Wort and Kava Kava*, that our bodies are equipped to handle, help in the weaning process from addictive substances.

• Use green superfoods. They are rich in chlorophyll, phytochemicals, antioxidants, vitamins, minerals, enzymes, etc. Superfoods help nourish the body, build immunity and help stave off cravings.

What does it feel like to withdraw from drugs or alcohol?

Breaking destructive habits is hard. Your body reacts when a substance it thinks it depends on is removed. The initial withdrawal phase is usually the most difficult part of the detox and can last from a day or two to a week or more. Withdrawal symptoms are the same as addiction symptoms, only worse and more frequent. You'll start getting chronic headaches, usually with diarrhea as your body tries to release toxins faster, and a lot of irritability. Some people experience hallucinations, disorientation or irrational thinking. Some go into depression. You'll probably sleep poorly, and your sleep will be interrupted during the night. Most people in withdrawal are sensitive to light and noise, hot and cold flashes, and sweating.

I encourage people to look at each episode of discomfort as a little victory on the road to recovery. Every day gets easier. One of the laws of the universe is that we don't have to fight the same battle twice. As your body dislodges and removes more toxins day by day, you have the satisfaction of knowing they are gone for good.

Some benefits you'll notice as your body responds to an addiction cleanse:

• Your mood will lift as your nerves heal.

• Memory and thinking will improve. Take ginkgo biloba extract for a month to help speed up your brain processes.

• Your skin will become clearer—less muddy; your eyes will become brighter.

• Digestion for most people improves right away

• Your immune response will noticeably improve, usually within a month.

Nutrition Plan

•Start with this 3 to 7 day nutrition plan.

The overwhelming majority of habitual drug and alcohol users suffer from malnutrition, metabolic upset and nutritional imbalances. The following drug detox diet not only helps remove alcohol and drug residues, but also helps rebuild a depleted system.

—On rising: a superfood/aloe drink gives energy and controls morning blood sugar drop: add 1 tsp. each to aloe vera juice: spirulina, bee pollen granules (for LGA), brewer's yeast; or use 1 TBS. of a superfood mix: Crystal Star ENERGY GREEN™ DRINK; Arise & Shine POWER UP; Green Foods GREEN MAGMA.

—Breakfast: make a mineral mix - 1 tsp. each: sesame seeds, wheat germ, bee pollen granules, brewer's yeast. Add to fresh fruit with yogurt; oatmeal or rice pilaf with maple syrup; whole grain cereal or granola with apple juice.

—Mid-morning: have fresh carrot juice or Super V-7 veggie juice: 2 carrots, 2 tomatoes, handful each spinach and parsley, 2 celery ribs, $\frac{1}{2}$ cucumber, $\frac{1}{2}$ bell pepper. Add 1 TBS. green superfood - Crystal Star ENERGY GREEN™ DRINK; Transitions EASY GREENS.

—Lunch: have a fresh veggie salad topped with almonds or sunflower seeds. Snip on sea vegetables. Snip on sea vegetables, 1 tsp. nutritional yeast, 1 tsp. flax or olive oil 1 tsp. lemon juice and Bragg's LIQUID AMINOS.

—Mid-afternoon: have a glass of carrot juice with 1 TBS. green superfood (see above); or Crystal Star SYSTEMS STRENGTH™, or a ginseng restorative tea.

—Dinner: have brown rice and steamed vegetables with chopped onions, nutritional yeast, snipped shiitake mushrooms.

—Before Bed: have a cup of miso soup with 1 TBS. sea vegetables and 1 tsp. pickled ginger.

Continuing Diet Notes: Eat magnesium-rich foods - green leafy and yellow vegetables, citrus fruits, whole grain cereals, fish, legumes. Eat potassium-rich foods - oranges, broccoli, green peppers, seafoods, sea vegetables, bananas, tomatoes. Eat chromium-rich foods - brewer's yeast, mushrooms, whole grains, seafoods and peas. Increase alkalinity with fresh foods. Cravings and withdrawal symptoms intensify in an acid body, from foods like meats, milk products, refined flours and sugars.

Herbs & Supplements

•Choose 2 to 3 cleansing boosters.

Cleansing support: Vale Ent. VALE'S PERMA-CLEAN. Liver support - the key to recovery from alcohol and drug abuse. *Alpha Lipoic Acid* - among the most powerful liver detoxifiers ever discovered. *Milk thistle seed, licorice and kudzu root* are key herbs: Planetary Formulas KUDZU CAPS; Gaia MILK THISTLE SEED extract; Crystal Star LIV-ALIVE™ TEA.

Aloe support: balances blood sugar, metabolism and hormonal system to help decrease cravings. AloeLife TERRY'S HERBAL ALOE DETOX PLUS.

Herbal support: Crystal Star WITHDRAWAL SUPPORT™ caps and DEPRESS-EX™ extract help overcome drug-related depression. Ginseng is a key: Y.S. ROYAL JELLY/GINSENG TEA; Crystal Star GINSENG SIX™. Zand ACTIVE HERBAL.

Buffered C Powder to overcome addictions: NutriCology BUFFERED C POWDER (beet source).

Antioxidant therapy: Jarrow Formulas ALPHA LIPOIC ACID or MRI ALPHA-LIPOIC ACID; Transformation Enzyme EXCELLZYME; Source Naturals COENZYME Q_{10} ULTRA POTENCY; Country Life SUPER 10 ANTIOXIDANT.

Vitamin therapy: C, E, beta-carotene, selenium bind with toxins and carry them out of the body: All One MULTIPLE VITAMINS, MINERALS, GREEN PHYTO BASE.

Amino acids: L-cysteine and glutathione help decrease toxicity of many drugs and chemicals, reduce cravings: Allergy Research THIODOX.

Enzyme support: cleans up cellular debris from drug therapy. Transformation Enzyme PUREZYME.

Green superfoods: Crystal Star ENERGY GREEN™ DRINK; Sun Wellness SUN CHLORELLA; Body Ecology VITALITY SUPERGREEN; Solgar EARTH SOURCE GREENS & MORE; Transformation Enzyme SUPER CELLZYME caps; Nature's Secret ULTIMATE GREEN tabs.

Bodywork Techniques

•Pick bodywork and relaxation techniques to accelerate and round out your cleanse.

Enema: especially important when detoxing from alcohol and drugs - take an enema the first and second day of your cleansing program. Irrigate: Or have a colonic for a more thorough colon cleanse.

Exercise: every day if possible. Exercise helps the movement of toxins out of the body - it also brings oxygen to the cells. Exercise also helps reduce the stress of detoxing from addictions. Take a walk every day of your cleanse, breathing deeply.

Guided imagery: give your body some active encouragement. Guided imagery is a relaxation technique to use frequently during an addictions detox. Actively imagine each gram of the addictive substance dislodging itself from your tissues, floating into your bloodstream and into your bladder or bowel for elimination. Make sure you visualize it leaving your body.

Flower remedies: Natural Labs ADDICTIONS.

Deep breathing exercise: Do deep breathing exercises on rising, and in the evening on retiring to clear the lungs and respiratory system, and to bring oxygen into the cells.

Hot and cold hydrotherapy: alternating hot and cold showers are effective. Spasmodic pain and cramping, circulation, muscle tone, bowel and bladder problems, system balance, relaxation, and energy all show improvement with hydrotherapy.

• Begin with a comfortably hot shower for three minutes. Follow with a sudden change to cold water for 2 minutes. Repeat this cycle three times, ending with cold. Follow with a full or partial massage, or a brisk towel rub and mild stretching exercises for best results.

Can't find a recommended product? Call the 800 number listed in Product Resources.

Do you need an arthritis cleanse for joints, connective tissue and immune system?

Arthritis is the country's number one crippling disease, affecting over 40 million Americans—80% of people over 50. When you add to that number of people suffering from **arthritis-like** diseases - gout, bursitis, tendonitis and lupus, and figure becomes staggering. Arthritis is inflammation of the joints, usually accompanied by changes in joint structure. But that's only part of the story. It isn't a simple disease in any form, affecting not only the bones and joints, but also the blood vessels (Reynaud's disease), kidneys, skin (psoriasis), eyes and brain. Because its causes are rooted in immune response as well as wear-and-tear effects, conventional medicine has not been able to address arthritis with even a small degree of success. Natural therapies, based in lifestyle and diet changes, however, work extremely well because they can address the causes of arthritis. In fact, diet improvement to normalize body chemistry is the single most beneficial thing you can do to control an arthritic condition. I have personally seen notable reduction of swelling, and deformity even in long-standing cases.

Arthritis is unique in its close ties to emotional health. Emotional stress frequently brings onset of the disease. Acid-causing, emotional resentments and negative obsessive-compulsive actions aggravate arthritis. Most arthritis sufferers have a marked inability to relax (relaxation techniques are essential to arthritis healing). Many have a negative attitude toward life that locks up the body's healing ability.

Although the focus of diagnosis has been on organic mineral (especially calcium) depletion as a cause of arthritis, I find that hormone imbalance and adrenal exhaustion are the keys to repair therapy. By far the greatest number of arthritis sufferers are menopausal women.

Is your body showing signs that it needs an arthritis cleanse?

—Do you notice marked stiffness and swelling in your fingers, shoulders or neck when the weather turns cold and damp?
—Are you unusually stiff when you get up in the morning, especially when the weather is damp?
—Have you started to notice bony bumps on your index fingers? Or bony spurs on any other joints?
—Are your joints starting to crack and pop?
—Are you anemic? Is your complexion unusually pale? Have you recently lost weight but weren't on a diet?
—Is your digestion poor? Do you have food allergies or intolerances?
—If you experience back or joint pain when you move, does it get worse with prolonged activity?
—Are you more than 20 pounds overweight and starting to feel the effects of the extra weight in your knees and hips?
—Do you have a lot of long-standing lung and bronchial congestion?
—Are you usually constipated? Do you suffer from ulcerative colitis?
—Do you take more than 6 aspirin a day on a regular basis? Are you on a long-term prescription of corticosteroid drugs? Either of these may eventually impair the body's own healing powers.

Pointers for best results from your arthritis cleanse:

•Numerous new studies are finding that osteoarthritis is repairable. Joint and connective tissue strength can be greatly increased with body chemistry improvement. Food allergies regularly contribute to osteoarthritis symptoms, so include fresh vegetables in your detox.

•**Avoid these foods during and after your detox:** fatty meat and dairy foods, wheat pastries that are also high in sugar and fat; nightshade foods like peppers, eggplant, tomatoes and potatoes; highly salted or spiced foods, caffeine, chocolate, colas and soda pop.

• Standard drug therapy with aspirin or NSAIDS drugs like MOTRIN suppress pain and inflammation, but may actually promote the progression of arthritis by damaging cartilage and inhibiting the ability of the body to repair normal collagen structures. A compound of **glucosamine sulfate and chondroitin sulfate,** body substances that stimulate the production of cartilage components. Products like Solgar GLUCOSAMINE CHONDROITIN COMPLEX work better than NSAIDS drugs without the side effects.

• If you have bumps on your knuckles, cherries and cherry juice are a specific food remedy. Take a mild herbal diuretic such as Crystal Star TINKLE CAPS™ to flush out released material.

• Accelerate your cleanse with a daily green drink and add enzyme therapy, like Rainbow Light ADVANCED ENZYME SYSTEM.

Benefits that you may notice as your body responds to the arthritis cleanse:

• Symptom reduction in inflammation and swelling is fairly rapid. When natural supplements are used along with the diet, some people experience relief within 24 hours. Remember, instead of dulling pain with drugs you are repairing damage in order to relieve pain.

• Regenerating flexibility takes longer—usually several months as cartilage and connective tissue rebuild, but some stiffness should subside within 2 to 3 weeks.

• As mucous membrane health improves, you should see better skin tone, digestive and bowel health (regularity) and eye moisture.

• Restoring your immune system is the last and best benefit to emanate from an arthritis detox.

An arthritis elimination sweat:

An arthritis sweat is an effective, ancient technique to help eliminate offending crystalline deposits in connective tissue and relieve stiffness. A surprising amount of arthritis-aggravating material can be eliminated via the skin. A sweat is also a good way to start an arthritis cleanse. Results increase when diaphoretic herbs like elder flowers, peppermint or yarrow are taken in a hot tea along with the bath.

Here's how to take the bath: *If you have a weak heart or hypertension, consult a health professional before trying an arthritis sweat bath.*

Use about 3 pounds of Epsom salts (or as directed for Dead Sea salts). Run hot bath water and add the salts. Let cool enough to get in; Try to stay in the bath for 15 to 20 minutes. Rub affected joints with a stiff brush in the water for 5 to 10 minutes On emerging, do not dry yourself. Instead, wrap up immediately in a clean sheet and go straight to bed, covering yourself with several blankets. The osmotic pressure of the Epsom salt solution absorbed by the sheet will draw off heavy perspiration, (protect your mattress with a sheet of plastic). The following morning the sheet will be stained with yellowish brown material excreted through the skin. Continue treatment once every two weeks until the sheet is no longer stained, a sign that the body is cleansed. Drink plenty of water throughout the procedure to prevent dehydration and loss of body salts. Improvement after the Epsom salt bath experience is notable.

Lack of water is linked to arthritis.

Chondroitin sulfate, a specific nutrient for arthritis, is the molecule in cartilage that attracts and holds water. Healthy joints are 85 to 90% water, but since cartilage doesn't have its own blood supply, chondroitin sulfate aids the "molecular sponge" that provides nourishment, waste removal and lubrication for healthy joints. Water helps restore healthy cartilage so it often relieves osteoarthritic symptoms. Including eight 8-oz. glasses of water daily in your arthritis healing diet is essential. Limit the use of alcoholic beverages since they are especially dehydrating.

Nutrition Plan

• **Start with this 3 to 7 day nutrition plan.**

—On Rising: take a glass of lemon juice and water, or a glass of fresh grapefruit juice. (Acidic citrus fruits help enzyme production to alkalize the body); or Crystal Star GREEN TEA CLEANSER™.

—Breakfast: take a potassium broth or essence (pg. 134); or a glass of carrot/beet/cucumber juice.

—Mid-morning: have apple or black cherry juice; or a green drink, like Sun Wellness CHLORELLA, Green Foods GREEN ESSENCE, Personal Best V-8 (pg. 138) or Crystal Star ENERGY GREEN™ drink.

—Lunch: have a cup of miso soup with sea veggies snipped on top, and a glass of fresh carrot juice with 1 teasp. Bragg's LIQUID AMINOS.

—Mid-afternoon: have another green drink, or alfalfa/mint tea, or Crystal Star CLEANSING & PURIFYING™ TEA.

—Dinner: have a glass of cranberry/apple, or papaya juice, or another glass of black cherry juice.

—Before Bed: take a glass of celery juice, or a cup of miso soup with 1 TBS. of nutritional yeast.

Note: Follow your detox with a fresh foods diet for 1 month. 1) Fresh fruits and vegetables, with lots of green leafy greens are rich in enzymes. 2) There is a link between a sulfur deficiency and arthritis. Eat sulfur-containing foods like broccoli, onions, cabbage and garlic. 3) Fiber keeps crystalline wastes flushed. Eat whole grains like rice and oats. 4) Bioflavonoids strengthen connective tissue. Eat (and drink) cranberries, grapes, papayas and citrus fruits, or Crystal Star BIOFLAVONOID, FIBER & C SUPPORT™ drink. 5) Have cold water fish like salmon for high Omega-3 oils twice a week.

Continuing Diet Notes: Mix 2 TBS. each: sunflower seeds, lecithin granules, brewer's yeast, wheat germ. Mix into yogurt, or sprinkle on fresh fruit or greens. Take 2 tsp. daily. Soy foods, like tofu, tempeh and miso can be a key diet factor for women. They are hormone balancing and immune stimulating with non-meat protein. Fiber foods with protein, like rice, oats, lentils and beans are a key factor for men. Use only olive or canola oil in cooking. Never fry your foods.

Herbs & Supplements

• **Choose 2 to 3 cleansing boosters.**

Cartilage protectives: Glucosamine sulfate and chrondroitin sulfate - Allergy Research MATRIX; Enzymatic Therapy GS-COMPLEX.

Herbal support: Crystal Star AR-EASE™, GREEN TEA CLEANSER™ each morning, and ADR-ACTIVE™ caps with EVENING PRIMROSE OIL 1000mg 2 daily. *Hawthorn, Siberian ginseng and ginkgo biloba* extracts.

Effective anti-inflammatories for arthritis: DLPA 750mg; Crystal Star ANTI-FLAM™ CAPS; Quercetin w/Bromelain; Omega-3 flax oil 3x daily; Allergy Research CURCUMIN/BROMELAIN; Premier Labs INFLAM-AWAY; Prevail MOBILE. Herbal Answers HERBAL ALOE FORCE.

Effective antioxidants for arthritis: CoQ$_{10}$ 60mg 3x daily; Grapeseed or white pine PCOs 50mg. 3x daily significantly reduce joint inflammation; Ester C 500mg with bioflavs for collagen synthesis. Biotec CELL GUARD; Jarrow ANTIOXIDANT OPTIMIZER; Enzymatic Therapy GRAPE SEED PHYTOSOME 100; NutriCology QUERCETIN 300.

Enzyme support: Transformation Enzyme PURE-ZYME (protease) carries protein-bound calcium; a protease deficiency lays the foundation for arthritis, osteoporosis and calcium-deficient diseases. Bitters herbs provide enzymes and stimulate bile production: BITTERS & LEMON CLEANSE™ extract.

Adrenal therapy sources: YS royal jelly/ginseng 2 tsp. daily; Enzymatic Therapy ADRENAL CORTEX COMPLEX; American Biologics SUB-ADRENE 3x daily. Chlorophyll sources to help stimulate cortisone: Solaray ALFA-JUICE caps; Crystal Star ENERGY GREEN™ DRINK; NutriCology PRO-GREENS; Wakunaga Kyo-Green; Body Ecology VITALITY SUPERGREEN; Vibrant Health GREEN VIBRANCE.

Bodywork Techniques

• **Pick bodywork and relaxation techniques to accelerate and round out your cleanse.**

Enema: take an enema the first, second and the last day of your arthritis cleanse to release toxins.

Exercise: A lack of exercise weakens muscles putting more stress on joints. A daily stretching program and yoga are my favorites for keeping skeletal muscles strong.

Bodywork therapies: Massage therapy relieves pain, improves the circulation and hastens elimination of harmful deposits.

—Hot and cold hydrotherapy, Epsom salts baths, chiropractic treatments and overheating therapy are all effective. (See bodywork section, page 30)

—Crystal Star ALKALIZING ENZYME™ herbal wrap normalizes body pH almost immediately.

—Use cayenne/ginger compresses on affected areas. Capsaicin ointment is also effective. Apply 3 to 4 times a day for at least 2 weeks.

Pain relief: Biochemics PAIN RELEAF gel, Capsaicin cream or Tiger Balm rub-on ointment. Add ginger to your daily diet; take bromelain 1500mg.

Acupressure pain relief: press the highest spot of the muscle between thumb and index finger. Press into the web muscle between the two fingers. Angle pressure toward the bone of the index finger. Press for 10 seconds at a time.

Effective local applications:

—Wakunaga FREEDOM ARTHRITIS RELIEF CREAM.

—Transitions PRO-GEST cream (women).

—Crystal Star ANTI-BIO™ gel with una da gato.

—B & T TRIFLORA gel.

—Biochemics PAIN RELEAF lotion.

—DMSO on clean skin as directed.

—Bioforce ARNICA LOTION.

Can't find a recommended product? Call the 800 number listed in Product Resources.

Does someone you know need an Alzheimer's or Parkinson's cleanse?

Alzheimer's disease is a progressive, degenerative condition that attacks the brain, forming neurofiber tangles and plaques that result in dementia symptoms—impaired memory, decreased intellectual and emotional function, and ultimately complete physical breakdown. It's a devastating, relentless assault that's rising at a rapid rate in industrialized countries worldwide. In the U.S. 10% of the population over sixty-five suffers from some dementia. Another 5% suffer from severe dementia. Increased oxidative damage from free-radicals plays a prominent role in the development of Alzheimer's. Contributing causes may include genetic factors, but like most degenerative diseases, environmental factors like exposure to harmful chemicals, aluminum or inorganic silicon are thought to be a key. Some Alzheimer's victims are really victims of too many drugs. Although orthodox medicine has been unable to make a difference in this destructive disease, natural therapies have been successful in slowing the deterioration of brain function.

Parkinson's disease, often a risk factor for Alzheimer's, is the progressive deterioration of specific nerve centers in the brain. The disease process changes the balance of acetylcholine and dopamine, two brain chemicals essential for transmission of nerve signals. The altered balance of these two neurotransmitters results in a lack of control of physical movements. Although the direct cause of Parkinson's is unknown, it is believed that a neurotoxin causes oxidative damage to the basal ganglia that control muscle tone.

What body signs indicate the need for an Alzheimer or Parkinson disease cleanse?

—Is there a noticeable loss of ability to think clearly or remember familiar names, places or events?
—Is there loss of touch with reality, impaired judgement, confusion, difficulty in completing thoughts or following directions?
—Are there clear, unexplained personality or behavior changes?
—Is there a slight tremor in the hands with numbness and tingling in the hands and feet?
—If you noticed a hand tremor, has it become more evident with shaking of the head as well?
—Is there slight dragging of the feet, pronounced with stress or fatigue? Has movement become increasingly difficult?
—If movement is lethargic, has speech also become slow and difficult to follow?
—Has the face lost expression (because of muscle rigidity)? Is there slight drooling? Is vision noticeably impaired?
—Is there unexplained depression? (supplementation may offer dramatic improvement)

Pointers for best results from your Alzheimer or Parkinson cleanse:

• Good nutrition is a key: Nutritional deficiencies are regularly present in Alzheimer's and Parkinson's patients. Some experts think lack of B-vitamins is a critical cause of Alzheimer's. Adding through diet or supplements can produce noticeable improvement.

• Oxidative damage is significant in the development and progression of both Alzheimer's and Parkinson's. An antioxidant-rich diet with plenty of fresh fruits and vegetables offers significant protection and can slow the progression of both conditions.

• Significant evidence over the last several decades shows that aluminum contributes to both Alzheimer's and Parkinson's. Considerably higher aluminum levels are found in the brains of those with Alzheimer's than in people with other types of dementia or in normal people. Do you regularly use aluminum pots and pans or aluminum foil in your cooking? Check on your water supply (aluminum may occur naturally in water, but it's added as alum). Preserved foods like relishes or condiments, antacids that are regularly taken, deodorants or baking powder are other aluminum culprits. Calcium citrate supplements appear to *increase* aluminum absorption.

Benefits you may notice as your body responds to the Alzheimer/Parkinson cleanse:

• A cleanse helps remove some of the scar-like deposits of proteins and cellular debris that compose Alzheimer's plaques. This toxin release brings a feeling of ease and sense of well being.

• Energy levels increase and circulation improves.

• Mental clarity increases and awareness heightens.

Continuing diet watchwords after the Alzheimer's/Parkinson's cleanse:

—Cognitive function is directly related to nutritional status - especially in the elderly. Good nutrition has a noticeable (sometimes rapid) positive effect on better mental function.

—Besides your focus on nutrient-rich foods, it is equally important to avoid foods that create toxic build-up — preserved meats like lunch meats, foods with coloring added, and most important, pesticide-sprayed fruits and vegetables. Especially avoid fatty, fried foods. Both too much fat and too many total calories are associated with Alzheimer's and Parkinson's, because both fat and total calories are associated with oxidative stress, and most fat leads to inflammation. Pesticides are full of environmental estrogens which disrupt the delicate hormone balance of the brain, and are thought to be implicated in Alzheimer's symptoms. Wash fruits and vegetables with a food wash (available in health food stores), or better yet, eat organically grown foods.

—A diet rich in magnesium is important in protecting against aluminum absorption. Good magnesium sources are dark green vegetables, seafoods and sea vegetables, whole grains, nuts, beans and seeds, tangy spices and cocoa.

—Antioxidant-rich foods are critical. More than any other food group they slow the progression of both Alzheimer's and Parkinson's. Focus especially on vitamin E and selenium-rich foods for antioxidant activity — wheat germ and wheat germ oil, sunflower seeds and oil, almonds, pecans, hazelnuts, whole grain cereals, legumes like soy products, peas and beans, seafoods and sea vegetables, broccoli, cabbage, garlic and onions. Note: Protease is a potent antioxidant enzyme nutrient. It prevents the formation of neurofibrillary tangles and amyloid plaques. Keep it in your supplement program.

—Boost your B-complex nutrients. Important food sources are soy foods, seafoods and sea vegetables, brewer's yeast, brown rice, nuts, poultry and leafy greens. Supplementing the diet with B_{12} (about 2500mcg daily and folic acid (400 to 800mg daily) have shown almost complete reversal in some Alzheimer's patients. I especially like food sources of these vitamins as they appear in bee pollen, royal jelly and sea vegetables. Prolonged B_{12} deficiency may lead to irreversible changes that will not respond to supplementation.

—Improving the diet with zinc-rich foods shows noticeable results in Alzheimer's patients, with positive progression in memory, understanding and communication. Good zinc food sources include brewer's yeast, beans, nuts, seeds, wheat germ and seafood.

—Try to limit prescription and over-the-counter drugs. A Johns Hopkins study reveals many Alzheimer's patients are really victims of too many drugs - most taking more than *6 different drugs simultaneously*. One-quarter of the medications were either unsafe or ineffective, and the side effects from both the drug interactions or the inappropriate medication affected brain neurotransmission. Most harmful were pain killers and sleeping pills that tended to leach acetylcholine from brain tissues, and diuretics which leached potassium needed by the brain. While it is sometimes necessary to take medication, drugs are so powerful that I feel it is critical for older people (indeed everyone) to be well informed about the drugs they are taking - dosage, side effects and interaction with other drugs.

—Dehydration contributes to Alzheimer's and Parkinson's. Drink plenty of water, ideally, eight 8-oz glasses daily.

Nutrition Plan

• **Start with this 2 to 4 day nutrition plan.**

Note: Eliminating or at least reducing toxicity from food, water and the environment is critical.

—On Rising: take an antioxidant rich fruit juice—grape, grapefruit, lemon and cherry - sources of bioflavonoids; or orange - source of selenium.

—Breakfast: have cranberry, grape or papaya juice; or mix in 1 TBS. Crystal Star Bioflavonoid, Fiber & C Support™ Drink for antioxidants; or have fresh cherries, bananas, oranges or strawberries with yogurt, and sprinkle on 2 tsp. daily of the following mix: Two TBS. each: sunflower seeds, lecithin granules, brewer's yeast and wheat germ.

—Mid-morning: have an antioxidant-rich vegetable juice: • Carrot, kale, parsley and spinach, sources of beta-carotene. • Kale, garlic, parsley, green pepper and spinach, sources of vitamin C, vitamin E and selenium (slows the progression of Alzheimer's and Parkinson's).

—Lunch: have a large dark green leafy salad with lemon/oil dressing (see Green Cuisine section); and/or a hot veggie broth or hearty veggie soup; with marinated tofu or tempeh in tamari sauce.

—Mid-afternoon: have a glass of fresh carrot juice or fresh apple juice. Add 1 TBS. of a green superfood such as Crystal Star Energy Green™ Drink, Green Kamut Green Kamut; Vibrant Health Green Vibrance.

—Dinner: have steamed brown rice and mixed steamed vegetables. Sprinkle with sea vegetables, 1 to 2 TBS. flax or olive oil, 1 tsp. liquid lecithin, 1 TBS. Bragg's Liquid Aminos and 1 TBS. nutritional yeast, sources of choline (a direct precursor of acetylcholine, the key neurotransmitter for memory) and B-complex (low levels linked to Alzheimer's).

—Before Bed: have a cup of green tea or Crystal Star Green Tea Cleanser™, rich in antioxidants.

Continuing Diet Notes: Excess meat protein and fat facilitate amyloid neurofiber tangle build-up. Reduce them in your diet to help both Alzheimer's and Parkinson's. Alzheimer's is linked to synthetic estrogens, like those injected into red meats and chickens. Eat organically grown foods when possible to avoid environmental estrogens from pesticides. Eat foods rich in antioxidants to feed the brain: include fresh vegetables, sea vegetables, whole grains, seeds, soy foods, and seafood.

Herbs & Supplements

• **Choose 2 to 3 cleansing boosters.**

Antioxidants: Free radicals destroy brain cells - antioxidants destroy free radicals - critical in overcoming oxidative damage to the brain to slow progression of Alzheimer's and Parkinson's. Biotec Cell Guard, NutriCology Quercetin 300, CoQ₁₀ 60mg 2x daily, L-acetyl-carnitine 500mg daily delays progression of Alzheimer's; phosphatidylserine for impaired mental function.

Antioxidant herbs: Ginkgo biloba extract treats Alzheimer's by normalizing acetylcholine receptors and increasing cholinergic transmission.

Enzymes: Oxidative damage and formation of amyloid plaques are the two main causes of Alzheimer's. Protease is a powerful antioxidant enzyme and prevents the formation of amyloid tangles. Transformation Enzyme PURE-ZYME. Note: Zinc links the tissues to antioxidant enzymes. Zinc deficiency can allow amyloid plaques.

Aloe vera support: Herbal Answers Herbal Aloe Force enhances immune response for Parkinson's and Alzheimer's, and helps regenerate tissue needed to correct damage to connective tissue.

Critical essential fatty acids for nerves and brain: 1 TBS. flaxseed oil per day; Evening Primrose Oil 4 - 6 daily; Nature's Secret Ultimate Oil.

Green superfoods are restoratives: Chlorella has the highest amounts of nucleic acids (RNA/DNA) of any food on earth. Crystal Star Energy Green™; NutriCology Pro-Greens; Sun Wellness Sun Chlorella; Body Ecology Vitality Supergreen.

Magnesium helps block aluminum absorption.
Silica prevents aluminum absorption.

Oral chelation: cleanses heavy metals - Hayestown Tricardia; Golden Pride Formula One.

Bodywork Techniques

• **Pick bodywork and relaxation techniques to accelerate and round out your cleanse.**

Enema: Take an enema at least once during your Alzheimer's or Parkinson's cleansing program to help release toxins out of the body.

Exercise: A steady moderate exercise regime lowers the risk of developing Alzheimer's. Daily mild exercise is also important for Parkinson's therapy. A brisk daily walk is highly recommended.

Exercise for brain cells: Keep your brain active and challenged with mentally creative activities. Use hot and cold hydrotherapy showers for brain and circulation stimulation.

Flower remedies: Natural Labs Forgetfulness for memory lapses and loss, wandering thoughts, lack of alertness and attentiveness, unconsciousness, senility and amnesia; Nelson Bach Rescue Remedy for stress.

Effective body work/therapies: Relaxation techniques like chiropractic treatment, massage therapy, acupuncture and acupressure have had notable success in reversing early Parkinson's and are helpful for Alzheimer's.

Special tip: Decrease prescription diuretics if possible. They leach potassium and nutrients needed by the brain.

Can't find a recommended product? Call the 800 number listed in Product Resources.

Do you need an allergy or asthma cleanse?

Allergies used to be defined as inappropriate immune responses to substances (like cat hair, or dust or wheat) that aren't normally harmful. Today, it's clear that the dramatic rise in allergies is due to substances that *are* harmful. Not only does the toxic overload from chemicals in our food and environment cause allergic reactions, it also impairs the body's immune response to them.

A strong immune system is critical in preventing or overcoming opportunistic diseases like herpes, candida albicans or chronic fatigue syndrome that have symptomatic allergic reactions. Immune system studies show that allergy-prone people produce an overabundance of complex proteins known as antibodies—which trigger special cells known as mast cells—which release inflammation-causing chemicals called histamines and leukotrienes throughout the body. A "histamine reaction" occurs when your body tries to neutralize the chemicals by a severe allergic reaction.

The substances that cause allergies are called allergens.

—**Allergies to environmental allergens like air pollutants, asbestos or heavy metals, and seasonal allergens to dust, pollen, spores and mold, are called Type 1 allergies.** This type of allergy often develops when the body has mucous accumulation that harbors the allergen irritants. Drugstore medications for environmental allergies only mask symptoms, often cause drowsiness and have a rebound effect. The more you use them, the more you need them. Steroid drugs for environmental allergies, especially if taken over a long period of time, depress immune defenses and impede allergen elimination. Allergens often interact in the bodies of allergy sufferers, both activating and aggravating other offending irritants. When this is the case, even the most powerful drugs do not relieve symptoms.

—**Allergies to chemicals and contaminant allergens are called Type 2 allergies.** Reactions to chemicals are frequently a defense mechanism, the body's attempt to isolate an offending substance by storing it in fatty tissue. An allergic reaction of this type only occurs after the second exposure to the irritant, as the body's inflammatory histamine response is alerted. Repeated exposures to the irritant set off massive free radical reactions as the body's contaminant toleration levels are reached, toxic overload results and a severe allergic reaction sets in. Chemical sensitivity also initiates other allergy reactions, so that the sufferer becomes allergic to nearly everything else. Common chemical/contaminant irritants vary, from a wide range of petrochemicals and estrogenic chemicals to combustion residues from household appliances and heating systems, to various kinds of sprays, paints and exhaust fumes. Other culprits include chlorine bleach, moth balls and insect repellents, dry cleaning chemicals, and clothes that have been chemically treated.

—**Allergies, intolerances and sensitivities to foods or food additives are also called Type 2 allergies,** and they're extremely widespread. In fact, they are the fastest growing form of allergic reactions in the U.S. today, as more people are more exposed to chemically altered foods. Food intolerances are often confused with food allergies. A **food allergy** is an antibody reaction, involving *an immune system response* to a food it views as a pathogen or parasite. Food allergies may be hereditary, with a child being twice as likely to develop allergies if one parent has them, or four times as likely if both parents have them. A **food intolerance** is an enzyme deficiency to digest a certain food. For example, people with a lactose intolerance experience the bloating, cramping and diarrhea of an allergy reaction. But the symptoms are really due to a deficiency of the enzyme lactase, which helps digest milk sugar. Common food intolerances include those to wheat, dairy foods, fruits, sugar, yeast, mushrooms, eggs, corn and greens. Although these foods may be healthy in themselves, they are often heavily sprayed or treated; in the case of animal products, also affected by antibiotics and hormones. **Food sensitivities** are similar to allergy reactions, but differ in that no antigen-specific antibodies are present. In general, they are not a permanent condition.

Conventional medical treatment for most allergies consists of antihistamines, steroids and desensitization shots. In obstinate cases, laser surgery may be used to vaporize mucous-forming nasal tissue. People with allergies know that these treatments seldom work because they don't get to the cause of the problem. At best they provide temporary relief of symptoms; At worst, they create side effects which may be worse than the allergy itself.

Is your body showing signs that it needs an allergy and asthma cleanse?

—Do you have chronic sinus congestion with itchy, watery nose and eyes? Do you get headaches with sneezing, coughing and scratchy throat? Does your face swell up, with itchy, rashy skin? Do you have trouble sleeping at night? Are you unusually tired? You may have a Type 1 seasonal allergy. Asthma is the most serious Type 1 allergy reaction. (Note: Spore and pollen allergens produce clogging and congestion as the body tries to seal them off from its regular processes, or tries to work around them. Extra mucous is formed as a shield around the offending substances, and we get the allergy symptoms of sinus clog, stuffiness, hayfever, headaches and watery, puffy eyes. Sometimes the body tries to throw this excess off through the skin, and we get skin irritation symptoms or scratchy sore throat.)

—Do you get unexplained migraine headaches? Are you frequently moody and depressed for no reason? Do friends and family tell you that your personality changes, that you are often space-y or that your memory is getting unusually bad? Do you have a child that's chronically hyperactive? You may have a Type 2 allergy to chemicals and contaminants.

—Do you get cyclical headaches with mental fuzziness after eating? Do you get heart palpitations, with sweating, rashes or puffiness around the eyes after eating? Does your abdomen become excessively swollen after eating with heartburn or stomach cramps? Have you gained significant weight even though your diet hasn't changed? Do you have a child that's irritable, flushed and hyperactive after eating? You may have an allergy, intolerance or sensitivity to certain foods or food additives, another kind of Type 2 allergy.

(Note: Regardless of the food, most food allergy symptoms are similar. Inflammation is generated by a release of histamines into tissue mast cells, walling off the affected body area until immune response agents can restore health. But this process takes time. If the body is re-exposed before health is renewed, inflammation and symptoms, especially mucous congestion become chronic.)

Pointers for best results from your allergy and asthma cleanse:

• An ample supply of water will expedite a mucous cleansing program. Drink 8-10 glasses of bottled water each day of your cleanse to lubricate and flush out allergens (can include herbal teas).

• Empowering your immune response is the key to overcoming allergies. I regularly recommend green superfoods because they are so rich in allergen neutralizers like chlorophyll, antioxidants, minerals and enzymes, and such powerful immune builders.

Benefits you may notice as your body responds to an allergy and asthma cleanse:

• Congestion will noticeably begin to clear in the body. Mucous from the lungs and throat will break up and be eliminated
• Respiratory inflammation will give way to relief as the cleanse progresses.
• Mucous from the colon is also often noticeably expelled.

Nutrition Plan

• **Start with this 3 to 7 day nutrition plan.**

The night before your allergy cleanse.....
—Have a green leafy salad for dinner to give your bowels a good sweeping.
The next day....
—On rising: take 2 squeezed lemons in water with 1 TBS. maple syrup; or take a glass of cranberry, apple, pineapple or grapefruit juice.
—Breakfast: have a vitamin E-rich drink (vitamin E has antihistamine activity): one handful spinach, 5 carrots, 4 asparagus spears (or mix Crystal Star Systems Strength™ Drink into hot water for an instant broth and add 1 tsp. nutritional yeast and a pinch of cayenne pepper).
—Mid-morning: have a glass of fresh carrot juice with 1 tsp. Bragg's Liquid Aminos added; or a cup of a congestion clearing tea, like Crystal Star X-Pec™ Tea, to aid mucous release, or Crystal Star Respr-Tea™, an aid oxygen uptake.
—Lunch: have a mixed vegetable juice, like V-8, or a potassium broth (page 134); or make this Mucous Cleansing Tonic by juicing: 4 carrots, 2 celery stalks, 2-3 sprigs watercress or parsley, 1 radish and 1 garlic clove.
—Mid-afternoon: have a veggie drink (page 138), or a packet of Sun Wellness Sun Chlorella granules in water; or a greens and sea vegetable mix, such as Crystal Star Energy Green™ Drink.
—Dinner: have a hot vegetable broth (page 153) with 1 TBS. nutritional yeast; or miso soup with sea veggies snipped on top; or a mixed fresh vegetable juice or fresh carrot juice with 1 TBS. of a green superfood mixed in.
—Before Bed: have a glass of apple juice or papaya/pineapple juice.

Herbs & Supplements

• **Choose 2 to 3 cleansing boosters.**

Antioxidants are a key: Crystal Star Anti-Oxidant Extract; Country Life Super 10 Antioxidant; Schiff Phytocharged Antioxidant; Ester C up to 5000mg daily with bioflavonoids, and CoQ$_{10}$ 30mg 3x daily helps the liver produce antihistamines: Vitamin E 400IU with selenium 200mcg; Quercetin up to 2000mg daily with bromelain; Nutricology Germanium 150mg with B$_{12}$ SL 2500mcg; Golden Pride Formula One oral chelation w. EDTA, 2 pkts daily.

Enzyme support: Bowel toxicity leads to a constant assault on the immune system. Use Transformation Enzyme Digestzyme with meals - especially helpful for food allergies. Other digestive formulas: Prevail Digestion Formula; Herbal Products and Development Power-Plus Enzymes; Rainbow Light Advanced Enzyme System.

Immune system herbal support: *panax ginseng, echinacea, ashwagandah, Siberian ginseng (eleuthero), goldenseal, licorice, ginger, astragalus, ligustrum, suma, yellow dock, dandelion and cayenne*. Immune formulas: Allergy Research Thiodox (*lipoic glutathione complex*); Silica for allergy immune enhancement - Flora Vegesil; Eidon Silica Mineral Supplement.

Green superfoods are potent immune builders: Crystal Star Energy Green™ Drink; NutriCology Pro-Greens; Vibrant Health Green Vibrance; Country Life Shiitake/Reishi Complex With Chlorella.

Adrenal support: Crystal Star Adrn-Active™ caps or extract; Planetary Schizandra Adrenal Support; Herbs, Etc. Adrenotonic.

Probiotics help maintain proper mucous levels, and boost the immune system: Nature's Path Flora-Lyte; Ethical Nutrients Intestinal Care; Jarrow Prod. Jarro-Dophilus + FOS.

Bodywork Techniques

• **Pick bodywork and relaxation techniques to accelerate and round out your cleanse.**

Enema: Take an enema the night before or the morning of your cleanse. Flushing the colon is one of the best ways to jump start a cleanse and allows a more expedient release of toxins. Irrigate: a colonic offers a more thorough colon cleanse.

Exercise: Exercise increases oxygen uptake. Take a daily walk with deep breathing exercises.

Body work: Acupuncture and chiropractic have both proven effective for allergies.

Acupressure points: •During an attack, press tip of nose hard or hollow above the center of upper lip as needed for relief. • Press underneath cheekbones beside nose, angling pressure upwards.

Stress & Relaxation techniques: Mental stress depresses immunity and aggravates allergies. Try this following calming technique:

—If your mind is racing and you're feeling anxious, shift your focus. Make a sincere effort to turn your attention to your breathing. It's the simplest form of concentrative meditation, the connection between the breath and one's state of mind, a basic principle of yoga relaxation.

—Consciously take slow, deep regular breaths, for at least one minute.

—To enhance the calming effect, recall a positive or pleasant past experience. Try to *feel* appreciation or love about the good things and people you have in your life. The effort to shift focus to this positive feeling helps to neutralize stress.

Flower remedies: Natural Labs Allergies/Asthma.

Avoid allergens: •Invest in an air filter. • Stop smoking and avoid secondary smoke. It magnifies all allergy reactions.

Continuing Diet Notes: Make sure your diet has plenty of organically grown fresh foods. Eat a fresh salad every day. I believe it's your best diet defense against allergy reactions. Cultured food, like yogurt, cottage cheese, miso and tofu help your body keep a good supply of friendly digestive flora. Green superfoods can be a key for extra rich concentrated nutrients to keep the immune system strong.

Can't find a recommended product? Call the 800 number listed in Product Resources.

Do you need a candida cleanse?

Candida albicans yeast is common, and normally lives harmlessly in the gastrointestinal tract and genito-urinary areas of the body. It's also found in the mouth (thrush), vagina (yeast infection) and on the skin. In the past, candida infection was regarded as a women's problem because of its connection to a vaginal yeast infection. Today, we know that both men and women are equally likely to develop candida. Candidiasis is really a state of inner imbalance, not a germ or bug. When immunity and resistance are low, the body loses its intestinal balance and candida yeasts multiply too rapidly, voraciously feeding on excess sugars and carbohydrates in the digestive tract. As an immune-compromised condition, candida is extremely hard to overcome. Unless the body's weakened defenses are given assistance, candida colonies will flourish throughout the body and keep releasing toxins into the bloodstream.

Watch out for these lifestyle factors that promote Candida infection: 1) Poor diet - especially excessive intake of sugar, starchy foods, yeasted breads and chemicalized foods. 2) Repeated use of antibiotics—long term use of antibiotics kill protective bacteria (that keep candida under control) as well as harmful bacteria. 3) Hormone medications like corticosteroid drugs and birth control pills. 4) A high stress life, too much alcohol, little rest.

Candida may infect virtually any part of the body. The most commonly involved sites include the nail beds, skin folds, feet, mouth, sinuses, ear canal, belly button, esophagus, intestine, vaginal tract and urethra. Candida also infects deep internal organs, which sometimes results in serious disease. Likely sites of infection include the thyroid and adrenal glands, kidneys, bladder, bowel, esophagus, uterus, lungs and bone marrow.

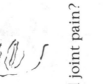

Is your body showing signs that it needs a candida cleanse?

—Do you have recurrent digestive problems, gas, bloating or flatulence?
—Do you have rectal itching, or chronic constipation alternating to diarrhea?
—Do you have a white coating on your tongue (thrush)?
—Have you been unusually irritable or depressed? Are you bothered by unexplained frequent headaches, muscle aches and joint pain?
—Do you feel sick all over, yet the cause cannot be found? Are the symptoms worse on damp, muggy days?
—Has your memory been noticeably poor? Are you finding it hard to concentrate or focus your thoughts?
—Do you have chronic vaginal yeast infections or frequent bladder infections?
—If you are a woman, do you have serious PMS or other menstrual problems? Do you have endometriosis?
—If you are a man, do you have abdominal pains, prostatitis, or loss of sexual interest?
—Do you have chronic fungal infections like ringworm, jock itch, nail fungus or athlete's foot?
—Do you have hives, psoriasis, eczema or chronic dermatitis?
—Do you catch frequent colds that take many weeks to go away?
—Are you bothered by erratic vision or spots before the eyes?
—Are you oversensitive to chemicals, tobacco, perfume or insecticides? Do you crave sugar, bread, or alcoholic beverages?
—Have you recently taken repeated rounds for 1 month or longer, of antibiotics or corticosteroid drugs, like Symycin, Panmycin, Decadron or Prednisone, or acne drugs?

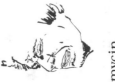

Getting rid of a candida yeast infection is not easy. The longer you wait to begin a detox and healing program, the harder the job becomes. I recommend staring now if you think you have candida. If you're unsure, call this number and get tested: Body Ecology (360-384-1238). Here's what you'll be doing on a candida cleanse:

• Killing the candida yeasts: The diet and supplement program will kill the yeasts. Avoid antibiotics, corticosteroid drugs and birth control pills, unless there is absolute medical need, so you don't get re-infected.

• Eliminating the dead yeasts from your body: The cleansing diet and cleansing products will release the dead yeasts and their waste from the body. Enemas or colonics will expedite their removal.

• Rebuilding your normal systemic environment and immune defenses: The program will strengthen your digestive system by enhancing its ability to assimilate nutrients. Afflicted organs, especially the liver, and glands will be strengthened. Metabolism will normalize and probiotic supplementation will promote friendly bacteria in the gastrointestinal tract.

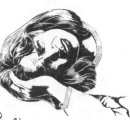

Pointers for best results from your candida cleanse:

—Drug therapy for candidiasis uses Nystatin, Ketaconazole and other antifungal products to try and kill the yeast invader. But this method only relieves the ill effects of candidiasis while the drug is being taken. And, of course, drugs do nothing to prevent recurrence. Many of the drugs further suppress the immune system. An effective program must not only kill the yeasts but also strengthen the body's own immune defense mechanisms to keep candida under control. Empowering your immune response is the real key to overcoming candida.

—Clinical testing is underway on candida. Early findings show that a program with plant enzyme therapy, probiotics, certain herbal extracts and organic minerals is clinically effective in treating and preventing candida.

—Drink 8-10 glasses of bottled water each day of your cleanse (can include herbal teas). Water lubricates and flushes wastes, toxins and dead yeast cells from the body. An ample supply of water will expedite a candida cleansing program.

Some benefits you'll notice as your body responds to a candida cleanse:

• Unpleasant symptoms like aversion to odors and allergy reactions will subside.
• You will be reestablishing the vitality of your colon, so alternating constipation and diarrhea will normalize.
• You'll start to regain your energy and stamina.
• Mental clarity will improve. You won't be feeling so "spaced-out."
• Sleep and the ability to rest will improve.
• Sugar cravings will begin to subside, but be careful... these cravings have a yo-yo reaction.
• The time line for feeling better varies widely. Some people feel better with one to two weeks; others take one to two months.

Then what? How do you keep candida yeast under control?

The whole healing-rebuilding process usually takes from 3-6 months for the yeast to be eliminated and friendly bacteria re-established. A strong immune system, a vital liver and robust colonies of friendly bacteria are critical to lasting control and prevention. The changes in

diet, habits and lifestyle are often radical. Some people feel better right away; others go through a rough "healing crisis." (Yeasts are living organisms - part of your body. Killing them off is traumatic. But most people with candidiasis infection are feeling so bad anyway, that the treatment and the knowledge that they are getting better, pulls them through the hard times. Be as gentle with your body as you can. Give yourself all the time you need. You want to get better quickly, but multiple therapies all at once can be psychologically quite stressful. Just stick to it and go at your own pace.

After your candida cleanse, keep your program going. Here are some watchwords:

• Eat plenty of beta-carotene-rich foods, and iodine and potassium-rich foods. They are most effective food nutrients against candida. My favorite food for these nutrients is sea vegetables - all kinds, in soups, on rice or a healthy pizza, or in a salad.

• Use raw sauerkraut in your diet. It is a superfood for conquering candida. Dr. Elson M. Haas, M.D., director of the Preventive Medical Center of Marin, CA; Gary Ross, M.D. of Health & Medical Clinic of San Francisco, CA; Dr. Paul Yanick, Director of Bio-Health Center, New Hope, PA, and Jack Tips, N.D., C.N.C. author of Conquer Candida, are just four of many candida experts who report that raw cultured vegetables (sauerkraut) is very helpful in controlling and conquering candida. Nutritional authors Patricia Bragg, Donna Gates and Klaus Kaufmann attest to amazing accounts of candida sufferers who report substantial improvement in their condition after eating raw sauerkraut. Use Rejuvenative Foods RAW SAUERKRAUT or VEGI-DELITE, or make the cultured vegetables yourself. To obtain a good raw sauerkraut recipe call BODY ECOLOGY 360-384-1238; E-mail bodyeco@aol.com; www.bodyecology.net.

• Eat three to four small, healthy meals a day. Provide your body with healing foods during periods of cleansing. But be careful not to overeat or you will divert your body's energy from cleansing to digestion.

• Eat alkalizing foods. A good rule of thumb is 80% alkaline-forming foods and 20% acid-forming foods. **Alkalizing foods are:** fresh, steamed, baked or grilled vegetables, sea veggies, brown rice, millet, quinoa, and amaranth grains, herbs and herb teas, sprouts and seeds (except sesame seeds), lemons, limes and unsweetened cranberries, cultured foods (like raw cultured vegetables, yogurt, kefir, organic apple cider vinegar), and soaked almonds. **Acid-forming foods are:** animal foods like beef, poultry, eggs, fish, and shellfish, buckwheat, and organic, unrefined oils,

• Limit or avoid these foods on a continuing basis to keep candida from coming back: Fruits (except those listed above). Acid-formers like sugary foods or sweeteners such as Saccharin or NutraSweet, soft drinks, wheat flour foods, beans, tofu, nuts and nut butters, wine or other alcoholic beverages, commercial vinegars or condiments. If you crave sweets, use the herb Stevia in your tea.

• Watch your food-combinations. Overgrowth of yeast will not disappear if you are combining foods that aren't compatible in the stomach. Instead, you'll get fermentation that produces sugars and alcohol and continue to feed the yeast. People with candidiasis are normally in a weak digestive state so good food combining becomes even more important.

Here are four general food-combining rules to follow: 1) Eat your fruits alone. 2) Eat protein foods like meats and grains with non-starchy vegetables or sea vegetables. 3) Eat starchy vegetables like potatoes with non-starchy vegetables or sea vegetables. 4) Don't combine a large amount of fat with protein foods like meat or grains. Large amounts of fat, especially refined oils, delay the secretion of hydrochloric acid needed to digest the protein. An example is mixing mayonnaise with tuna or chicken. If you make this combination into a sandwich with bread, you'll be making it even more difficult to digest. Use an oil-free or miso dressing to make tuna, egg or chicken salad. Eat it with a vegetable salad instead of with bread.

Need a test to see if you have Candida? Call Body Ecology (360-384-1238).

Nutrition Plan

• **Start with this 3 to 7 day nutrition plan.**

To overcome a candida yeast infection, your diet must simultaneously nourish your body while starving candida of the foods that support its growth.

—On rising: take 2 tsp. cranberry concentrate, with 1 tsp. cider vinegar and 1 tsp. maple syrup in water; or a fiber cleanser like AloeLife FIBERMATE or Crystal Star FIBER & HERBS COLON CLEANSE™, or a cup of Crystal Star GREEN TEA CLEANSER™.

—Breakfast: have a vegetable omelette with broccoli; or scrambled eggs with onion, shiitake mushrooms and red pepper; or brown rice with onions and carrots; or oatmeal with 1 TBS. Bragg's LIQUID AMINOS; or cream of buckwheat sweetened with stevia and sauteed veggies.

—Mid-morning: have a vegetable drink (page 138) with Sun Wellness CHLORELLA or Green Foods GREEN MAGMA; or Crystal Star SYSTEMS STRENGTH™; or a cup of miso soup with sea veggies; and a cup of pau d' arco, echinacea or chamomile tea.

—Lunch: have a fresh green salad with lemon/coconut, olive or flax oil dressing and seafood, chicken or turkey; or a vegetable or miso soup with sea veggies; or steamed veggies with brown rice.

—Mid-afternoon: have potato corn chowder with crackers; or some raw veggies dipped in lemon/coconut, olive, or flax oil dressing; or mineral water and hard boiled egg with sea vegetable seasoning.

—Dinner: have broiled fish or chicken with raw sauerkraut or green beans; or steamed vegetables or baked potato sprinkled with sea vegetables and Bragg's LIQUID AMINOS; or a vegetable stir fry with brown rice, sea veggies and miso soup.

—Before Bed: chamomile tea, Crystal Star AFTER MEAL ENZ™ extract drops in water, or miso soup.

Herbs & Supplements

• **Choose 2 to 3 cleansing boosters.**

Cleansing support formula: Gaia Herbs 2 week CANDIDA SUPREME VITAL CLEANSE.

Powerful candida fighters:

1) Enzyme support: Plant protease supplements help your body's own enzymes to destroy candida and strengthen your defenses. Transformation Enzyme PUREZYME. Add *Milk Thistle Seed extract* to accelerate liver regeneration

2) Probiotics keep Candida under control: Friendly bacteria battle candida and detoxify. Rejuvenative Foods VEGI-DELITE; Body Ecology Eco RENEW; Professional Nutr. DOCTOR-DOPHILUS+FOS; Solgar ABC DOPHILUS POWDER (also use as a douche); Futurebiotics LONGEST LIVING ACIDOPHILUS +.

3) Oregano oil: essential oil with amazing antimicrobial powers, strongly inhibits growth of candida albicans. North American Herb & Spice OIL OF OREGANO or OREGAMAX. Use only as directed.

4) Olive leaf extract: stimulates phagocytosis of all types of pathogenic microfungi and bacteria. NutriCology PROLIVE.

5) Coconut oil: rich source of caprylic acid, a potent anti-fungal. Has 50% lauric acid - a disease-fighting fatty acid. Body Ecology COCONUT OIL.

6) Reishi mushrooms support immunity, discourage infection: Crystal Star REISHI-GINSENG EXTRACT; New Chapter REISHI 5 EXTRACT; Country Life SHIITAKE/REISHI COMPLEX WITH CHLORELLA.

Candida cleansing formulas: Crystal Star CANDEX™; Nature's Secret CANDISTROY; Rainbow Light CANDIDA CLEANSE; Futurebiotics A.Y.

Green superfoods - potent immune builders: Crystal Star ENERGY GREEN™; Body Ecology VITALITY SUPER GREEN; Vibrant Health GREEN VIBRANCE.

Bodywork Techniques

• **Pick bodywork and relaxation techniques to accelerate and round out your cleanse.**

Enema: Take an enema the night before or the morning of your cleanse. Flushing the colon is one of the best ways to jump start a cleanse; it allows a more expedient release of dead yeast cells and toxins from the body. Irrigate: Have at least one colonic once during your cleanse for best results.

Exercise: Take a brisk walk for more body oxygen, and a positive mind and outlook. They are essential to overcome candida body stress. Try a good hearty laugh every day.

Rest: Candida infection often means interrupted sleep patterns.

Flower remedies: Natural Labs Deva Flower CLEANSING REMEDY or FEARFULNESS (dread seems to be the primary emotion described by candida and chronic fatigue syndrome victims); Nelson Bach RESCUE REMEDY (for stress).

Effective vaginal treatment: use one or more.
• Soak infected areas in tea tree oil solution. Use in water as a vaginal douche.
• Nutribiotic GRAPEFRUIT SEED EXTRACT as a vaginal douche or enema.
• Garlic douche or vaginal insertion.
• Acidophilus capsule insertions, or sprinkle powder on a tampon and insert.
• Make up a garlic, echinacea, myrrh solution in a squirt bottle and wash perineum after defecating to keep from reinfecting.

Nail fungus soak: Pau d' Arco tea.

For thrush (yeast infection of the mouth): use tea tree oil, homeopathic *thuja*, Nature's Pharmacy MYR-E-CAL, and BLACK WALNUT extract. Disinfect toothbrush with 3% hydrogen peroxide frequently.

Note: Brewer's yeast does not cause or aggravate candida albicans yeast overgrowth. It is one of the best immune-enhancing foods available. While it is well known that candida yeasts feed on dietary sugars, it is not well known that the yeasts also need minerals, and they deplete the minerals from our bodies. Restricting sugar in your permanent diet is esential. Supplement minerals to shore up mineral defiencies caused by the yeast - Nature's Path TRACE-LYTE; Arise & Shine ALKALIZER.

Can't find a recommended product? Call the 800 number listed in Product Resources.

Can detoxification foods possibly
be delicious?

You bet they can!
This "Green Cuisine" section is full
of recipes to cleanse your body,
gratify your taste buds
and satisfy your soul.

Green Cuisine

What is green cuisine?

The recipes in this section have been carefully targeted and tested for a wide variety of cleansing, purifying and detoxification needs.

Each recipe has effective detoxification ability. Many are high in vitamins C, B-complex and minerals to neutralize the effects of pesticides, environmental pollutants and heavy metals, as well as toxins from drugs, caffeine and nicotine.

Cleansing foods should be organically grown and eaten fresh for best results. Only fresh foods and juices retain the full complement of nutrients and plant enzymes that Mother Nature offers.

•**Fruits and fruit juices** eliminate wastes quickly and help reduce cravings for sweets.

•**Fresh vegetable juices** carry off excess body acids, and are rich in vitamins, minerals and enzymes that satisfy the body's nutrient requirements with less food.

•**Chlorophyll-rich foods,** like leafy greens and green superfoods like spirulina, chlorella, and barley grass help stabilize and maintain the acid/alkaline balance of the body and also have anti-infective properties. Since chlorophyll has a molecular structure close to our own plasma, drinking them is like giving yourself a mini transfusion. They especially help clear the skin, cleanse the kidneys, and clean and build the blood.

•**Herb teas and mineral drinks** provide energy and cleansing at the same time, without having to take in solid food for fuel.

•**Sea plants** act as the ocean's purifiers and they perform much the same for the human body, also largely made up of salt water. Sea plant chemical composition is so close to human plasma, that it can help balance your body at the cellular level. Sea vegetables alkalize and purify the blood from the effects of a modern diet. They strengthen the body against illness caused by environmental toxins. Their benefits for a healing diet against serious disease rival the healing powers of their land-based cousins broccoli and cabbage. They reduce stores of excess fluid and fat, and work to transform toxic metals (including radiation), into harmless salts that the body can eliminate. In fact, the natural iodine in sea vegetables reduces by almost 80% radioactive iodine-131 in the thyroid.

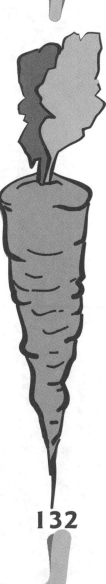

132

Sea vegetables have superior nutritional content. As one of nature's richest sources of proteins, complex carbohydrates, minerals and vitamins, they transmit those nutrients to your body. Ounce for ounce sea vegetables are higher in vitamins and minerals than any other food group except herbs. They are almost the only non-animal source of Vitamin B_{12}, necessary for cell development and nerve function. Sea vegetables are a superior source of vegetable protein. They provide full-spectrum concentrations of all the carotenes, chlorophyll, enzymes, amino acids and fiber. Their mineral balance is a natural tranquilizer for sound nerve structure and good metabolism. The distinctive salty taste is not just "salt," but a balanced, chelated combination of sodium, potassium, calcium, magnesium, phosphorus, iron and trace minerals. They convert *inorganic* ocean minerals into *organic* mineral salts that combine with amino acids (an ideal way for our bodies to get nutrients for structural building blocks). In fact, sea vegetables contain all the necessary trace elements for life, many of which are depleted in the earth's land-based soil.

How do you use green cuisine?

Our bodies are designed to be self-healing organisms. Healing is allowed to occur through cleansing. Cleansing foods and juices can optimize your detox program. In fact, they are crucial to its success in three ways:

• They keep your body chemistry balanced and your body processes stable while you detox, so you don't become uncomfortable. Don't forget that Mother Nature is cleaning house during a detox cleanse. You may eliminate accumulated poisons and wastes quite rapidly, causing headaches, slight nausea and weakness as your body purges. (These reactions are usually only temporary and disappear along with the waste and toxins.)

• They regulate the speed of your detox so your body doesn't cleanse too fast or dump too many toxins into your bloodstream all at once that your body can't handle. Green cuisine keeps you from re-poisoning yourself during the detox process.

• They support your nutrition and energy levels while you detox, so you don't become too hungry or too tired. New healthy tissue starts building right away when the detoxification juices are taken in. Gland secretions stimulate the immune system during a cleanse to set up a disease defense environment.

Remember these easy diet watchwords as you use green cuisine:

—The day before you begin your detox, eat green salads and fresh fruits, and drink plenty of healthy liquids, so that the upcoming body chemistry changes will not be uncomfortable. A gentle herbal laxative taken the night before can be beneficial.

—Avoid all dairy products and cooked foods during a cleansing fast.

—Drink 6 to 8 eight oz. glasses of bottled water daily to keep your body continually flushing out the toxins your tissues are releasing.

Detoxification Drinks

Detoxification drinks have a powerful effect on the body's recuperative powers because of their rich, easily absorbed nutrients. Fresh juices contain proteins, carbohydrates, chlorophyll, mineral electrolytes and healing aromatic oils. But most importantly, fresh juice therapy makes available to every cell in our bodies large amounts of plant enzymes, an integral part of the healing and restoration process.

Nothing gets done in our bodies without enzymes. They are the activity components of life. Digestive function, assimilation and elimination are all instigated or assisted by enzymes. Enzymes cause every chemical reaction in our bodies. They play a vital part in breaking down foreign matter (like toxins) as well as food. Enzymes and mineral electrolytes (which restore peristaltic bowel activity) are major contributors to moving toxins out of the body instead of building up and poisoning us. When your diet is full of cooked foods without enzymes, or low residue, processed foods (which have a higher tendency to stagnate and putrefy), the process of internal decay develops far more rapidly.

Should you get a juicer?

Juicers are expensive appliances, but they can really boost the nutrient power of your cleansing drinks. A good juicer essentially *predigests* fresh fruits and vegetables for almost immediate assimilation by your body. Juicer juices can accelerate your cleanse and noticeably boost your energy level. A juicer can juice *all* of a fruit or vegetable (even rinds, stems, peels, seeds) to give you up to 95% of the plant's food and nutritive value.

Champion, JuiceMan and Acme are all good juicers for a detox program.

POTASSIUM JUICE

This is the single most effective juice for cleansing, neutralizing acids and rebuilding the body. It is a blood and body tonic that provides rapid energy and system balance.
For one 12-oz. glass:

Juice in the juicer 3 CARROTS, 3 STALKS CELERY, $^1/_2$ BUNCH SPINACH, and $^1/_2$ BUNCH PARSLEY.
—Add 1 to 2 teasp. Bragg's LIQUID AMINOS if desired.

POTASSIUM ESSENCE BROTH

If you don't have a juicer, make a potassium broth in a soup pot. While not as concentrated or pure, it is still an excellent source of energy, minerals and electrolytes.

For a 2 day supply: Cover with water in a soup pot 3 to 4 CARROTS, 3 STALKS CELERY, $^1/_2$ BUNCH PARSLEY, 2 POTATOES with skins, $^1/_2$ HEAD CABBAGE, 1 ONION, and $^1/_2$ BUNCH BROCCOLI.
—Simmer covered 30 minutes. Strain and discard solids.
—Add 2 teasp. Bragg's LIQUID AMINOS or 1 teasp. MISO. Store in the fridge, covered.

Cleansing Fruit Drinks

Fruit juices are like a quick car wash for your body. Their high water and sugar content speeds up metabolism to release wastes quickly. Their alkalizing effects help reduce cravings for sweets. Still, because of their fast assimilation, pesticides, sprays and chemicals on fruits can enter your body rapidly. So, eat organically grown fruits whenever possible. Wash fruit well if commercially grown. Fruits and fruit juices have their best nutritional effects when taken alone. Eat them before noon for best energy conversion and cleansing benefits.

BLOOD BUILDER
A blood purifying drink with iron enrichment.
For 4 large drinks:

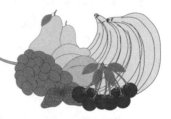

Juice 2 bunches GRAPES or 2 cups GRAPE JUICE, 6 ORANGES or 2 cups ORANGE JUICE, and 8 LEMONS peeled or 1 cup LEMON JUICE.
— Stir in: 2 cups WATER and 1/4 cup HONEY.

GINGER/LEMON CLEANSE FOR ALLERGIES
For 2 drinks (a day's supply):

1-inch slice FRESH GINGER ROOT, 1 FRESH LEMON, 6 CARROTS with tops, and 1 APPLE, seeded.

STOMACH CLEANSER & BREATH REFRESHER
For 2 drinks:

Juice 1 bunch GRAPES, 1 basket STRAWBERRIES, 3 APPLES, cored, and 4 sprigs FRESH MINT.

DIURETIC MELON MIX
A good morning drink with diuretic properties. Take on an empty stomach, 3x daily.
For 1 quart:

Juice 3 cups WATERMELON CUBES, 2 cups PERSIAN MELON CUBES, and 2 cups HONEYDEW CUBES.

HEMORRHOID & VARICOSE VEIN TONIC
For 1 drink:

Juice 1 cup CHERRIES pitted, 1 bunch GREEN GRAPES, 1/4 PINEAPPLE with skin, 1/2 APPLE, seeded, and 1/4-inch slice GINGER ROOT.

BLADDER INFECTION CLEANSER
For 2 drinks:

Juice 3 to 4 APPLES, and $\frac{1}{2}$ cup CRANBERRIES.

GINGER AID FOR PROSTATE ENLARGEMENT
For 2 drinks:

Juice $\frac{1}{2}$ LEMON, $\frac{1}{2}$-inch slice FRESH GINGER ROOT, and 1 bunch GREEN GRAPES
—Fill glass with SPARKLING WATER.

ARTHRITIS & BURSITIS RELIEF
For 1 drink:

Juice 2 to 3 ORANGES, peeled, $\frac{1}{4}$ PINEAPPLE, with skin, and $\frac{1}{2}$ APPLE, seeded.

CONSTIPATION CLEANSER
For 1 drink:

Juice 1 firm PAPAYA, $\frac{1}{4}$-inch slice GINGER ROOT, and 1 PEAR

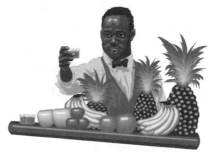

ACNE FIGHTER
For 1 drink:

Juice 2 slices PINEAPPLE with skin, $\frac{1}{2}$ CUCUMBER, $\frac{1}{2}$ APPLE, and $\frac{1}{4}$-inch slice GINGER ROOT.

APPLE CLEANSE FOR MUCOUS CONGESTION
For 1 drink:

Juice 2 large APPLES, seeded, and $\frac{1}{2}$ teasp. grated HORSERADISH

Note: Other good cleansing fruit juices include:
- —black cherry juice for gouty conditions
- —cranberry juice for bladder and kidney infections
- —grape and citrus juices for high blood pressure
- —celery for nerves
- —canteloupe for allergies

Green Drinks, Vegetable Juices & Blood Tonics

I believe green drinks are critical to the success of every cleansing program. The molecular composition of chlorophyll is so close to that of human hemoglobin that these drinks can act as "mini-transfusions" for the blood, and tonics for the brain and immune system.

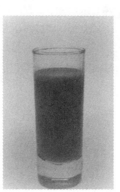

They are an excellent nutrient source of vitamins, minerals, proteins and enzymes. They contain large amounts of vitamins C, B_1, B_2, B_3, pantothenic acid, folic acid, carotene and choline. They are high in minerals, like potassium, calcium, magnesium, iron, copper, phosphorus and manganese. They are full of enzymes for digestion and assimilation, some containing over 1,000 of the known enzymes necessary for human cell response and growth. Green drinks also have anti-infective properties, carry off acid wastes, neutralize body pH, and are excellent for mucous cleansing. They can help clear the skin, cleanse the kidneys, and purify and build the blood.

Green drinks and vegetable juices are potent fuel in maintaining good health, yet don't come burdened by the fats that accompany animal products. Those included here have been used with therapeutic success for many years. You can have confidence in their nutritional healing and regenerative ability.

Chlorophyll is the key to green therapy.

The most therapeutic ingredient of all fresh green plants and green superfoods (like chlorella and spirulina), is chlorophyll. Chlorophyll is the pigment that plants use to carry out the process of photosynthesis — absorbing light energy from the sun, then converting it into earth and plant energy. This energy is transferred into our cells and blood when we eat chlorophyll-rich greens.

Chlorophyll is the basic component of the "blood" of plants. The chlorophyll molecule is also remarkably similar to human plasma, except that it carries magnesium in its center instead of iron. Green foods help human bodies build red blood cells. In essence, eating any of the chlorophyll-rich foods is almost like giving yourself a little transfusion to help treat illness, enhance immunity and sustain well-being. They have a synergistic effect when added to a normal diet. The green superfoods are valuable in almost all of the healing diets.

Chlorophyll is a primary aid for organ detoxification, particularly the liver. It helps to neutralize and remove drug deposits from the body, purify the blood and counteract acids and toxins in the system. Even the medical community is seeing chlorophyll as a possible means of removing heavy metal build-up, because it can bind with several heavy metals and help eliminate them. Because of its detoxifying and anti-bacterial qualities, chlorophyll has proven to be a valuable remedy in the treatment of colds, rhinitis, inner-ear infections and inflammation.

A new U.S. Army study reveals that a chlorophyll-rich diet can double the lifespan of animals exposed to lethal radiation. Chlorophyll is now being considered (since the days of Agent Orange and Gulf War Syndrome) as a health protector against some chemical warfare weapons.

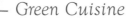

PERSONAL BEST V-8
A high vitamin/mineral drink for normalizing body balance. A good daily blend even when you're not cleansing.
For 6 glasses:

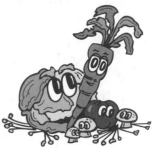

Juice 6 to 8 Tomatoes (or 4 cups Tomato Juice), 3 to 4 Green Onions with tops, 1/2 Green Pepper, 2 Carrots, 2 Stalks Celery with leaves, 1/2 Bunch Spinach, washed, 1/2 Bunch Parsley, 2 Lemons, peeled, (or 4 TBS. Lemon Juice).
—Add 2 teasp. Bragg's Liquid Aminos and 1/2 teasp. ground celery seed.

IMMUNE ENHANCER
For 2 drinks:

Juice 1/2 Bunch Parsley, 1 Garlic Clove, 6 Carrots, 3 Stalks Celery with leaves, 1 Large Tomato, 1 Red Bell Pepper, a dash of Hot Pepper Sauce (or Cayenne Pepper), 4 Romaine Leaves, 1 Stalk Broccoli.
—Add 1 teasp. Miso Paste mixed with a little water.

HEALTHY MARY TONIC
A virgin mary is really a healthy green drink when you make it fresh.
For 4 drinks:

Juice 3 cups water, 1/2 Green Bell Pepper, 2 Large Tomatoes, 2 Celery Stalks with leaves, 1 Green Onion with tops, and 1 handful Fresh Parsley.
—Add 1 TBS. crumbled, dry Sea Veggies, (any kind), or 1 teasp. Kelp Powder.

CLEANSING ENERGY TONIC
A good afternoon pick-me-up juice during a 3 to 7 day cleanse.
For 2 drinks:

Juice 4 cups Mixed Sprouts (especially Alfalfa, Buckwheat, Sunflower and Mung), 1 large Carrot, 1 Stalk Celery with leaves, 1/2 Cucumber, 1 Green Onion, and 2 TBS. Raw Sauerkraut.

KIDNEY FLUSH
A purifying kidney cleanser and diuretic, with high potassium and other minerals.
For four 8-oz. glasses:

Juice 4 Carrots with tops, 1 Cucumber with skin, 4 Beets with tops, 1 handful Spinach Leaves, and 4 Celery Stalks with leaves.
—Add 2 teasp. Bragg's Liquid Aminos.

CANDIDA YEAST CLEANSER
For 2 drinks:

Juice 1 Bunch Parsley, 2 Cloves Garlic, 6 Carrots, 2 Stalks Celery, and 3 Kale or Collard Leaves.
—Add 1 teasp. Miso Paste mixed with a little water.

BLOOD TONIC
This is an amazingly simple, but effective Chinese medicine restorative for women after childbirth, people with anemia, or those suffering blood loss from surgery.
For 8 drinks:

Simmer 35 Black Dates and 5 slices Fresh Ginger in 8 cups Water.
—Stir in 1 teasp. Royal Jelly (or 1 TBS. royal jelly mixed with honey) and 1 TBS. Sesame Tahini. Sip throughout the day for several weeks.

DAILY CARROT JUICE CLEANSE
For 2 large drinks:

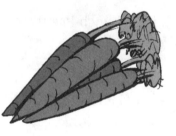

Juice 4 Carrots, ¹/₂ Cucumber, 2 Stalks Celery with leaves, and 1 TBS. chopped Dry Dulse.

INTENSE PARSLEY CLEANSE
For 2 large drinks (a day's supply):

Juice 1 bunch Parsley, 6 Carrots with tops, and ¹/₂ Apple, seeded.

PROSTATE SEDIMENT CLEANSER
For 2 large drinks (a day's supply):

Juice 2 large handfuls mixed dark green leaves, especially Spinach, Kale, Collards and Dandelion leaves, and 3 Large Tomatoes.

SKIN CLEANSING TONIC
Deep greens to cleanse, nourish and tone skin tissue from the inside.
For 1 drink:

Juice 1 Cucumber with skin, ¹/₂ bunch Fresh Parsley, 1 4-oz. tub Alfalfa Sprouts, and 3 to 4 Sprigs Fresh Mint.

EXCESS BODY FLUID, WATER RETENTION CLEANSER

For 1 large drink:

Juice 1 Cucumber, 1 Beet, ½ Apple, seeded, and 4 Carrots with tops.
—Add a 2-inch piece fresh Daikon Radish or soak a few slivers of dried Daikon and add.

HIGH BLOOD PRESSURE REDUCER

For 1 large calcium/magnesium drink:

Juice 2 Garlic Cloves, 1 handful Parsley, 1 Cucumber, 4 Carrots with tops, and 2 Stalks Celery with leaves.

REMOVE THE COBWEBS BRAIN BOOSTER

For 1 large drink:

Juice 1 bunch Parsley, 4 Carrots, a 1-inch piece fresh or preserved Burdock or Ginseng Root, and 2 Stalks Celery.

ARTHRITIS RELIEF DETOX

For 1 large drink:

Juice a large handful Spinach, a large handful Parsley, a large handful Watercress, 5 Carrots with tops, 3 Radishes.
—Add 1 TBS. Bragg's Liquid Aminos.

BLADDER INFECTION DETOX

For 2 drinks (a day's supply):

Juice 3 Broccoli Flowerets, 1 Garlic Clove, 2 Large Tomatoes, 2 Stalks Celery with leaves, and 1 Green Bell Pepper.

HEMORRHOIDS & VARICOSE VEINS DRINK

Vitamin C, calcium and bioflavonoids boost collagen production which helps new more elastic tissue to form.
For 2 large drinks (a day's supply):

Juice 3 handfuls of dark greens — Kale Leaves, Parsley, Spinach, or Watercress, 5 Carrots with tops, 1 Green Bell Pepper and 2 Tomatoes.

REDUCE HIGH CHOLESTEROL
For 2 drinks:

I large handful PARSLEY, 5 CARROTS with tops, 2 APPLES, and ¹/₂ TUB ALFALFA SPROUTS.

DIABETES BALANCER
For 1 large drink:

Juice 3 ROMAINE LETTUCE LEAVES, 5 CARROTS with tops, 2 handfuls FRESH GREEN BEANS, and 2 BRUSSELS SPROUT HEADS.
—Add I teasp. MISO PASTE dissolved in water and stir.

GENTLE CLEANSE FOR CROHN'S DISEASE & COLITIS
For 2 large drinks:

Juice 3 handfuls greens — I SPINACH, I PARSLEY, and I KALE or COLLARDS; 3 BEETS with tops, 5 CARROTS, ¹/₂ GREEN PEPPER, and ¹/₂ APPLE, seeded.

OVERWEIGHT DETOX
For 1 drink:

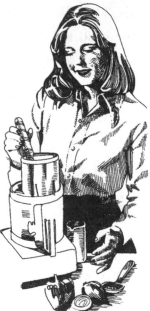

Juice I large handful dark greens like SPINACH, KALE or PARSLEY, I STALK CELERY with leaves, I CARROT, I BELL PEPPER, I TOMATO, and I BROCCOLI FLOWERET.
—Add I TBS. dry SEA VEGGIES (any type)

DIVERTICULITIS DETOX
For 2 large drinks (a day's supply):

Juice I large handful PARSLEY, ¹/₄ head GREEN CABBAGE, 2 large TOMATOES, 4 CARROTS with tops, I GARLIC CLOVE and 2 stalks CELERY with leaves.

STRESS CLEANSE
For 1 drink:

Juice I small handful each PARSLEY and WATERCRESS, 2 STALKS CELERY, I CARROT, ¹/₂ RED BELL PEPPER, I TOMATO and I BROCCOLI FLOWERET.

CONSTIPATION CLEANSE
For 2 large drinks (a day's supply):

Juice ¹/₄ head G REEN C ABBAGE, 3 stalks C ELERY with leaves, and 5 C ARROTS with tops.

PSORIASIS & ECZEMA CLEANSE
For 1 large drink:

Juice 1 T OMATO, 1 C UCUMBER, 2 S TALKS C ELERY, and 1 handful each: P ARSLEY and W ATERCRESS.

MAGNESIUM MIGRAINE CLEANSE
For 1 large drink:

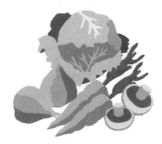

Juice 1 G ARLIC C LOVE, 1 handful P ARSLEY, 5 C ARROTS, 2 S TALKS C ELERY, with tops.

HIGH PROTEIN SPROUT COCKTAIL
This high protein juice is particularly good for ending a fast.
For 2 drinks:

Juice 3 cored A PPLES with skin, 1 tub (4 oz.) A LFALFA S PROUTS and 6 S PRIGS F RESH M INT.

Enzyme therapy drinks

Plant enzymes are the key to longterm results from detoxing with fresh plant juices. Enzymes are the cornerstone of health because they are the foundation elements of the immune system. Plant enzymes allow our bodies to use the full array of plant nutrients, including the main components of anti-aging—antioxidants to fight free radicals, and keep immunity strong.

Enzymes operate on both chemical and biological levels.

Chemically, they are workhorses that drive metabolism to use the nutrients we take in.

Biologically, they are our life energy. Without enzyme energy, we would be a pile of lifeless chemical substances.

Each of us is born with a battery charge of enzyme energy at birth. As we age, our internal enzyme stores are naturally depleted. A new study shows that a 60 year old has 50% fewer enzymes than a 30 year old. The faster you use up your enzyme supply—the shorter your life. Much of the anti-aging research in the natural healing world is about boosting enzyme supply to delay the aging process.

There are three categories of enzymes:

1) **Metabolic enzymes,** which repair cells and tissues and are involved in the healing process, are needed for every chemical reaction that takes place in the human body.

Note: Enzyme supplements taken in between meals (when there isn't food to digest), function as metabolic enzymes, absorbed directly into the body to repair and heal.

2) **Our own digestive enzymes** assimilate our food and nutrients. Human digestive enzymes are stronger than any of the body's other enzymes, and more concentrated than any other enzyme combination found in nature. A very good thing, since our processed, over-cooked, nutrient-poor diets demand a great deal of enzymatic work!

3) **Fresh plant enzymes** start food digestion and enhance our own digestive enzymes. All foods in their natural state contain the enzymes required to digest them. All food, whether plant or animal, has its own enzymes that serve it in life. When eaten, these become the property of the eater and are now *its* food enzymes, and begin immediately to work for the eater's digestive benefit. Humans cannot independently assimilate food— our bodies must have the help of the food itself. Only whole food enzymes give your body what it needs to work properly. The best plant enzyme sources for humans are bananas, mangos, sprouts, papayas, avocados and pineapples.

How does plant enzyme therapy work?

Enzyme therapy uses metabolic enzymes to stimulate immune response. The link between enzymes and our immune system comes from lymphocytes, or white blood cells. Immune organs, like the thymus and lymph nodes, keep a constant level of white blood cells circulating through the body to attack foreign invader cells. When body toxins are detected, white blood cells attack them and essentially digest them by secreting enzymes on their surfaces.

Some diseases, such as cancer, leukemia, anemia and heart disease can even be diagnosed by measuring the amount and activity of certain enzymes in the blood and body fluids.

So far, enzyme therapy has been most helpful in conditions like heart disease, tumor malignancies, skin problems, low and high blood sugar, stomach and colon pain, eye diseases and headaches. Some enzymes clean wounds, dissolve blood clots and control allergic reactions to drugs.

Plant enzymes help us to heal faster. Certain enzymes, particularly proteolytic enzymes or proteases, shorten the inflammatory process during healing by breaking up debris in the injured area and stimulating our own healing enzyme activity without suppressing the immune system (unlike cortisone or hydrocortisone drugs). Proteolytic enzymes, like bromelain from pineapples, are used as anti-inflammatory agents for sports injuries like sprains, and respiratory problems where they help unclog. They can also boost healing from degenerative diseases and surgery, reducing swelling and pain for a more rapid recovery.

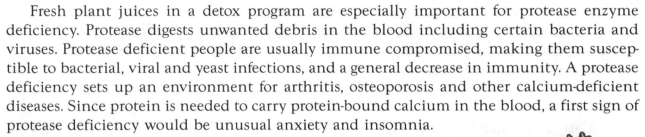

Fresh plant juices in a detox program are especially important for protease enzyme deficiency. Protease digests unwanted debris in the blood including certain bacteria and viruses. Protease deficient people are usually immune compromised, making them susceptible to bacterial, viral and yeast infections, and a general decrease in immunity. A protease deficiency sets up an environment for arthritis, osteoporosis and other calcium-deficient diseases. Since protein is needed to carry protein-bound calcium in the blood, a first sign of protease deficiency would be unusual anxiety and insomnia.

Protease deficiency also leads to inadequate protein digestion which leads to hypoglycemia resulting in moodiness, mood swing and irritability.

Do you have enough enzymes?

Enzyme depletion, lack of energy, disease and aging all go hand in hand. The first signs of enzyme deficiency are fatigue, premature aging and weight gain. Unless we do something to stop the one-way-flow of enzyme energy out of the body, our digestive and eliminative capacities weaken, obesity, and chronic illness set in and lifespan shortens.

Most nutrient deficiency problems as we age result not from the lack of the nutrients themselves, but from the body's inability to absorb them. Eating junk foods and over-cooked foods without enzymes means the pancreas and the liver have to use their enzyme stores. As a result, reserve enzymes for metabolic processes are pulled from their normal work, to digest your food.

But even this substitute measure doesn't make up for the missing enzymes that should be in the food, because the body needs that food's enzymes to break itself down correctly so it can deliver its own nutrients (Nature provides for everything).

Enzyme deficiency means we end up with undigested food in the blood. So, white blood cell immune defenses are pulled from their jobs to take care of the undigested food and the immune system takes a dive. It's a perfect environment for disease. Eating enzyme-rich foods takes care of this unhealthy cascade of reactions before it ever starts.

How can we maximize daily enzyme benefits?

I believe Nature intended us to eat a largely plant-based diet with fresh foods that have plenty of plant enzymes. It is not necessary to always eat raw foods. But it is important to have a large percentage of your overall diet be enzyme-rich. Clearly, as you increase consumption of fresh foods, the enzymatic activity within your body also increases.

WARNING: Enzyme protection and enzyme therapy are dramatically affected by the use of a microwave oven because microwaving destroys enzymes.

Enzymes are extremely sensitive to heat. Even low degrees of heat can destroy food enzymes and greatly reduce digestive ability. Heat above 120° F. completely destroys them. Enzymes are also destroyed by substances like tobacco, alcohol, caffeine, fluorides, chlorine in drinking water, air pollution, chemical additives and many medicines.

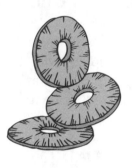

GOLDEN ENZYME DRINK
A drink specifically for healing enzyme properties.
For 2 drinks:

Juice enough pineapple for 1 1/2 to 2 cups PINEAPPLE JUICE,
4 CARROTS, 1 teasp. HONEY.

EVER GREEN ENZYME DRINK
A personal favorite for taste, mucous release and enzyme action.
For 1 drink:

Juice 1 APPLE, cored, 1 tub (4 oz.) ALFALFA SPROUTS, 1/2 FRESH PINEAPPLE, skinned/cored, 3 small handfuls FRESH MINT and 1 teasp. SPIRULINA GRANULES.

GOOD DIGESTION PUNCH
Natural sources of papain and bromelain for enzyme, ginger to break up stomach acids.
For 2 drinks:

Juice 1 PAPAYA, peeled/seeded, 1 PINEAPPLE, skinned/cored, 1/4-inch FRESH GINGER, peeled.

ENZYME COOLER
An intestinal cleanser to help lower cholesterol and allow better assimilation of foods.
For 2 large drinks:

Juice 1 APPLE, cored, or 1/2 cup APPLE JUICE, 2 LEMONS, peeled, or 1/4 cup LEMON JUICE, and 1 PINEAPPLE, skinned and cored, or 1 1/2 cups PINEAPPLE JUICE.

FRUIT & ALOE STOMACH & DIGESTIVE CLEANSER
For one 8-oz. glass:

Whirl in the blender, 1 APPLE cored, 2 TBS. ALOE VERA JUICE and 1/4 teasp. GROUND GINGER.
—Add enough WATER to make 8-oz.

VEGETABLE & VINEGAR STOMACH/DIGESTIVE CLEANSER
For one 8-oz. glass:

Juice 1/2 CUCUMBER with skin, 2 TBS. APPLE CIDER VINEGAR and 1/4 teasp. GROUND GINGER.
    —Add enough WATER to make 8-oz.

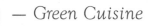

MINERAL RICH CLEANSING BROTH
For 6 cups of broth:

Put in a large soup pot with 1½ qts. WATER. Add 1 large ONION, chopped, 3 sliced CARROTS, 2 POTATOES cubed, 1 cup FRESH PARSLEY, chopped, 2 STALKS CELERY with tops.
—Bring to boil; reduce heat; simmer 30 minutes. Strain; add 1 TBS. Bragg's LIQUID AMINOS.

PURIFYING DAIKON & SCALLION BROTH
A clear cleansing drink with bladder/kidney cleansing activity.
For one bowl:

Heat gently together for 5 minutes, 4 cups VEGETABLE BROTH, one 6-inch piece DAIKON RADISH, peeled and cut in matchstick pieces, and 2 SCALLIONS, with tops.
—Stir in 1 TBS. TAMARI or 1 TBS. Bragg's LIQUID AMINOS, 1 TBS. FRESH CILANTRO leaves and ½ teasp. PEPPER.

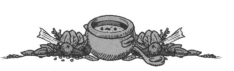

MINERAL-RICH AMINOS DRINK
A complete, balanced food-source vitamin/mineral electrolyte drink — rich in greens, amino acids and enzyme precursors. Use for detoxification, or after illness or a hospital stay.
Enough for 8 drinks:

Whirl ingredients in the blender, then mix about 2 TBS. of the powder into 2 cups of hot water for 1 drink. Let flavors bloom for 5 minutes before drinking. Sip over a half hour period for best assimilation.

4 to 6 packets MISO SOUP POWDER (Edwards & Son Co. makes a good one), 1 TBS. crumbled DRY SEA VEGETABLES (any type), ½ cup SOY PROTEIN POWDER, 1 packet INSTANT GINSENG TEA, 2 TBS. BEE POLLEN GRANULES, 1 teasp. SPIRULINA OR CHLORELLA GRANULES, 1 TBS. BREWER'S YEAST FLAKES, 1 teasp. ACIDOPHILUS POWDER, 2 TBS. FRESH PARSLEY LEAF.
—Add 1 teasp. Bragg's LIQUID AMINOS to each drink if desired.

CHINESE WEIGHT MANAGEMENT SOUP
A detox recipe for a weight loss liquid diet. Take 2 to 4 cups daily to eliminate congested fluids, break down blood fats and activate the intestines.

Tie herbs in a muslin bag: 2-oz. ASTRAGALUS, 2-oz. PORIA, 12 TO 18 pitted RED DATES, 2-oz. fresh chopped GINGER. Simmer with ½ cup BARLEY for one hour in 7 cups VEGETABLE STOCK.
—Add 3 CELERY STALKS, diced with leaves, 3 BEETS, sliced in matchstick, 3 CLOVES GARLIC, minced, 12 SHIITAKE MUSHROOMS, soaked and sliced, and simmer for another 20 minutes. Remove herb bag. Add ½ cup FRESH WATERCRESS LEAVES or SUNFLOWER SPROUTS and serve.

SPRING CLEANING ENZYME SOUP

For 8 cups soup:

Simmer washed chopped greens: 2 cups Fresh Nettle Tops, 1 cup Fresh Watercress Leaves, $\frac{1}{2}$ cup Fresh Dandelion Leaves, in pot with 2 cups Water.
—Saute 1 large minced Onion in 2 TBS. Olive Oil. Add 2 Carrots diced, 2 Turnips diced, 3 TBS. Miso Paste and 6 cups Water. Simmer 30 min. Add 1 cup Sunflower Sprouts.

PINEAPPLE/PAPAYA ENZYME SALAD

For 4 large salads:

Toss together half a Pineapple peeled and chunked, 1 cup Blueberries, 1 cup Strawberries, 1 cup Blackberries, 1 cup Raspberries
—Use the enzyme dressing below if desired.

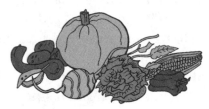

ENZYME DRESSING

For 4 large salads:

Blend in the blender 1 cup Lemon or Plain Yogurt, or Kefir Cheese, 1 TBS. Lime Juice, 1 TBS. Lemon Juice, 1 teasp. Ginger Syrup, or $\frac{1}{2}$ teasp. Ginger Powder, and $\frac{1}{4}$ teasp. Tamari.

CONSTIPATION CLEANSING ENZYME SALAD

For 2 salads:

Mix together lightly in a bowl, 1 firm chunked Papaya, 3 TBS. minced Crystallized Ginger, 1 chunked Pear, 1 cup Raspberries, $\frac{1}{2}$ cup Raspberry Vinegar mixed with $\frac{1}{2}$ cup Water.

SPRING BITTERS SALAD

For 6 salads:

Toss together $\frac{1}{2}$ cup Dandelion Leaves, $\frac{1}{2}$ cup Spinach Leaves, 4 cups Red Leaf Lettuce, $\frac{1}{2}$ cup Fresh Parsley, 1 cup mixed wild greens like Chicory, Borage, Violet Leaves, Sorrel, and Beet Greens, $\frac{1}{2}$ cup mixed tips of Chives, Fennel, Mint, Tarragon and Yarrow.
—Add 1 Tomato, chopped, 1 cup Alfalfa Sprouts, 1 Leek, white portion chopped.

AFTER DINNER ENZYME DIGESTIVE TEA

Steep 2 parts Peppermint, 2 parts Hibiscus, 1 part Papaya Leaf and 1 part Rosemary.

Herb Teas For Detoxification

Herb teas and high mineral drinks during a liquid diet can provide energy and cleansing without having to take in solid proteins or carbohydrates for fuel. Herbal teas are the most time-honored of all natural healing mediums. Essentially body balancers, teas have mild cleansing and flushing properties, and are easily absorbed by the system. The important volatile oils in herbs are released by the hot brewing water, and when taken in small sips throughout the cleansing process, they flood the tissues with concentrated nutritional support to accelerate regeneration, and the release of toxic waste. In general, herbs are more effective when taken together in combination than when used singly.

How to take herbal teas for best results in your detox program:

1) Use a glass, ceramic or earthenware pot. Stainless steel is acceptable, but aluminum negates the herbal effects, and the metal may wash into the tea and into your body.

2) Pack a small tea ball with loose herbs.

3) Bring 3 cups of cold water to a boil. Remove from heat. Add herbs, and steep covered (10 to 15 minutes for a leaf and flower tea, 20 to 25 minutes for a root and bark tea).

4) Keep lid tightly closed during steeping and storage. Volatile herbal oils are the most valuable part of the drink, and will escape if left uncovered.

5) Drink teas in small sips over a long period of time rather than all at once, to allow the tissues to absorb as much of the medicinal value as possible.

6) Take 2 to3 cups of tea daily for best medicinal effects.

A tea combination for blood cleansing might include: *red clover, hawthorn, pau d'arco, nettles, sage, alfalfa, milk thistle seed, echinacea, horsetail, gotu kola and lemongrass.*

A tea combination for mucous cleansing might include: *mullein, comfrey, ephedra, marshmallow, pleurisy root, rose hips, calendula, boneset, ginger, peppermint and fennel seed.*

A tea combination for cleansing the bowel and digestive system might include: *senna leaf, papaya leaf, fennel seed, peppermint, lemon balm, parsley, calendula, hibiscus and ginger.*

A tea combination for gentle bladder and kidney flushing might include: *uva ursi, juniper berries, ginger and parsley.*

A tea combination for clearing sinuses might include: *marshmallow, rose hips, mullein and fenugreek.*

A tea combination for clearing a stress headache might include: *rosemary, spearmint or peppermint, catnip and chamomile.*

A tea combination for removing congestion from chest and sinuses might include: *marshmallow root, mullein, rose hips and fenugreek seed.*

Santé
TEAPOT

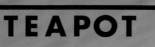

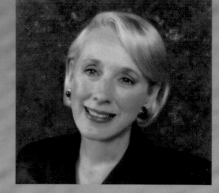

Dear Friends,

I have long believed that herbs have **a unique healing spirit** – they are a path to the universe – an eye of the needle through which we can glimpse the wonders of creation. Herbs are complex, and filled with ancestral memory. Indeed, herbs have been with us throughout our entire history adapting to the Earth's changes, as has mankind. Ancient healers discovered **the powerful healing properties of herbs.** Herbs have been widely accepted by different cultures for centuries.

Herbs are foundation nutrients, nourishing and enhancing the body's basic elements – the brain, glands and hormones. Herbal medicinal teas are subtle, gentle essences – they combine with our bodies, much in the same way that food does.

Herbal medicinal teas are easily absorbed by everyone - children, the elderly, even our pets! Inhaling the soothing vapors and sipping the warm herbal steep throughout the day is a wonderful way to transport the healing power of herbs into the body.

The boiling hot water used to brew herbal medicinal tea releases the healing powers of the herbs and unfolds their full potency. Using the right teapot and the right brewing method is as important as the tea itself for harnessing maximum healing benefits.

I had been looking for the perfect teapot for years – I finally found it. **Santé is not just beautifully designed and functional, it is the perfect teapot for brewing medicinal teas.** The unique, stainless steel sieve lets the tea leaves float and develop freely, allowing the herbs to release their full healing properties. Both the glass bowl and its stainless steel frame, as well as the stainless steel sieve are dishwasher safe and easy to clean. There is never any leftover tea residue or lingering flavor. My favorite feature of Santé is the integrated warmer wich keeps the tea at the perfect temperature for sipping over several hours. Another invaluable feature is the timer – it alerts you to the perfect steeping time, and can be reset to let you know when it is time for another cup of that healing herbal tea.

To your health!

Linda Page

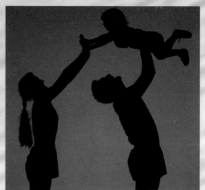

Santé -
for health's sake!

The complete Santé teapot collection:

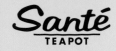
Santé
TEAPOT

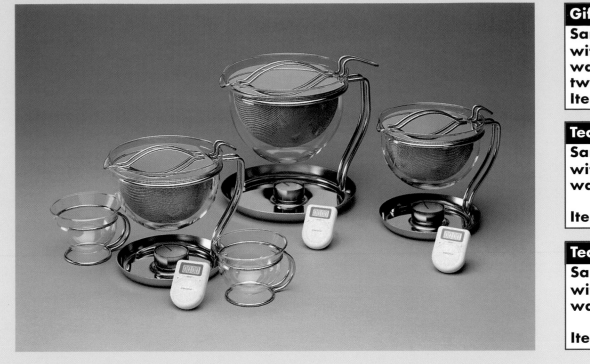

Gift set: Tea for me
Santé 22 oz
with integrated
warmer, timer and
two glass cups
Item # 45015

Tea for 2 or more
Santé 45 oz
with integrated
warmer and timer

Item # 45045

Tea for me
Santé 22 oz
with integrated
warmer and timer

Item # 45022

Stands: stainless steel **Lids/strainers:** stainless steel **Teapots:** heat-resistant Duran glass

How to use your Santé teapot:

Always use loose tea, not tea bags. When herbs are cut for tea bags, facets are created on the herb structure, which results in a substantial loss of essential healing oils.

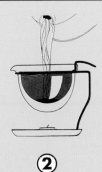

① Use 2 heaping tea-spoons of herbs for the small (22 ounces) and 3 heaping tea-spoons for the large pot (45 ounces). Place the herbs in Santé´s stainless steel sieve, and watch the herbs unfold freely, as they release their medi-cinal properties, and evolve to their highest potency.

② Use filtered water or pure spring water for increased herbal strength and effecti-veness. In a tea kettle, bring water to a gent-le boil. Pour over the herbs, replace the lid, light the warmer candle and start the steeping process.

③ Now is the time to set the timer. Generally, you want to steep the tea according to the formula or desired fla-vor and strength - as a rule, 10 minutes for a leaf/flower tea; 20 minutes for a root/bark tea. Be sure to keep the lid on your teapot to prevent es-sential oils from es-caping.

④ When your Santé tea timer goes off, remove the sieve and replace the cover. Try the used herbs on your potted plants or in your gar-den - they are a great fertilizer!

⑤ Your tea will stay at the perfect tempera-ture as it steeps and as you drink it through-out the day. One-half to 1 cup taken 3 or 4 times over a few hours allows for gentle, continual absorption of the medicinal brew. R e m e m b e r : breathe-in the healing vapors as you sip the soothing tea.

Caution: Do not light candle unless there is liquid in the pot. Extinguish candle when the pot is empty.

> "Herbs have been meeting people's medical needs for thousands of years. Herbal teas are the most basic of all natural healing mediums. They are easily absorbed by the body. We need only to use them with thanksgiving and wisdom."

**Linda Page,
N.D., Ph.D.**

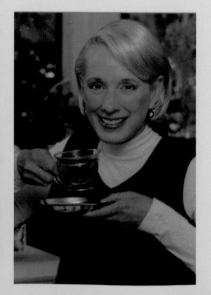

Santé , for health's sake!
by mono

Order your favorite Santé - Tea set now

By Phone (toll free):   888 - Santé 19
By Fax: 404 - 355 6708
By Mail: **mono** Santé
                                     P.O. Box 20217
                                     Atlanta, GA 30325
By Internet: www.healthyhealing.com
                                     CODE H 1198

Quantity   Gift set: Tea for me, Santé 22 oz with integrated warmer, timer and two glass cups
45015 $ 134.95

Quantity   Tea for two or more, Santé 45 oz with integrated warmer and timer
45045 $ 134.95

Quantity   Tea for me, Santé 22 oz with integrated warmer and timer
45022 $ 99.95

Total $ _____ + local tax $ _____ + shipping &

handling within the US $ 7.50

Total due $ _____

Please select your payment option:

☐ Enclosed is my check for $_____
☐ Please bill my
    ☐ Visa Card
    ☐ Master Card
    ☐ American Express
Card # _____ Exp. Date _____

Ship to:

Name _____
Street _____
City _____ State _____
Country _____ Phone _____
Fax _____ Zip _____

Signature _____

Enjoy your *Santé* , for health's sake!
TEAPOT

Name _____

Address _____

State _____

Place
Stamp
Here

mono Santé
P.O. Box 20217
Atlanta, GA 30325

Santé
TEAPOT

Linda Page,

N.D., Ph.D. has been working with herbs for ov‹ 25 years, and is a leading expert on herbal healing. Following a life threatenin illness Dr. Page regained her health through the use of natural therapies and herbal healing - she has dedicated her life to teaching people about the curative power of herk

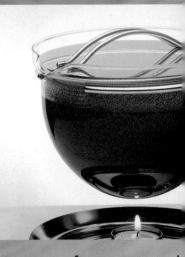

For more information on th benefits of herbal healing visit:

www.healthyhealing.com

mono Santé
P.O. Box 20217
Atlanta, GA 30325
888 - Santé 19
Code H 1198

A tea combination for releasing body energy might include: *gotu kola, peppermint, red clover and cloves.*

A tea combination for warming against aches and chills might include: *wild cherry bark, licorice root, rose hips and cinnamon.*

A tea combination for restoring bowel and colon regularity might include: *fennel seed, flax seed, fenugreek seed, licorice root, burdock root and spearmint.*

A tea combination for loosening lung congestion might include: *ginger root, cinnamon, cloves, lemon peel and cardamom pods.*

I think my favorite herb tea for a good detox is **GREEN TEA**, an unfermented tea rich in flavonoids with antioxidant and anti-allergen activity. Green tea has a long history in the Orient as a beneficial body cleanser. Its anti-oxidant polyphenols do not interfere with iron or protein absorption, and as with other plant antioxidants, like beta carotene and vitamin C, green tea polyphenols work at the molecular level, combatting free radical damage to protect against degenerative disease.

HOMEMADE GINGER ALE FOR CLEANSING & DIGESTION

This is an original nineteen-twenties home remedy tea for both children and adults. It works amazingly well to settle the stomach, and help elimination during a cold, flu or fever. I like it better than today's ginger ale. Use it as part if your liquid intake during a detox.
For 1 quart:

Bring 3 cups WATER to a boil and simmer for 5 minutes. Add 2 teasp. fresh grated GINGER ROOT, I teasp. dry RED RASPBERRY LEAVES, 1 teasp. dry SASSAFRAS ROOT , chopped, and 1 teasp. dry SARSAPARILLA ROOT, broken.
—Let steep for 15 minutes. Strain and add 1 cup SPARKLING WATER, like Evian or Calistoga just before serving. Add 3 fresh lemon slices if desired.

ROOTBEER REVITALIZER

Here's the old-fashioned version of a popular favorite. Decidedly delicious medicine for cleansing and digestion.
For 1 quart add 4 TBS. of the following dry blend:

Combine in a large pot: 3-oz. dry SASSAFRAS BARK, broken, 2 teasp. fresh grated GINGER ROOT, 2-oz. dry SARSAPARILLA ROOT, 1 TBS. ground CINNAMON, 1-oz. dry DANDELION ROOT, 2 teasp. ORANGE PEEL, 1-oz. dry BURDOCK ROOT.
—Add 4 TBS. dry mixture. Simmer for 15 to 20 minutes.

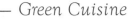
Cleansing Broths & Hot Tonics

Clear broths are a very satisfying form of nutrition during a cleansing fast. They are simple, easy, inexpensive, can be taken hot or cold, and provide a means of "eating" and being with others at mealtime without going off a liquid detox program. This is more important than it might appear, since solid food, taken after the body has released all its solid waste, but before the cleanse is over, will drastically reduce your diet's success. Broths are also alkalizing and help balance body pH.

Hot tonics are neither broths nor teas, but unique hot combinations of vegetables, fruits and spices with purifying and energizing properties. The ingredients provide noticeable synergistic activity when taken together — with more medicinal benefits than the single ingredients alone. Take them morning and evening for best results.

PURIFYING CLEAR BROTH

Rich in potassium and minerals.
For 6 cups:

Sauté in 2 TBS. Canola or Olive Oil: $^1/_4$ cup chopped Celery, $^1/_4$ cup Daikon Radish, $^1/_4$ cup chopped Leeks, $^1/_2$ cup Broccoli chopped.
—Add 6 cups Rich Vegetable Stock, 2 TBS. Fresh Snipped Lemon Peel, 2 teasp. Bragg's Liquid Aminos, $^1/_4$ cup snipped Parsley, and $^1/_4$ cup grated Carrots.
—Heat for 1 minute, then serve hot.

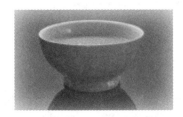

RICE PURIFYING SOUP

A good start to a macrobiotic cleansing diet.
For 6 cups:

Toast in a large pan until aromatic (about 5 minutes), $^2/_3$ cup Lentils, $^2/_3$ cup Split Peas, $^2/_3$ cup Brown Rice and 2 Cloves Garlic minced.
—Add 1 Onion, chopped, 1 Carrot, chopped, 1 Stalk Celery, chopped, 3 cups Onion Or Veggie Broth, 3 cups Water, 1 teasp. Cayenne Pepper, $^1/_2$ teasp. Lemon Pepper and $^1/_2$ teasp. Ginger Powder. Cook over low heat for 1 hr. stirring occasionally.

ONION & MISO BROTH

A therapeutic broth with antibiotic and immune-enhancing properties.
For 6 small bowls of broth:

Sauté 1 chopped Onion in $^1/_2$ teasp. Sesame Oil for 5 minutes. Add 1 Stalk Celery with leaves; sauté for 2 minutes. Add 1-qt. Vegetable Stock. Cover and simmer 10 minutes.
—Add 4 TBS. Miso and 2 Green Onions with tops. Remove from heat; whirl in blender.

GARLIC TONIC BROTH
Enough for 6 cups broth:

Bring to a boil, lower heat and simmer for 20 minutes: 6 cups WATER, 2 small HEADS GARLIC, I LARGE ONION, peeled, quartered, 2 STALKS CELERY, diagonal cut, ¹/₂ teasp. CURRY POWDER, I BAY LEAF, pinch SAFFRON THREADS, ¹/₂ cup chopped FRESH PARSLEY, ¹/₂ teasp. dry SAGE, and snipped dry or granulated SEA VEGETABLES to taste.
—Let cool slightly, remove bay leaf and puree in blender.

REVITALIZING TONIC
A good drink for an addiction purifying program or any kind of hangover. Effective hot or cold. Works every time.
Enough for 8 drinks:

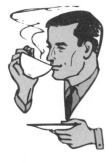

Whirl in the blender I ¹/₂ cups WATER, I cup chopped ONIONS, 2 STALKS CELERY chopped, I BUNCH PARSLEY chopped, 2 TBS. chopped fresh or dried BASIL, 2 teasp. HOT PEPPER SAUCE, I teasp. ROSEMARY LEAVES, ¹/₂ teasp. FENNEL SEEDS, and 2 teasp. Bragg's LIQUID AMINOS.
—Pour into a large pot with 48-oz. Knudsen's SPICY VEGGIE JUICE. Bring to a boil and simmer for 30 minutes. Use hot or cool.

IMMUNE PROTECTION BROTH
For 6 large servings (a week's supply):

Soak I-oz. dry REISHI MUSHROOMS, I-oz. dry SHIITAKE MUSHROOMS, 4 TBS. dry snipped SEA VEGETABLES (any kind), I-oz. ASTRAGALUS BARK and I-inch piece GINGER ROOT in water to cover. When soft, sliver mushrooms (save soaking water); discard astragalus and ginger.
—Simmer 8 cups WATER, add soaking water, 4 TBS. organic PEARLED BARLEY, 4 TBS. organic BROWN RICE and 2 cups chopped ORGANIC VEGETABLES (any kind). Simmer 30 minutes.

MISO, GREEN TEA AND MUSHROOM BROTH
For 2 large servings:

Steep 2 TBS. GREEN TEA LEAVES, a 2-inch piece LEMONGRASS, 2 TBS. snipped SEA VEGETABLES in I cup WATER. Add 3 cups dry shiitake mushrooms, soaked and slivered (save mushroom soaking water)
—Sizzle I large GARLIC CLOVE, minced, and ¹/₂ SMALL ONION, diced in I tsp OLIVE OIL, and I teasp. SESAME OIL. Add 3 cups VEGETABLE STOCK, bring to a boil and add ¹/₄ cup shredded CARROTS. Add I TBS. MISO PASTE, MUSHROOM SOAKING WATER and CAYENNE PEPPER to taste.
—Cook five minutes. Add tea, simmer gently 5 minutes.

CHINESE MEDICINE DEEP DETOX STEW

A traditional stew to enhance immunity, reduce cholesterol and regulate blood pressure.
For 4 bowls:

Soak, the slivers of 15 SHIITAKE MUSHROOMS and 1-oz. BLACK FUNGUS (save soaking water).
—Sauté 3 cloves GARLIC, 2 LEEKS and 4 TBS. SESAME SEEDS in 2 TBS. SESAME OIL for 5 minutes. Add 2 BURDOCK ROOTS, chopped, 2-oz. dry HIJIKI SEAWEED for 5 minutes more.
—Add mushrooms and soaking water to 6 cups water. Add 1 bunch chopped BOK CHOY, 1 small can LYCII BERRIES, and 6 TBS. WHITE MISO. Let simmer for several minutes to blend.

MINERAL BALANCE SOUP

This detox soup from Japan has anti-viral, anti-diabetic and anti-aging properties.
For 2 bowls:

Cover with water in a pot: $1/4$ DAIKON RADISH, chopped with leaves, $1/4$ large BURDOCK ROOT, 1 CARROT, 2 dry SHIITAKE MUSHROOMS, soaked and slivered (save soaking water).
—Add soaking water. Simmer for one hour.

IMMUNE BOOSTER SOUP

For 4 drinks:

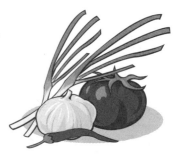

Sauté in 2 TBS. OLIVE OIL 5 minutes til aromatic: 1 LEEK, $1/2$ cup sliced SCALLIONS, $1/2$ cup diced FENNEL and 6 GARLIC CLOVES minced.
—Add 6 cups VEGETABLE STOCK, 1 cup GREEN CABBAGE and 1 cup BROCCOLI FLORETS; simmer for 10 minutes.
—Add 2 cups FROZEN PEAS, 4 cups DARK GREEN LEAVES (kale, collards, spinach, chard, etc.), $1/2$ cup FRESH PARSLEY and 2 teasp. ASTRAGALUS extract. Simmer 5 minutes.
—Add 4 TBS snipped SEA VEGETABLES and season with CAYENNE to taste.

ANTIOXIDANT GINGER SOUP

For 4 drinks:

Sauté in 3 TBS. OLIVE OIL 5 minutes til aromatic: 2 TBS. minced GARLIC, 2 TBS. minced GINGER ROOT and 2 ONIONS, chopped. Add 2 lbs. chopped CARROTS and 4 cups VEGETABLE STOCK. Simmer for 40 minutes. Add 1 TBS. grated ORANGE ZEST and 1 $1/2$ cups ORANGE JUICE.
—Remove solids with a slotted spoon. Puree in the blender and return them to the pot with other liquid.
—Add zest and orange juice.
—Season with CAYENNE PEPPER and snipped or granulated SEA VEGETABLES to taste.

CIRCULATION STIMULANT
For 4 drinks:

Heat 15 minutes: 1 cup CRANBERRY JUICE, 1 cup ORANGE JUICE, 2 TBS. HONEY, 6 CLOVES, 6 CARDAMOM PODS, 1 CINNAMON STICK, 4 TBS. RAISINS, 4 TBS. ALMONDS, chopped, and 1 teasp. VANILLA.
—Remove cloves, cardamom and cinnamon stick. Serve hot.

HERB & VEGETABLE IMMUNE ENHANCING BROTH
For 4 cups of broth:

Heat 3 cups homemade VEGETABLE STOCK in a soup pot.
—Add and heat gently: 2 TBS. MISO dissolved in 1 cup WATER, 1 TBS. BREWER'S YEAST FLAKES, 2 TBS. chopped GREEN ONIONS, $\frac{1}{2}$ cup TOMATO JUICE and $\frac{1}{2}$ teasp. each: dry BASIL, THYME, SAVORY and MARJORAM.

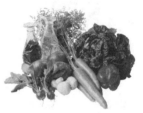

WOMEN'S BLOOD TONIC
This Chinese herb blood-nourisher is a long term tonic for meno-pausal women. The herbs can be bought in a health food store.
For 6 large bowls:

Heat 8 cups VEGETABLE STOCK. Add 1-oz. DONG QUAI ROOT, 1-oz. ASTRAGALUS, $\frac{1}{2}$-oz. PORIA MUSH-ROOM, 1 oz. WILD YAM ROOT, 8 BLACK DATES, 16 RED DATES. and heat for 30 minutes.
—Discard herbs. Add 2 TBS TAMARI or Bragg LIQUID AMINOS.

ALKALIZING APPLE BROTH
This broth alkalizes body pH, gives a spicy energy lift and helps lower serum cholesterol.
For 4 drinks:

Sauté $\frac{1}{2}$ chopped RED ONION and 2 CLOVES GARLIC minced in 1 teasp. CANOLA OIL til soft.
—While sautéing, blend in the blender, 1 SMALL RED BELL PEPPER, 2 TART APPLES, cored, 1 LEMON partially peeled, 2 TBS. PARSLEY and 2 cups Knudsen's VERY VEGGIE-SPICY (or any good spicy tomato juice). Add onion mix to blender and puree. Heat gently.

SPRING CLEANSE CARROT SOUP
For 6 bowls:

In a soup pot, sauté 1 LARGE ONION, minced in 2 TBS. OLIVE OIL until translucent.
—Add 8 cups water place 1 cup dry NETTLES or WATERCRESS, $\frac{1}{2}$ cup dry YELLOW DOCK ROOT, $\frac{1}{2}$ cup fresh DANDELION LEAVES, 4 CARROTS, diced and 3 TBS. WHITE MISO. Cook 30 min.

Sea vegetables can boost every detox program.

Sea vegetables and marine superfoods like spirulina and chlorella are a veritable medicine chest of premium nutrition. Ounce for ounce sea weeds are higher in essential nutrients than any other food group. They are vigorous sources of proteins, enzymes, antioxidants and amino acids with whole cell availability. Sea plants offer your body basic building blocks for acid/alkaline balance, regulate body fluid osmosis, strengthen nerves synapses, digestive and circulatory activity, help reduce cholesterol and regulate blood sugar levels.

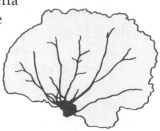

They are especially rich in minerals like iodine and potassium (with all forty-four trace minerals), and chlorophyll, have substantial amounts of beta carotene, B vitamins (the only vegetarian source of measureable B-12), essential fatty acids, octacosonal for tissue oxygenation and soluble fiber.

MINERAL RICH ENERGY GREEN

Helps build strong teeth, bones, nails and hair. A good choice for a weight loss cleanse.
For 4 drinks:

Mix up in the blender: $^1/_2$ cup AMAZAKE RICE DRINK, $^1/_2$ cup OATS, 2 TBS. BEE POLLEN GRANULES, I packet INSTANT GINSENG TEA GRANULES, 2 Packets BARLEY GRASS OR CHLORELLA GRANULES, 2 TBS. GOTU KOLA HERB, 2 TBS. ALFALFA LEAF, I TBS. DANDELION LEAF, I TBS. crumbled DULSE, and I teasp. VITAMIN C CRYSTALS with BIOFLAVONOIDS.

—Then mix 2 TBS. into 2 cups of hot water per drink. Let flavors bloom for 5 minutes before drinking. Add I teasp. LEMON JUICE or I teasp. Bragg's LIQUID AMINOS if desired.

WATERCRESS & SEA VEGGIE BROTH

For 2 bowls:

Blend ingredients to a smooth consistency: $^1/_2$ Cup WATER, I cup chopped WATERCRESS, I cup chopped MIXED GREENS, 4 TBS. GREEN ONION minced, $^1/_2$ cup SUNFLOWER SPROUTS and $^1/_4$ teasp. cayenne pepper. Heat gently and serve.

BASIC SEA VEGGIE MISO SPECIAL

Two tablespoons dry minced sea veggies daily is a therapeutic dose.
For about 4 bowls:

Bring 4 cups WATER to a simmer. Add 4 TBS. WHITE MISO, 2 chopped GREEN ONIONS, 8-oz. firm TOFU in small cubes, and 6 TBS. dry snipped WAKAME. Simmer for 2 minutes. Remove from heat and add $^1/_2$ cup SOY MOZZARELLA CHEESE in small cubes. Sprinkle on 3 teasp. BREWER'S YEAST FLAKES. Let flavors bloom 30 seconds and serve.

MINERAL-RICH ALKALIZING ENZYME SOUP

An exceptional source of minerals, trace minerals and enzymes for good assimilation.
For 4 soups:

Put the following vegetables in a pot with 1 1/2 quarts of cold water: 2 POTATOES chunked, 1 ONION chunked, 2 CARROTS sliced, 1 STALK CELERY with leaves sliced, 1 cup FRESH PARSLEY packed, and 4 TBS. chopped dry DULSE. Simmer for 30 minutes. Strain and take hot or cold.
—Add 2 TBS. soaked flax seed or oat bran if there is chronic constipation.
—Add 1 teasp. Bragg's LIQUID AMINOS to each drink if desired.

FRESH CORN AND ARAME SOUP

For 6 servings:

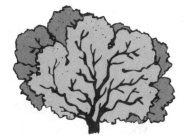

Blender blend 4 cups fresh CORN KERNELS, 1 cup WATER, 1 cup chopped ALMONDS, 1 AVOCADO, 4 TBS. dry snipped ARAME SEAWEED, 1/2 bunch fresh CILANTRO chopped, 3 teasp. CUMIN SEEDS, 1 TBS. LEMON PEPPER, and 1 teasp. GARLIC POWDER.

HIGH VITAMIN C GAZPACHO

For 6 servings:

In one cup water in a soup pot simmer 2 CLOVES GARLIC til aromatic. Add 4 large TOMATOES or 3 cups TOMATO JUICE, 4 GREEN ONIONS with tops, 1/2 GREEN PEPPER diced, 1/2 CUCUMBER diced, 2 TBS. crumbled dry SEA VEGETABLES (any kind), 4 SPRIGS PARSLEY, 2 TBS. LEMON JUICE and 1 teasp. Bragg's LIQUID AMINOS.

Drinks to clear congestion, and cold or flu infection

These drinks are specifically designed to help clear toxins and infective organisms from your system. They work extremely well—in some cases almost immediately. Use them when you're feeling toxic or run down, or to help you recover from a "hanging on" illness.

COLD DEFENSE CLEANSER

Make this broth the minute you feel a cold coming on. Drink in small sips.
Heat gently for 2 drinks:

Heat 1 1/2 cups WATER. Stir in 1 TBS. HONEY, 1 teasp. GARLIC POWDER, 1/2 teasp. CAYENNE, 1 teasp. GROUND GINGER and 1 TBS. LEMON JUICE. Off heat, add 3 TBS. BRANDY.

COLDS & FLU CONGESTION TONIC

This drink really opens up nasal and sinus passages fast. Very potent.
For 2 drinks:

Toast in a pan until aromatic, 4 Cloves Minced Garlic, $\frac{1}{2}$ teasp. Cumin Seeds, $\frac{1}{4}$ teasp. Black Pepper, and $\frac{1}{2}$ teasp. Hot Mustard Powder. Stir in 1 TBS. Flax Oil. Toast a little more.
—Add 1 cup Water, 1 cup Cooked Split Peas or 1 cup Frozen Peas, 1 TBS. fresh Cilantro, 1 teasp. Turmeric, $\frac{1}{2}$ teasp. Sesame Salt, or $\frac{1}{2}$ teasp. ground Coriander. Simmer gently 5 min.

VITAMIN C IMMUNE BOOSTER FOR COLDS & FLU

For 1 drink:

Juice or blender blend 1-inch slice Ginger Root or 1 TBS. crystallized ginger, 1 Apricot, pitted, $\frac{1}{2}$ Lemon, peeled, 3 teasp. Vitamin C Crystals, and 3 Carrots.

MUCOUS CLEANSING BROTH

Your grandmother was right. Chicken broth really does clear chest congestion fast.
For 4 bowls:

Use 1-qt. homemade Chicken Stock (boil down bones, skin and trimmings from 1 fryer in 2-qts. water, and skim off fat).
In a large pot, sauté 3 Cloves Garlic minced, 1 teasp. Horseradish, and 1 pinch Cayenne for 5 minutes until aromatic.
—Add Chicken Stock and simmer for 10 minutes. Top with Nutmeg and snipped Parsley.

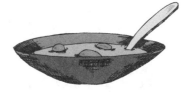

CHINESE CLEAR HEALING CHICKEN SOUP

All over the world, people find that chicken soup really works.
For 2 large bowls of broth:

Bring to a simmer 3 to 4 cups strained homemade Chicken Broth, $\frac{1}{2}$ cup Bean Sprouts. Add 1 cup shredded Chicken, $\frac{1}{2}$ cup Carrots, in thin matchsticks, 2 thin slices Ginger, 2 TBS. Tamari and simmer for 10 minutes.
—Add $\frac{1}{2}$ cup fresh Pea Pods and $\frac{1}{2}$ cup shredded Chinese Cabbage. Heat for 3 minutes.

ANTI-RHINO COLD FIGHTING TEA

Brew 1 teaspoon Chamomile Flowers. Add 1 dropperful each of Echinacea and Goldenseal Extract, and a 2-inch piece Ginger Root, skinned and sliced thinly. Brew for ten minutes, strain.

Cool spring and summer soups for easy cleansing

Chilled soups are easy to make, refreshing and light.... they're really a liquid salad. They are ideal for cleansing, packed with digestion-friendly plant enzymes for nourishment and energy. Don't worry if you don't have every ingredient in a recipe on hand. It's almost impossible to make a mistake. Just substitute something you like that's fresh and handy.

GAZPACHO

This soup makes a great salad dressing, too.
For 2 bowls:

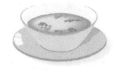

Blender blend to retain a slightly chunky texture: 2 large Tomatoes cubed, 1 Scallion, 1 cup Alfalfa Sprouts, 1 Celery Stalk with leaves, $\frac{1}{2}$ Lemon peeled, 1 teasp. Tamari, 1 pinch each Basil and Oregano (fresh or dried), $\frac{1}{2}$ Avocado, and 1 pinch Cayenne.

HIGH MINERAL SOUP

For 2 to 3 large bowls:

Blend 1 large Tomato, 2 Stalks Celery chopped, 3 Green Cabbage Leaves, $\frac{1}{2}$ Small Cucumber, 6 large Spinach Leaves, $\frac{1}{4}$ small Beet, 1 small Green Onion, 1 teasp. Vegetable Salt, and Water to thin. Top with 1 TBS. crumbled, toasted Dulse or crunchy Sea Palm.

HIGH ENERGY SOUP

For 2 to 3 large bowls:

Blender til smooth 4 chunked Carrots, $\frac{1}{2}$ bunch Spinach, 1 small Jicama peeled and chunked, 1 large Tomato, 1 Stalk Celery chunked, 1 4-oz. tub Alfalfa Sprouts, and 1 handful fresh Parsley. Add a little Water to thin and a dash of Hot Pepper Sauce to spice.

GARDEN VEGGIES & GREENS SOUP

For 6 large bowls:

Blend the broth: 3 cups Carrot Juice, 6 Celery Stalks, 1 Avocado and 1 Lemon peeled.
—Add the veggies: 1 Summer Squash grated, 2 to 3 Celery Stalks diced, 2 to 3 Ears Fresh Corn cut off cob, and 1 cup finely chopped Arugula, Frisee, Radicchio or Parsley Leaves.

CARROT ALMOND SOUP

Blend 3 cups Carrot Juice, 1 cup Almonds, 1 Red Bell Pepper, $\frac{1}{2}$ bunch Dill Weed, 1 teasp. Lemon Juice, and $\frac{1}{4}$ teasp. Garlic Powder.

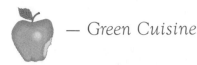

HIGH PROTEIN SOUP
For 2 to 3 large bowls:

Blend smooth 1 cup mixed NUTS and SEEDS, 1 cup grated mixed VEGETABLES (summer squash, zucchini, carrots, celery, peas, etc.), 1 cup MUNG or ALFALFA SPROUTS, 3 TBS. ONION minced, $^{1}/_{2}$ teasp. GARLIC POWDER, 1 teasp. TAMARI, $^{1}/_{4}$ teasp. CAYENNE PEPPER, and 1 to 2 cups WATER to thin to desired consistency.

INFECTION STOPPER SOUP
For 2 bowls:

Sizzle 2 to 3 GARLIC CLOVES in a pan til aromatic. Add 1 cup chopped mixed KALE, COLLARDS and SPINACH LEAVES, 1 large TOMATO, 2 STALKS CELERY and 1 TBS. BALSAMIC VINEGAR.
—Heat gently, then blender blend smooth.

ARTHRITIS RELIEF ASPARAGUS SOUP
Serves 4:

Blender blend 1 cup whole ALMONDS, 2 cups fresh ASPARAGUS (save tips for topping), 1 small handful PARSLEY, 2 cups leafy SALAD GREENS, 2 stalks CELERY, and 1 CLOVE GARLIC.
—Float on ASPARAGUS tips to top soup.

WATERMELON DIURETIC SOUP
Serves 6:

Puree in the blender: 1 6-lb. WATERMELON, 1 LIME and 1 LEMON partially peeled, $^{2}/_{3}$ cup BLUEBERRIES, $^{1}/_{2}$ cup diced FENNEL BULB, $^{1}/_{2}$ cup chopped MINT, a 1-inch piece peeled, sliced GINGER ROOT or 1 TBS. chopped CRYSTALLIZED GINGER, and 1 RED CHILE PEPPER.

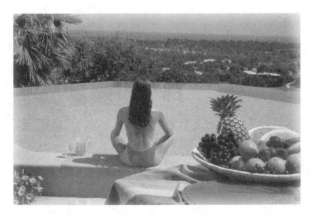

Energizing Morning Protein Drinks

Morning nutrients are more than just early fuel. They are a key factor in a healing diet. Ideally, the body needs to get about one third of its daily nutrients in the morning. The nutrients you take on rising, at breakfast and mid-morning, lay the foundation for the day's improvement in body chemistry balance. Healing progress can be noticeably accelerated through conscious attention to the nutritional content of the foods you eat before noon.

Here's why:

• Detoxification and blood purification can be stimulated for the next 24 hour period.

• Liver can be better encouraged to metabolize fats and form healthy red blood cells.

• The body's glycogen supply can be maximized in the morning hours for better sugar tolerance and energy use. If you have hypoglycemia, a good solid breakfast is almost a must.

• Broad spectrum enzyme production can be established through the pancreas for increased assimilation of nutrients and better tolerance of food sensitivities.

• Brain and memory functions make maximum use of fuel in the morning, especially after a restful night. Consider a morning protein drink for the health of your head.

• Morning is the day's best opportunity to get high fiber foods like whole grains and fruits, for regularity and body balance.

• Metabolism is at its highest in the morning to burn up calories. A low-fat, high energy morning drink can help keep you away from junk foods and unconscious nibbling all day.

My Personal Favorite

I especially like brown rice in the morning. It is an efficient source of protein and B vitamins that particularly well for a brown rice cleanse or a spring cleanse.

I always sprinkle my brown rice with at least 2 tablespoons (usually more) of snipped dry sea vegetables. I usually top it with about a cup of fresh shredded carrots and romaine lettuce. I often stir in about 2 TBS sesame seeds and sprinkle the whole thing with tamari sauce. It's my perfect breakfast.

NON-DAIRY MORNING PROTEIN DRINK

You must have protein to heal. The new breed of light, vegetarian protein drinks like this one are a wonderful way to get protein without meat or bulk or excess fat. These drinks obtain protein from several sources so that a balance with carbohydrates and minerals is achieved, and a real energy boost felt.

For 2 drinks:

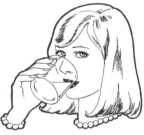

Blend together I cup STRAWBERRIES or KIWI sliced, I BANANA sliced, I cup PAPAYA or PINEAPPLE chunked, 8-oz. SOFT TOFU or I cup AMAZAKE RICE DRINK, 2 TBS. MAPLE SYRUP, I cup ORGANIC APPLE JUICE, I teasp. VANILLA, I TBS. toasted WHEAT GERM, and $^1/_2$ teasp. GINGER POWDER or I TBS. CRYSTALIZED GINGER.

MORNING MEAL REPLACEMENT
Effective non-dairy protein.
For 2 drinks:

Blender blend 1 cup Strawberries or Kiwi sliced, 2 TBS. Sweet Cloud Syrup or Barley Malt, 1 Banana sliced, 1 cup Papaya chunked, 1 cup Pineapple/Coconut Juice, 8-oz. Soft Tofu (or 1 cup Amazake Rice Drink), 2 teasp. Vanilla and 2 TBS. toasted Wheat Germ.

MORNING ORANGE SHAKE
For 2 drinks:

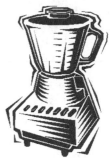

Blender blend 2 Oranges peeled with a little rind left on, 1 Frozen Banana chunked, 2 TBS. Yogurt, 1/4 cup Orange Juice, and 1 teasp. Vanilla.

NON-DAIRY MORNING PROTEIN
For 2 drinks:

Blender blend 1 cup Strawberries sliced, 1 Banana sliced, 1 cup Pineapple chunked, 8-oz. Soft Tofu, 2 TBS. Maple Syrup, 1 TBS. Crystallized Ginger and 2 TBS. toasted Wheat Germ.

MORNING FIBER DRINK
Also good to take in the evening for morning regularity. Make up the dry mx, then take 1 heaping teaspoon in water or juice in the morning and at bedtime. Store airtight.

Blender blend 1/2 cup Oat or Rice Bran, 1/3 cup Flax Seed, 3 TBS. Psyllium Husk Powder, 2 TBS. Fennel Seed, and 2 TBS. Acidophilus Powder.

MORNING PROTEIN IMMUNE ENHANCER
For 1 drink:

Blender blend 3 Pineapple Rings, 4-oz. Soymilk (or 1/2 cup Almonds and 1/2 cup Water), 1 Banana, 3 TBS. Protein Powder (or 1 TBS. Brewer's Yeast.)

DE-STRESS MORNING SHAKE
For 2 drinks:

Blend 1 pint each Strawberries and Blackberries, 1 Banana, 1/2 Pear, 2-oz. Tofu, 1 TBS. Brewer's Yeast.

Simple Raw Salads & Dressings For Cleansing

A simple fruit or vegetable salad is the best way to begin and end a liquid detox diet. A small salad the night before prepares your body and starts the cleansing process. A salad on the last night of a fast begins the enzymatic and systol/diastole activity of digestion again. Use the following salads any time you want to put less strain on your digestive system.

Fruit salads to take until noon:

Fruits are wonderful for a quick system wash and cleanse. Their high natural water and sugar content speeds up metabolism to release wastes rapidly. Fresh fruit has an alkalizing effect in the body, and is high in vitamins and nutrients. The way that you eat fruits is as important as which fruits you eat. Eat fruits alone or with other fruits for their best healing and nutritional effects. With a few exceptions, eat fruits before noon to take advantage of your body's best energy conversion and cleansing benefits.

MORNING FRESH FRUITS & YOGURT

For 4 salads:

Chop together in a bowl: 1 BANANA, 1 PEACH or PEAR, 1 APPLE, $\frac{1}{4}$ FRESH PINEAPPLE, 1 ORANGE.
—Mix in 2 TBS. RAISINS, 2 TBS. TOASTED SUNFLOWER SEEDS, and $\frac{1}{2}$ cup LEMON/LIME YOGURT.
—Top with 2 TBS. GINGER GRANOLA if desired.

PINEAPPLE ENZYME SUNDAE

For 6 salads:

Toss in a bowl: 3 cups chopped FRESH PINEAPPLE or MANGOES, 3 cups chopped APPLES or APRICOTS, 12 fresh STRAWBERRIES or CHERRIES, and 6 TBS. chopped ALMONDS.

MID-MORNING FRUIT TREAT

For 4 salads:

Chop together in a bowl: 4 BANANAS, 2 PEARS, 3 cups GREEN GRAPES, 2 PEACHES, and 4 NECTARINES. For a sauce, blend 2 cups of the fruit with 1 cup RAISINS. Top with 4 TBS. COCONUT SHREDS.

SPRING CLEANSE SALAD

For 2 salads:

Chop together in a bowl: 1 PEACH, 1 NECTARINE, 1 APRICOT, and 12 CHERRIES pitted.

MORNING MELON SALAD

For best digestion, activity and cleansing results, eat melons alone.
For 4 salads:

Remove rinds and cube melons in a bowl: $1/2$ Honeydew, $1/2$ Casaba, $1/2$ Cantaloupe, and $1/2$ Persian Melon
—Make a sauce by blending a portion of the melon mix and pour over if desired.

MORNING CITRUS MIX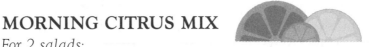

For 2 salads:

Chop together in a bowl: 2 Oranges peeled, 2 cups fresh Pineapple Chunks, 1 Grapefruit, 1 Kiwi peeled, and 2 cups Red & Black Seedless Grapes.

Keep sauces and dressings simple for body cleansing fruit salads. I make them in the blender and pour them over the fruit just before I'm ready to eat.

BASIC FRUIT CREAMS

Blender blend 1 or 2 small pieces of the same fruit you used in salad. Add 1 TBS. Honey. For a thin sauce, add about $1/2$ cup Water. For thicker sauce, add 1 Banana or $1/2$ Avocado.

APPLE-AVOCADO CREAM

Makes about 2 cups:

Blend 2 Golden Delicious Apples, 1 - 2 Avocados, $1/2$ cup Apple Juice and 1 TBS. Honey.

PINEAPPLE WHIP DRESSING

Blend $1/4$ Fresh Pineapple, 2 to 3 Bananas sliced.

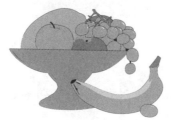

A fresh vegetable salad is one of Mother Nature's "superfoods."

Massive new research is validating what natural healers have known for decades. The more fruits and vegetables you eat, the less your risk of disease. Even for cancer, people who eat plenty of vegetables have half the risk of people who eat few vegetables.

Most studies show that even moderate amounts of vegetables make a big difference. Eating certain fresh vegetables twice a day, instead of twice a week, can cut the risk of lung cancer by 75%, even in smokers. The evidence is so overwhelming that some researchers are beginning to view fruits and vegetables as powerful preventive "drugs" that could substantially wipe out the scourge of cancer. What an about-face this has been for cancer study!

The healing power of vegetables works both raw and cooked. It is not always true that raw vegetables are better. Even though several fragile anticancer agents, like indoles and vitamin C, are destroyed by heat, a little heat makes beta carotene *more easily* absorbed. I frequently recommend lightly cooked vegetables because their action is gentler, especially if your body is very ill or your digestion is impaired.

What is a serving of fresh vegetables? One serving is about $^1/_2$ cup of cooked or chopped vegetables, 1 cup of leafy vegetables, or 6-ounces of vegetable juice. Only 10% of Americans eat that much every day.

SHREDDED SALAD SUPREME

To me, grated or shredded veggies have much more flavor — probably more of their "essence" is released during the grating process.
For 1 large salad:

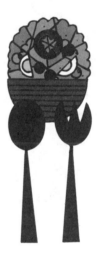

1 cup each CARROTS, CABBAGE and ZUCCHINI, grated, 2 GREEN ONIONS in matchsticks, 1 handful FRESH PARSLEY, 3 TBS. TOASTED SESAME SEEDS.
—Use with MUSTARD GARLIC SAUCE (page 167), if desired.

EVERGREEN SALAD

For 2 salads:

Mix 2 cups fine chopped mixed GREENS (romaine, endive, chicory, spinach), 1 small handful each WATERCRESS LEAVES, PARSLEY and CHIVES minced, and 2 Cup GREEN ONIONS, minced.
—Mix together juice of $^1/_2$ LEMON, 1 TBS. DIJON MUSTARD, 1 TBS. SESAME SEEDS, and 1 TBS. TOASTED SESAME OIL. Pour over salad.

LETTUCE & LEMON POTPOURRI

Make a mix of your favorite lettuces. Then mix together 2 TBS. FRESH LEMON JUICE 1 TBS. FRESH LIME JUICE, 1 teasp. HONEY, 1 teasp. ITALIAN HERBS, a pinch of CRACKED PEPPER and 1 TBS. OLIVE OIL. Toss with the lettuces until they glisten.

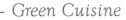
CUCUMBER BODY FLUSHING SALAD
For 6 large salads:

Slice and divide on salad plates 2 large CUCUMBERS and 3 large TOMATOES, $^1/_2$ cup CELERY sliced, and 1 RED PEPPER, finely chopped.
—Blend for a dressing: 1 CLOVE GARLIC, 2 TBS. fresh CHIVES chopped, $^1/_2$ LEMON, and 2 teasp. minced dry SEA VEGETABLES (any type).

FRESH GOULASH SALAD
For 4 salads:

Toss together 1 cup diced TOMATOES, 1 cup shredded or diced ZUCCHINI, 1 cup fresh CORN KERNELS, $^1/_4$ cup chopped BELL PEPPER, $^1/_4$ cup chopped GREEN ONION, pinches of THYME, OREGANO and MARJORAM.
—Make a fresh goulash sauce. Blend 1 TOMATO, 1 pinch CAYENNE PEPPER, 4 TBS. SUNFLOWER SEEDS, and juice of $^1/_2$ LEMON. Pour over the salad.

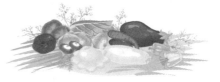

GUACAMOLE SALAD
For 2 to 4 salads:

Mash 1 ripe AVOCADO with the juice of 1 FRESH LEMON, and 1 teasp. GRANULATED DULSE.
—Mix with 2 TOMATOES diced, $^1/_2$ RED PEPPER diced, 1 TBS. ONION minced.

SPINACH & SPROUT SALAD
An excellent protein and greens salad to end a detox cleanse.
For 2 salads:

Wash and toss together 1 small bunch FRESH SPINACH LEAVES, 8-oz. fresh MUNG BEAN SPROUTS, and 2 CAKES TOFU diced or 4-oz. fresh sliced MUSHROOMS
—Toss with 2 TBS. TOASTED SESAME OIL, 2 TBS. BROWN RICE VINEGAR, 2 teasp. TAMARI, 2 teasp. minced CRYSTALLIZED GINGER (or $^1/_4$ teasp. GINGER POWDER) and 1 teasp. SESAME SALT. Chill.

MUSHROOMS AND GREENS
Toss all ingredients and add a dressing of your choice. Dark, chlorophyll-rich greens are delicious with mushrooms. Try watercress and mushrooms, too.
For 2 to 4 salads:

Toss together with 4 TBS. BALSAMIC VINEGAR: 2 Cups shredded SPINACH LEAVES, 4 TBS. minced GREEN ONIONS, 2 BEETS with tops in matchsticks, and 2 cups thin-sliced MUSHROOMS.

SPROUTS GALORE
For 6 salads:

Combine 4 cups MUNG and LENTIL BEAN SPROUTS, 4 TBS. TAMARI or Bragg's LIQUID AMINOS, 2 TBS. finely chopped GREEN ONIONS, ¹/₂ CLOVE GARLIC chopped, 2 TBS. OLIVE OIL, and 2 teasp. KELP.

SPROUTS PLUS
For 2 salads:

Toss together 1 tub ALFALFA SPROUTS, 2 cups GRATED CARROTS, 1 cup minced CELERY.

SESAME-MUSHROOM MEDLEY
For 6 salads:

Toss together everything in a bowl: 1 lb. MUSHROOMS sliced, 1 RED BELL PEPPER diced, 1 bunch SCALLIONS sliced, 1 teasp. CORIANDER, 2 TBS. TOASTED SESAME OIL, pinch CAYENNE PEPPER, and 3 TBS. each toasted BLACK and WHITE SESAME SEEDS.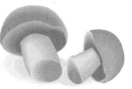
—Drizzle on 1 TBS. TAMARI, juice of 2 LIMES and 1 TB. MIRIN OR SAKE WINE.

MAKE A RAINBOW SALAD
Serve this salad on a round platter with each veggie in concentric "rainbow color arcs."
For 6 salads:

Prepare each vegetable separately. Thin-slice 2 cups PURPLE CABBAGE and 2 cups BROCCOFLOWER. Grate (or shred in a Salad Shooter) 3 small ZUCCHINI, 2 LARGE BEETS, 4 CARROTS, 3 small CROOKNECK SQUASH.
—Toss 3 TBS. toasted SESAME SEEDS, 3 TBS. TOASTED SESAME OIL, 2 TBS. TAMARI and 1 teasp. GARLIC POWDER in a small bowl.

WILD SPRING HERB AND FLOWER SALAD
For 6 salads:

Toss together ¹/₂ head ROMAINE LETTUCE, ¹/₂ head RED LEAF LETTUCE, ¹/₂ head FRISEE LETTUCE, ¹/₃ cup young NASTURTIUM LEAVES, ¹/₂ cup ARUGULA LEAVES ¹/₄ cup SWEET VIOLET FLOWERS, ¹/₃ cup SWEET VIOLET LEAVES, ¹/₄ cup FRESH DANDELION LEAVES, ¹/₄ cup ORANGE MINT LEAVES, ¹/₄ cup LEMON BALM LEAVES, and sprinkles of snipped DILL WEED and toasted SEA VEGETABLES.
—Drizzle with 3 TBS. OLIVE OIL and 2 TBS. BALSAMIC VINEGAR.

FOUR MUSHROOM IMMUNE BOOSTING SALAD

For 6 salads:

Sizzle for 3 minutes I TB. Olive or Sesame Oil with 2 Garlic Cloves minced and 2 teasp. minced Pickled Ginger. Add 3-oz. Oyster Mushrooms, 3-oz. Shiitake Mushrooms, 3 oz. Reishi Mushrooms, and 3-oz. Portobellas (or 3 oz. Maitake Mushrooms), and 2 TBS. Balsamic Vinegar. Sizzle 4 minutes.
—Add ¹/₄ cup Tamari, ¹/₄ cup Seasoned Stock and simmer 2 minutes.
—Finely slice I head Belgian Endive, ¹/₂ head Red Leaf Lettuce, ¹/₂ head Endive, I head Raddichio. Divide between salad plates and pile on mushroom mix.

SWEET & SOUR CUCUMBERS

For one salad:

Slice I Cucumber and ¹/₄ cup Red Onion.
—Mix together the dressing: 2 teasp. Olive Oil, 2 teasp. Honey, 3 teasp. Raspberry Vinegar.
—Chill, and top with I tablespoon of Plain or Lemon Yogurt.

SWEET & SOUR MIXED SALAD

For one large salad:

Slice I Cucumber and ¹/₂ Green or Red Bell Pepper very thin.
—Heat together until aromatic: 3 thin slices Red Onion, I teasp. Honey, ¹/₄ cup Tarragon Vinegar, and I teasp. fresh (or dried) Daikon Radish. Toss with veggies. Serve on lettuce.
—Stir together the dressing: 6 TBS. Olive Oil, 4 TBS. Lime Juice, 4 TBS. Tomato Juice, and I teasp. Sesame Salt. Toss with veggies. Delicious!

CARROT & LEMON SALAD

For 2 salads:

Grate 2 cups Carrots. Toss with 2 TBS. Raisins, and 2 teasp. Fresh Mint minced
—Mix together 2 TBS. Lemon Juice, I ¹/₂ TBS. Canola Oil, ¹/₄ teasp. 5 Spice Powder, 2 teasp. Fresh Parsley minced, and I pinch Stevia Leaf. Spoon over carrots.

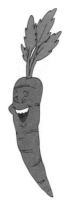

CARROT & CABBAGE SLAW

For 2 salads:

Whirl ¹/₂ head Chinese Cabbage and I Carrot in a food processor. Cover and chill.
—Mix the dressing 2 teasp. Honey, 3 TBS. Tarragon Vinegar, I teasp. Crystallized Ginger minced, I Green Onion minced with tops, ¹/₄ teasp. Sesame Salt. Toss with veggies and chill to marinate.

Simple sauces and dressings for your cleansing veggie salads.

Make fresh, right before serving if you can for best taste and nutrition.

BASIC VEGETABLE SAUCE

Almost every vegetable, or mix of veggies, can be blended with seasonings to make a low fat, cleansing dressing for salads. Options: Use avocado to bind after liquefying other ingredients. Add a little water into blender to help blend mixture.

Blend I VEGETABLE chopped, I TBS. granulated DULSE and I TBS. TAMARI, I TBS. OLIVE OIL —Optional: I teasp, GARLIC, GINGER or powdered MUSTARD.

MUSTARD GARLIC SAUCE

Blend ¹/₂ cup WALNUTS, 2 TBS. TAHINI, I TBS. DIJON MUSTARD, I LEMON, peeled, I teasp. GARLIC minced, I teasp. TAMARI, and WATER to thin slightly.

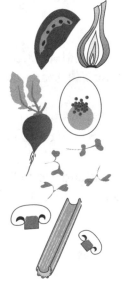

LOW FAT NORTHERN ITALIAN

For 1 salad:

Whisk together I TBS. fresh chopped PARSLEY, 2 teasp. WINE VINEGAR, pinch GARLIC/LEMON SEASONING, 2 teasp. LEMON JUICE, 2 teasp. OLIVE OIL, and I TBS. WATER or WHITE WINE.

AVOCADO DRESSING

Blend 3 AVOCADOS, ¹/₂ cup CELERY, ¹/₂ cup RED BELL PEPPER, ¹/₂ LEMON peeled, ¹/₂ cup chopped SCALLIONS, ¹/₂ cup PARSLEY, I teasp. GARLIC HERB SEASONING, and a little WATER to blend.

SOUTHWEST GUACAMOLE SAUCE

Blend 2 AVOCADOS, 6 to 8 DRIED TOMATOES, cut into pieces, 2 GREEN ONIONS, I LEMON peeled, I clove fresh GARLIC, I TBS. TAMARI, and WATER to blend.

ZUCCHINI SAUCE

Blend I medium ZUCCHINI grated, I small peeled JICAMA, ¹/₂ medium TOMATO, ¹/₂ AVOCADO, 2 SCALLIONS, ¹/₂ RED BELL PEPPER, I TBS. fresh minced BASIL, I clove GARLIC, I TBS. OLIVE OIL, ¹/₂ teasp. VEGETABLE SALT, I TBS. TAMARI, and 4 TBS. WATER.

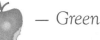

TAHINI & LEMON DRESSING

Blend 1 cup Tahini, 1 Lemon peeled, 1 clove fresh Garlic, 1 TBS. Honey, 1 sprig each fresh Basil and Thyme.

COOL MINT DRESSING

Blend 8 Mint Leaves, 2 teasp. Lemon Juice, 1 Cucumber, 2 TBS. Sesame Oil, and 1 TBS. Tamari.

GINGER-FLAXSEED DRESSING
For 2 cups:

Blend 1 Cucumber chopped, $\frac{1}{2}$ cup Sunflower Seeds, 1 TBS. Flax Seeds, 1 TBS. fresh grated Ginger, 1 teasp. Sesame Oil, and 1 $\frac{1}{2}$ cups Water.

SUNFLOWER SEED CREAM

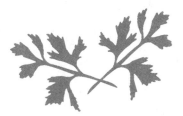

Blend 1 cup Sunflower Seeds, $\frac{1}{2}$ Lemon peeled, $\frac{1}{2}$ teasp. Tamari, $\frac{1}{2}$ teasp. Dulse, 1 sprig each fresh Basil and Sage, and 2 to 4 TBS. Water.

NO OIL TAMARI LEMON
For 1 salad:

Whisk in a bowl 2 TBS. Lemon Juice, 1 TBS. Tamari, 1 TBS. Honey, 1 teasp. Sesame Seeds, and 1 teasp minced Crystallized Ginger.

HONEY - MUSTARD DRESSING

Blend 2 TBS. Olive Oil, 1 teasp. Dijon Mustard, 1 TBS. Cider Vinegar, 1 teasp. Dried Dill, 1 teasp. Honey, and $\frac{1}{4}$ teasp. Lemon Pepper. Chill.

ORIGINAL HONEY FRENCH
For 6 salads:

Whisk together 1 cup Balsamic Vinegar, 2 TBS. Honey, 1 pinch Dry Mustard, 2 pinches Lemon Pepper, and 4 TBS. Canola Oil.

GINGER LEMON/LIME DRESSING

For 4 salads:

Whisk 1 cup LEMON YOGURT, 1 TBS. LIME JUICE, 1 TBS. LEMON JUICE, and $\frac{1}{2}$ teasp. GINGER POWDER.

HERBS & LEMON DRESSING

For 1 salad:

Whisk together 1 teasp. RASPBERRY VINEGAR, 1 teasp. LEMON JUICE, 1 TBS. FRESH PARSLEY chopped, 2 teasp. OLIVE OIL, $\frac{1}{4}$ teasp. DIJON MUSTARD, 1 teasp. FRESH BASIL minced, $\frac{1}{4}$ teasp. LEMON PEPPER, $\frac{1}{4}$ teasp. dry TARRAGON, $\frac{1}{4}$ teasp. dry OREGANO, and $\frac{1}{4}$ teasp. HONEY.

IMMUNE ENHANCING VINEGAR

This vinegar, rich with immune-boosting herbs, strengthens your system as it adds zip to salads. Both fresh and dried work. Warm the vinegar to help to release the herbal benefits. Except for the peppers, amounts of individual herbs aren't important; just fill the jar with what you have on hand. Use as you would any vinegar.

Pack a clean jar full of ECHINACEA LEAVES, SHIITAKE MUSHROOMS, ASTRAGALUS CHIPS, THYME, BASIL and SAGE LEAVES, 6 GARLIC CLOVES and 2 whole dry CAYENNE PEPPERS. Pour BROWN RICE or APPLE CIDER VINEGAR over herbs to cover. Let stand 4 to 6 weeks.

Salads With Sea Vegetables

Sea vegetables are natural cleansing superfoods. Their high antioxidant qualities make sea vegetables effective toxin scavengers that can help detoxify both the digestive and eliminative tracts. I try to eat them every day, and since I believe in a green salad every day, too, sea veggies and salads have become a staple combination in my lifestyle. Dried sea vegetables can be soaked in water and reconstituted before adding to a salad. Roasted nori or dulse flakes are a tasty, crunchy sprinkle on a salad before serving. They are also wonderful as part of a low-fat, nutritious salad dressing.

SESAME SEA VEGGIE VINAIGRETTE

For 3 salads:

Mix together $\frac{1}{4}$ cup TAMARI, 3 TBS. BROWN RICE VINEGAR, 1 teasp. each BLACK SESAME SEEDS and WHITE SESAME SEEDS, 1 TBS. TOASTED SESAME OIL, 1 TBS. SAKE, 2 teasp. HONEY, pinch GRANULATED DULSE.

WAKAME SALAD PICKLES

Use this recipe as an appetizer condiment or as a "pickle" garnish for any salad.

Soak I cup or $^1/_2$-oz. dried WAKAME until tender. Drain. Cut into quarter-inch strips.
—Mix $^1/_2$ teasp. TOASTED SESAME OIL, $^1/_4$ cup THIN SLICED RED ONION), I teasp. minced CRYSTALLIZED GINGER, and I teasp. HONEY and add to the WAKAME.

MARINATED SEA PALM WITH ROASTED RED PEPPERS

A perfect topper for salads, vegetables, grains, grilled salmon and swordfish.

Soak I-oz. dry SEA PALM FRONDS until tender. Drain.
—Mix 4 TBS. BALSAMIC VINEGAR, 2 roasted RED BELL PEPPERS thin-sliced (bottled okay), 2 teasp. LEMON PEPPER, 4 CLOVES GARLIC minced, $^1/_2$ cup SESAME OIL, 2 TBS. fresh minced MIXED HERBS (like rosemary, basil and thyme), 3 TBS. HONEY, and 2 TBS. crystallized GINGER ROOT minced.
—Pour over SEA PALM and let marinate for about 4 hours before serving.

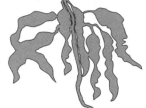

WATERCRESS AND HERB SALAD

Mix I bunch WATERCRESS SPRIGS, I bunch fresh PARSLEY, I teasp. minced GAR-LIC, I cup fresh BASIL LEAVES chopped, 2 TBS. dry snipped NORI or SEA PALM, 2 TBS. minced fresh TARRAGON, I TBS. minced fresh SAGE LEAVES, 2 TBS minced fresh MARJORAM LEAVES, 2 TBS. OLIVE OIL, $^1/_4$ teasp. CAYENNE PEPPER, I TBS. fresh LEMON JUICE, and I $^1/_2$ TBS. WATER.

SESAME NORI NO-OIL SALAD DRESSING

A delicious recipe to introduce sea vegetables—as a condiment for a low-fat diet.

Combine in a jar and shake vigorously to blend: I cup snipped TOASTED NORI SHEETS, 4 TBS. BROWN RICE VINEGAR, 3 TBS. pan roasted SESAME SEEDS, I cup ONION or MUSHROOM BROTH, and I teasp. TAMARI or BRAGG's LIQUID AMINOS. Serve over vegetable or rice salads, or ramen noodles.

SEA VEGGIE SOUP AND SALAD SPRINKLE SUPREME

This blend is a flavor enhancer, and a nutritional part of any recipe. Crumble into a bowl; then just barely blend in the blender, so that there are still sizeable chunks of the sea vegetables. They expand in any recipe with liquid, and when heated, return to the beautiful green color they had in the ocean. Use freely as a seasoning on salads, soups and rice.

Heat in a dry pan, $^3/_4$ cup chopped dried DULSE, $^1/_2$ cup dried chopped NORI or SEA PALM, $^1/_4$ cup chopped dried WAKAME, $^1/_4$ cup chopped dried KOMBU, $^1/_4$ cup chopped toasted WALNUTS, and $^1/_2$ cup toasted SESAME SEEDS.

Sea vegetable main dishes for a detox diet:

Modern science is validating many of the traditional benefits of sea plants, especially in relation to their algin content. In fact, the alginic acids in sea vegetables perform a dual miracle. First, algin absorbs toxins from the digestive tract in much the same way that a water softener removes the hardness from tap water. It binds with the ions of toxic heavy metals which are then converted to harmless salts. The salts are insoluble in the intestine and are excreted, so less toxins enter the circulatory system. Second, algin also chelates radioactive matter present in the human body and binds it for elimination via the large intestine. Algin compounds are also thought to be responsible for much of the success of seaweeds in the treatment of obesity, asthma, atherosclerosis and blood purifying.

Still, even though scientists know that algin compounds in seaweeds directly counteract carcinogens, most researchers believe that sea plants primarily boost the body's immune system, allowing it to combat the carcinogens itself.

Sun-dried, packaged sea vegetables retain almost all of their health advantages. The recipes here can be used over a lifetime as part of your immune-boosting detox maintenance plan.

I can't think of a seaweed I don't like... so I've offered a sampling to give you an idea of their great variety and taste. They're good in soups, with cooked vegetables, over hot rice, even in sandwiches.

Nori:

The popularity of sushi has introduced many Americans to the sweetness of nori. But this delicate sea vegetable with its distinctive nutty taste is far more versatile. Nori (and its American cousin, laver) is the highest in B-complex vitamins, as well as vitamin C and E.

Nori, and its American counterpart *laver*, is easy to roast. Spread the dried plant on a baking sheet, sprinkle with teriyaki sauce and bake at 300° for 5 to 8 minutes until crisp but not burned.

HIGH PROTEIN SPROUTED NORI ROLLS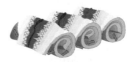

Blender blend a nut and seed mixture: 2 cups ALMONDS and 1 cup SUNFLOWER or SESAME SEEDS, $^1/_2$ teasp. SESAME OIL, 1 LEMON peeled, 1 TBS. fresh chopped GINGER (or PICKLED GINGER), and 3 TBS. TAMARI. Add a little water if needed to blend.

—Lay out 6 to 10 TOASTED NORI SHEETS. Spread nut-seed mixture over sheets. Spread 3 cups ALFALFA or SUNFLOWER SPROUTS across nut and seed mix, forming a line down the edge of the sheet.

—Cut 1 CARROT, 1 AVOCADO and 1 CUCUMBER into long thin sticks and place lengthwise across nori. Roll up like a burrito. Then eat like a burrito, or cut in 2" thick rolls and decorate with fresh BASIL LEAVES, SWEET-HOT MUSTARD or a dab of WASABI SAUCE.

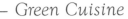

SUSHI MAIN DISH SALAD

California maki in a bowl—with the same great taste of sushi rolls.
For 4 salads:

Toast 1 cup BROWN RICE, or WILD and BROWN RICE mixed in a dry pan til aromatic.
—Add 2 cups WATER or LIGHT MISO BROTH. Bring to a boil, cover and simmer 30 minutes until all liquid is absorbed. Remove from heat.
—Mix and toss in a bowl: 1 AVOCADO chopped, 3 SCALLIONS minced, 1 cup KING CRAB PIECES, 2 TBS. BROWN RICE VINEGAR and a pinch WASABI POWDER. Crumble a toasted NORI SHEET over the top.

Serve with a dab of **HOT MUSTARD DRESSING**:
Mix 4 teasp. CHINESE HOT MUSTARD, 1 TB. TAMARI, pinch WASABI PWDR., 2 TBS. TOASTED SESAME OIL.

Sea Palm:

Sea palm is a rare ocean vegetable that looks like a miniature palm tree attached to the rocks on the California coast. It lives in the pounding surf of the shoreline, bending and waving in the tides instead of the winds. It has become very popular in California healthy food recipes for its sweet taste and versatility.

Sea palm is delicious. Mix SEA PALM FRONDS in a bowl with chopped ALMONDS or SUNFLOWER or PUMPKIN SEEDS and 2 TBS. TERIYAKI SAUCE. Roast in a 325° oven for 8 to 10 minutes until dry and crunchy. Then sprinkle the mix over a pizza or rice and roast it in. Yum!

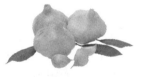

SEA PALM & TOFU CASSEROLE

For 6 servings:

Soak 1-oz. dried SEA PALM FRONDS in water. Drain and cut in 2-inch lengths. Place in a pan with a little water, cover and simmer for 20 minutes until tender.
—Mash 1 lbs. TOFU with the tender sea vegetables and toss with 1 teasp. dry BASIL and 1 teasp. dry OREGANO.
—Make the sauce: dice 1 large ONION and 1 1/2 lbs. CARROTS. Sauté in 2 TBS. CANOLA OIL or ONION BROTH for 10 minutes. Remove from heat and puree in the blender with 3 TBS. UMEBOSHI PASTE or SWEET AND SOUR SAUCE. Toss with palm fronds; mix in a skillet to heat.
—Make the topping: puree 1/3 cup toasted SESAME SEEDS in the blender with 1 teasp. TAMARI, 6 SPRIGS FRESH PARSLEY and enough WATER to make a thick sauce. Spread on tofu mixture in the skillet, and cook for 5 more minutes to heat. Serve hot.

Ocean Ribbons:

Ocean ribbons are a brown sea plant, thin and delicate like Japanese Kombu, but noticeably sweeter and more tender. They grow on the outermost reaches of the rocky inter-

tidal zone among sea palm and mussel beds, looking like a glistening miniature willow trees overhanging the water at low tide. You can watch ocean ribbons keep the environment clean. Branching off the woody trunk of a mature ocean ribbon plant, over 500 blades sweep its rock face clear of other organisms in the thrashing tidal surges. I like ribbons best with vegetables, in light soups and as a pickled side dish or topping for rice.

OCEAN RIBBONS PICKLES

For 4 servings:

Soak 6 strips OCEAN RIBBONS in cold water for 15 minutes, then chop in 3-inch pieces. Slice 1 RED ONION very thin in crescents. Slice thinly 1 long EUROPEAN CUCUMBER. Layer veggies in a flat bowl and cover with equal parts MIRIN, TAMARI and UME PLUM VINEGAR. Press with a weight for 3 hours. Toss and serve.

DEEP DETOX STEW

This is a variation on a Traditional Chinese Medicine immune-supporting stew. It helps reduce cholesterol, regulate blood pressure and aid fat digestion.

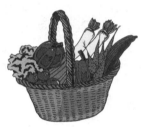

For 6 bowls:

Soak til soft, about 20 minutes: 18 dried SHIITAKE MUSHROOMS, half a 3-oz package of dried BLACK FUNGUS or REISHI MUSHROOMS, and 2-oz. dried OCEAN RIBBONS SEAWEED in 6 cups WATER. Save soaking water. Sliver mushrooms and ribbons.

—Roast $1/4$ cup each BLACK and WHITE SESAME SEEDS in a dry skillet. Combine with $1/3$ cup miso and 3 TBS. of the mushroom-seaweed stock. Set aside.

—Slice thinly the white and pale green parts of 2 LEEKS and wash. Matchstick-cut 1 fresh BURDOCK ROOT and 1 DAIKON RADISH. Thinly cut 1 BUNCH BOK CHOY.

—Sizzle LEEKS and 3 CLOVES GARLIC in 2 TBS. SESAME OIL for several minutes until aromatic. Add burdock and daikon roots and mushroom-seaweed soaking water. Cover, and let stew 10 minutes until burdock is tender. Mix in MISO-SESAME paste, and add bok choy, mushrooms and ocean ribbons. Cover and cook a few minutes until bok choy is tender. Season with 1 TBS. TAMARI.

Wakame:

Wakame, and it's American cousin *alaria*, are mild and smooth, excellent with rice, black beans and cous-cous. Wakame's heavyweight minerals, enzymes and fiber, but light-weight texture and flavor, make it perfect for cleansing soups and salads.
I like to roast wakame before I use it in a grain or pizza recipe. Just snip bite-sized pieces and roast for 3 to 5 minutes at 300°. Use right from the package for soups. Blanch wakame for 20 minutes in hot water before using in a salad. Then cut out midribs and toss with your greens. Pan-fry as a snack in a little toasted sesame oil and tamari until dark green and crisp.

QUICK WAKAME SUCCOTASH
For 4 servings:

Soak 1-oz. dried WAKAME in water for 30 minutes. Drain and steam for 10 minutes until tender. Snip into 1-inch pieces, removing the tough stems. Cook a 10-oz. package of frozen SUCCOTASH VEGETABLES and 1 CUBE TOFU crumbled in a pan according to package directions.

—Sauté 1 thin-sliced RED ONION in 2 teasp. CANOLA OIL until fragrant. Toss with vegetables and wakame. Add and toss 2 TBS. minced CHIVES and 2 TBS. UMEBOSHI PLUM or BROWN RICE VINEGAR, and let marinate for 3 to 4 hours before serving.

MILLET SALAD WITH WAKAME
For 4 salads:

Roast 1 cup MILLET in a dry pan until aromatic. Add 2 $\frac{1}{2}$ cups WATER and cover. Cook 25 minutes. Remove from heat and fluff.

—Snip $\frac{1}{2}$ cup WAKAME pieces into hot water. Blanch 3 minutes. Remove with a slotted spoon. Keep water hot and dice in $\frac{1}{2}$ cup CARROTS, $\frac{1}{4}$ cup CELERY, $\frac{1}{3}$ cup DAIKON RADISH. Blanch 5 minutes and drain. Season with LEMON PEPPER. Add $\frac{1}{2}$ cup snipped FRESH PARSLEY, $\frac{1}{2}$ cup diced CUCUMBER, a handful of DRY ROASTED ALMONDS. Toss all together with millet, and serve on lettuce with:

SESAME MISO DRESSING:
For 1$\frac{1}{2}$ cups dressing:

Blender blend a scant $\frac{1}{3}$ cup plain SESAME OIL, 1 TBS. LIGHT MISO, 2 TBS. TOASTED SESAME OIL, 2 TBS. BROWN RICE VINEGAR, $\frac{1}{2}$ teasp. VEGGIE SALT, 1 TBS. LEMON JUICE, 3 TBS. SESAME SEEDS toasted, dashes CAYENNE or HOT PEPPER SAUCE.

Kelp and Kombu:
Kelp and kombu is an all-purpose sea veggies. It's delicious in soups in place of chicken or beef stock—especially on a cleansing diet. Just put a strip in for flavor as you make the soup. Then, remove or chop in when the soup is ready. You don't have to add salt if you use kelp. Its minerals provide a salty flavor by themselves. Kelp and kombu are extra good with beans because natural glutamates tenderizes them.

KELP & HONEY BITS SNACK
Soak dried kelp or kombu pieces in water until soft. Drain and snip into bite size pieces to fill $\frac{1}{2}$ cup. Bring $\frac{1}{4}$ cup HONEY and $\frac{1}{2}$ cup WATER to a boil. Reduce heat, add sea vegetables and simmer until liquid is evaporated, about an hour. Spread 1 cup SESAME SEEDS, or GROUND ALMONDS on a baking sheet and arrange sea vegetables on top, turning with tongs to coat. Bake in a 300°F oven for 30 minutes.

COUSCOUS, RED LENTILS & KELP
A delicious low fat, high protein cleansing meal.
For 6 servings:

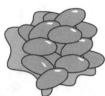

Bring 1 ¹/₄ cups WATER to a boil. Add 1 cup COUSCOUS, 2 TBS. CANOLA OIL and a 5-inch piece of KELP. Stir, cover and remove from heat. Allow to stand 5 minutes. Fluff with a fork.

—Remove kelp from couscous, mince and sauté with ¹/₂ cup chopped LEEKS, (white parts only) for 5 minutes in 2 TBS. ONION BROTH.

—Add 2 cups VEGETABLE STOCK and 1 cup RED LENTILS and 1 chopped TOMATO. Stir in 1 teasp. TAMARI, 1 teasp. BASMATI VINEGAR, 1 teasp. GARLIC/LEMON SEASONING and dashes CAYENNE. Reduce heat, cover and simmer for 20 minutes.

KOMBU SALAD WITH VINEGAR SAUCE
For 4 salads:

Snip a handful of dried of KOMBU (or WAKAME) into 1-inch lengths. Soak for 1 hour in RICE VINEGAR or LEMON JUICE. (Acidity tenderizes the sea vegetables). Rinse, drain, set aside.

—Peel and halve 1 EUROPEAN-TYPE CUCUMBER and cut into matchsticks. Sprinkle with SEA SALT and put in a colander over a pan to drain for 30 minutes. Squeeze out any remaining excess water and set aside.

—Toss CUCUMBER and KOMBU with 8-oz. CORN NIBLETS and then mix the salad with:

VINEGAR SAUCE:

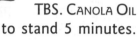

Mix together 1 TBS. BROWN RICE VINEGAR, 1 teasp. CHILI POWDER or 2 to 3 dashes of HOT PEPPER SAUCE, 1 crushed CLOVE GARLIC, 1 TBS. HONEY, 1 TBS. pan-roasted SESAME SEEDS, and ¹/₂ bunch GREEN ONIONS with tops, finely chopped.
—Serve on tiny appetizer plates.

Dulse:
Dulse has a nutty, seafood-bacon taste, so it's great in dips, sandwiches, soups, salads and stir-fries. A rich red seaweed, it's a good source of iron, B vitamins, plant protein and fiber. Cooking with dulse is a treat. You can pan-fry it in a oil-sprayed pan until the pieces turn brownish and crisp like chips. You can dry-roast the pieces in a 300° oven until they turn greenish - not black (burned). Then crumble the crispy pieces onto grains, soups, pizza and popcorn.

I love roasted dulse ground in the blender with walnuts, dried tomatoes and dry basil. Mmmmmm - I use it as a condiment on lots of steamed veggie dishes.

Dulse can be used like bacon bits in sandwiches, chip dips, soups and stir fries.

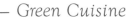

— Green Cuisine

BROWN RICE, DULSE & TOFU

The protein complementarity of brown rice, dulse and tofu is good for a healing diet.
For 8 servings:

Soak 8 dried SHIITAKE MUSHROOMS and a small handful DRIED DULSE in WATER to cover. Sliver both when soft and set aside. Reserve soaking water.

—Dry roast 1$\frac{1}{3}$ cups BROWN RICE in a pan; then cook in 2$\frac{1}{2}$ cups WATER (4 cups cooked).

—Sauté 2 cubed CAKES TOFU in 2 TBS. SESAME OIL in a skillet, and add to rice.

—Add 1 TBS. SESAME OIL to skillet and sauté 2 minced CLOVES GARLIC and 1 chopped ONION until translucent. Add 1 teasp. BREWER'S YEAST FLAKES, 1 teasp. CUMIN POWDER, 1 teasp. SESAME SEEDS, and $\frac{1}{4}$ teasp. LEMON PEPPER until spices are fragrant. Mix into rice.

—Add and sauté until color changes 2 CARROTS, 2 STALKS CELERY and 2 ZUCCHINI chopped, chopped, 1 GREEN BELL PEPPER in matchsticks, the MUSHROOMS and DULSE.

—Add mushroom soaking water and steam-braise for 5 minutes. Vegetables should be just tender crisp, not completely cooked. Add to rice and tofu. Season with HERB SALT.

BROWN RICE, DULSE & GREENS CLASSIC

For 6 main dish servings:

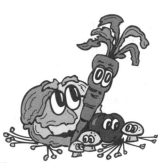

Have ready 4 cups cooked BROWN RICE. Toast $\frac{1}{2}$ cup chopped WALNUTS, $\frac{1}{4}$ cup chopped DULSE and 2 TBS. SESAME SEEDS in a 300° oven for 8 minutes.

—Shred or finely chop 1 cup each ROMAINE LETTUCE, CHINESE NAPPA CABBAGE, BOK CHOY, SPINACH LEAVES, 1 CARROT diced, and 1 slice ONION chopped.

—Preheat a large wok. Add 3 to 4 TBS. SESAME OIL, $\frac{1}{2}$ teasp. fresh MINCED GINGER and 1 minced CLOVE GARLIC. Heat until fragrant. Add carrots and onion and sauté for 5 minutes.

—Add the greens and toss just until color changes. Add 1$\frac{1}{2}$ cups BEAN SPROUTS or SUNFLOWER SPROUTS. Toss to coat and heat. Add brown rice and mix briefly. Turn off heat.

—Make a well in the center and add 1 EGG (optional). Toss for 3 minutes until hot and set. Turn onto large serving platter. Top with WALNUTS, DULSE, SESAME SEEDS, SESAME SALT and 1 TB. TAMARI.

BLACK-BEAN & DULSE CHILI

For 6 bowls:

Soak $\frac{1}{2}$-oz. SHIITAKE MUSHROOMS, $\frac{1}{2}$-oz. BLACK FUNGUS MUSHROOMS and $\frac{1}{2}$ oz. dry DULSE in water to cover. Drain, save soaking water and sliver mushrooms and dulse. Chop finely 2-inch piece DAIKON RADISH, 1 CLOVE GARLIC minced and 1-inch FRESH GINGER.

—Simmer $\frac{1}{2}$ cup BLACK BEANS, 6 cups VEGETABLE STOCK, the mushrooms, dulse and herbs, 2 TBS. ground PASILLI CHILI, 1 teasp. ground CHILI NEGRO and 1 teasp. HERB SALT for 1 hour.

—Add 1 cup fresh STRING BEANS until bubbly and fragrant.

—Top with $\frac{1}{2}$ cup TOASTED PUMPKIN SEEDS and $\frac{1}{2}$ cup fresh MINCED CILANTRO.

Want to know more about the herbs in your detox program?

This chapter includes herbs from all types and traditions of body cleansing methods.

Materia Medica
of detoxification herbs

This *materia medica* is a short, quick-look catalogue of notable herbs for detoxification and cleansing. While many of the herbs have a wide range of therapeutic activity, the elements discussed in this listing are those that specifically relate to their cleansing activity.

• **Agrimony,** *Agrimonia eupatoria,* Family: *Rosaceae*
Common Names: sticklewort, cocklebur, church steeples, philanthropos, burr marigold, agrimonia (Sp), egrimony (Gr), eupatoire des ancines (Fr).
Traditional Use: Used in Greek and Roman times, and in the Middle Ages as an herb for liver cleansing, often with mugwort and vinegar. Agrimony-honey tea was effective for jaundice. It was in continuous use throughout Renaissance Europe for the ague (flu). Native Americans used agrimony as a cleanser and strengthener of the liver and blood.
Medicinal Parts: root, leaves
Preparation Forms: tea, extract, capsules, poultice, skin or eye wash. OK for children and for long term use. Agrimony ointment shrinks bleeding hemorrhoids, and is effective in a uterine bolus to arrest bleeding; leaves may be used as an anal suppository with cocoa butter. Dosage: tea: 3 cups daily; extract: 1-3 ml 3x daily; child: fractional dose depending on age.
Nutrition Profile: high in tannins, flavonoids, polysaccharides, vitamins B and K, iron and thiamine.
Herbal Healing Actions: a bitters tonic with superior astringent properties that contract and harden tissue; an anti-inflammatory, analgesic, hemostatic and vermifuge; an antiviral that works well with other anti-infective herbs. A cardiotonic tonic. Reduces cholesterol.
Cleansing Properties & Detox Activity: Works chiefly to cleanse and strengthen the liver, especially as a spring tonic where its "bitters" stimulation wakes up digestive secretions. A valuable remedy for urinary incontinence and cystitis. A diuretic that allows fluids to pass more readily through the kidneys. A good stomach tonic for acidity and gastric ulcers (hemostatic to help curtail ulcer bleeding). Helps arrest bleeding from the uterus (a sign of cervical cancer). Helpful for diarrhea (especially child diarrhea and child pinworms), flaccid bowel and bladder tissue, and as a suppository for hemorrhoids. A vaginal cleanser - soak cotton balls in a strong tea and insert into the vagina overnight once a week to treat trichomonas vaginitis with itching. May be taken as a tea by breast-feeding mothers to dose their babies. A childhood suppository for tapeworms and diarrhea is effective.
Safety Precautions: Should not be used when you are constipated.
Synergy With Other Herbs: 1) A cleansing douche: equal parts *agrimony, mullein* and *slippery elm.* 2) A hemostatic to stop bleeding: equal parts *agrimony, cinnamon bark* and *yarrow* (add *bilberry* for more astringency and *marshmallow root* for inflammation).

• **Alfalfa,** *Medicago sativa,* Family: *Leguminoseae*
Common Names: buffalo herb (Iraq), mielga (Spain), mu su, purple medic, sai pi ka (China).
Traditional Use: Discovered in North Africa by the Arabs, who called it the "father of all foods." Native Americans used alfalfa as a green vegetable to alleviate jaundice and encourage blood clotting. Early Chinese physicians and Ayurvedic physicians of India used alfalfa to treat digestive disorders, ulcers, as a diuretic and in treatment of arthritis.
Medicinal Parts: leaves, flowering tops and seeds.

Preparation Forms: tea, tincture, extract, capsules and sprouts Dosage: tea: 6 oz. 3x daily; tincture: 5-10 drops 3x daily; extract: $^{1}/_{2}$ to 1 tsp. 3x daily; capsules: 2 caps 3-4 times daily with meals.

Nutrition Profile: a highly nutritive herb, rich in vitamin C (can even counteract scurvy), carotenes, vitamin K, amino acids, octacosonal and a full spectrum of minerals and trace minerals; an excellent source of fiber and chlorophyll with a balance of elements almost identical to human hemoglobin. One of the world's richest mineral foods, pulling up earth sources from root depths as great as 130 feet!

Herbal Healing Actions: a laxative, natural diuretic, and anti-hemorrhaging agent.

Cleansing Properties & Detox Activity: Alfalfa binds and neutralizes a wide range of carcinogenic agents in the colon, and is a proven nutritive for colon cancer prevention.. As a green superfood, alfalfa helps neutralize allergens, overcome anemia and jaundice, and balance over-acidity. It is used therapeutically for arthritis, bursitis and gout, stimulating removal of inorganic mineral deposits from the blood. As a blood clotting agent, it counteracts internal bleeding from ulcers. It is an estrogen precursor for menopause. Alfalfa is beneficial for indigestion, in reducing blood sugar levels, in lowering cholesterol and in the prevention of tooth decay. It is a healer for a wide range of intestinal and skin disorders, liver problems, breath and body odor, even morning sickness.

Safety Precautions: none in common use

Synergy With Other Herbs: With *pau d' arco* and mineral-rich herbs like *carrot root* to help detoxify, rebuild and restore foundation body strength. With *dandelion* for better digestion and to detoxify the liver. With *yucca* to help relieve pain and inflammation of arthritis.

• **Aloe Vera,** *Aloe barbadensis, Aloe vera,* Family: *Liliaceae*

Common Names: burn plant, medicine plant, lily of the desert, aloes des jardins (Haiti), aloes do cabo (Brazil), cape aloes, zabila (Mexico, Venezuela), bitter aloes, hepatic or horse aloes (U.S.).

Traditional Use: Originating in Africa, aloe vera's healing and cleansing powers are referenced in almost every healing tradition, both ancient and modern. Some therapeutic recommendations are as old as 3500 years. Its purging action was highly valued in ancient herbal therapy. Known in ancient Greece and Egypt, and protected since the 4th century B.C., aloe was so prized that Aristotle persuaded Alexander the Great to wage war against the Island of Xocotra to obtain aloe for his soldiers' wounds. Cleopatra attributed her irresistible skin to the use of aloe. The Chinese used aloe for stomach ailments and skin disorders and to strengthen digestion. As early as 700 A.D. aloe was a treatment for sinusitis, eczema, dizziness, red eyes and constipation.

Medicinal Parts: bottom leaves yield the most gel with the most healing potential.

Preparation Forms: juice, gel, poultice (esp. with comfrey), capsules. Dosage: external: cover affected area 3x a day; internal: 1 TSP. of juice 3x daily as a cathartic. Effective in ridding children of roundworms by injection: 10 grains to 3-oz of water.

Nutrition Profile: Aloe has medicinal amounts of protein for healing, almost 18% dietary fiber, up to 5% of 22 amino acids and all B complex vitamins. Aloe contains active enzymes for enzyme therapy. Skin-building nutrients include vitamin E, selenium and silicon.

Herbal Healing Actions: a laxative, stomach and liver tonic, blood cleanser, antiseptic, emollient, vermifuge and antioxidant with free-radical scavenging effects. Has antibacterial, anti-tumor and antifungal properties; inhibits replication of herpes and the HIV virus. Has active anti-diabetic compounds; and salicylates with anti-inflammatory, pain-killing characteristics. Its enzyme carboxpeptidase hydrolyzes the inflammatory mediators responsible for burn wound fluid leakage. Contains magnesium lactate which inhibits histamine reactions that cause skin itching and irritation.

Cleansing Properties & Detox Activity: Aloe juice penetrates injured tissue, relieving pain through anti-inflammatory activity; dilates capillaries to increase blood supply to an injured area. Aloe is a colon, bowel and digestive cleanser. Both aloe vera gel and juice are beneficial for gastrointestinal complaints, like diverticulitis, peptic, gastric or duodenal ulcers, Crohn's disease and ulcerative colitis. Aloe treats liver

symptoms like jaundice and cirrhosis. (Tests on liver cirrhosis show that after six months of aloe treatment normal liver enzymes are achieved.) Aloe also contains a substance which inhibits liver cancer. Because of its blood cleansing qualities, drug detoxing patients treated with aloe have fewer complications than those given regular therapy. Synergistic with vitamin C in treating arthritis, aloe helps prevent or slow tissue breakdown and reduce inflammation.

Safety Precautions: Evaporated aloe concentrate is a purgative; large doses can cause rectal piles. Don't take internally during pregnancy or nursing (it will purge the suckling child).

Synergy With Other Herbs: A tea of *aloe, fennel, catnip* and *St. John's wort* cleanses the liver and reduces stomach cramping. As a poultice: with *comfrey* (50:50). With *ginger* as a liver tonic.

• **Astragalus,** *Astragalus membranaceous (Huang chi)*, Family: *Leguminosae*
Common Names: yellow vetch, milk vetch, locoweed, poison vetch and bok kee.
Medicinal Parts: root
Preparation Forms: liquid and powdered extract, tea. Dosage: for health maintenance: 2 capsules 3x daily at mealtime; for recovery from illness: 4 capsules 4x daily.
Traditional Use: An ancient remedy, used in China for 2000 years to strengthen immunity, boost respiratory health, accelerate wound healing and increase energy. 4,000 years ago, Shen-nong, the ruler of China, credited Astragalus as a first class herb in the oldest herbal reference book known, *Shen'nong Bencaojing*. Astragalus is still considered "the superior tonic" in Traditional Chinese Medicine.
Nutrition Profile: high in flavonoids, amino acids and trace minerals including selenium. Rich in key nutrients like folic acid, calcium, iron and potassium. Immuno-active polysaccharides are responsible for its amazing immune-defense power.
Herbal Healing Actions: Immune stimulating adaptogen (especially for nerve and hormone systems), a strong chi tonic, vasodilator and antiviral. A liver protecting and toning herb, its primary use is in immune resistance building, even against the immune-suppressing effects of cancer drugs and radiation. Antioxidant, adaptogen qualities prevent cellular damage from free radicals.
Cleansing Properties & Detox Activity: Astragalus is a toning diuretic in kidney inflammation formulas. It nourishes exhausted adrenals to combat fatigue. It is a strong antiviral agent, producing extra interferon in the body. Promotes the regeneration of bronchi cells after a viral infection. Astragalus stimulates immune system white blood cell activity to help destroy invading microorganisms. Damaged immune system cells taken from cancer patients have been restored to full function in tests with Astragalus extract. Astragalus also increases the number of stem cells in bone marrow and lymphatic tissue to stimulate their development into immune cells. Astragalus is especially useful in the rebuilding and maintaining stages of a cleanse to increase disease resistance against repeated infections.

Vasodilating properties help significantly lower blood pressure, reduce excess fluid retention, and improve circulation. Chinese experts use astragalus as a valuable anticlotting agent in preventing coronary heart disease and to strengthen heartbeat.
Safety Precautions: Do not take if you have an acute disease, high fever or severe inflammation.
Synergy With Other Herbs: For anemia: a tea with equal parts *astragalus* and *angelica*, 2 cups daily. For cold and numbness: a tea with 2 parts *astragalus bark* and 1 part *cinnamon bark*, 1 cup twice a day. In combination with *ligustrum* to boost the immune system.

• **Barberry,** *Berberis vulgaris*, Family: *Berberidaceae*
Common Names: agracejo (Sp), amberparis (Turk), barberry, epine vinette (Fr), sowberry, jaundice berry, pepperidge bush, guild tree, woodsour, maiden barberry.
Medicinal Parts: bark of stem and root, and berries.
Preparation Forms: The tea is a valuable astringent for swollen spleen and chronic, inflamed stom-

ach problems taken 3x a day in tablespoons before meals. Dosage: Barberry is a "bitters" herb, take in small doses. Capsules: 2, 3x a day; tincture: $^1/_2$ to 1 tsp.; tea: 2-3 TBS. 3x a day; extract: 10-20 drops every 3-4 hours (extract has the widest range of effects).

Traditional Use: Barberry was regarded in folk medicine as a more valuable liver remedy than either goldenseal or Oregon grape. It was a popular traditional treatment for all forms of abdominal inflammation. Employed the Far East as an anti-diarrheal and anti-infective herb, as long as 3000 years ago. Native Americans used the root tea as a blood tonic, cough medicine, for kidney ailments and to arrest hemorrhaging. In Ayurvedic medicine it is used with turmeric to regulate liver and digestion.

Nutrition Profile: rich in vitamin C and fiber, the root has about 6.6% protein. Has measureable B vitamins, and the minerals calcium, chromium, cobalt, magnesium, potassium, selenium and silicon.

Herbal Healing Actions: Berberine, the most notable ingredient, is a strong antiseptic, and a potent activator of macrophages, cells responsible for destroying bacteria, viruses, yeast and tumor cells. Barberry is a laxative stimulant, blood purifier, diuretic, bitter tonic, and astringent.

Cleansing Properties & Detox Activity: Barberry's bitters compounds improve digestion, stimulate bile production, dilate blood vessels and have a mild laxative effect for cleansing. Anti-microbial against a wide range of organisms, including *candida albicans* yeast, and several intestinal parasites. Diarrhea is a common symptom of *candidiasis*—barberry has remarkable anti-diarrhea activity even in severe cases.

Barberry's astringent compounds tighten and shrink inflamed tissues. In the upper digestive organs, (liver, stomach and duodenum), barberry's bitters break up and remove morbid matter from the intestinal tract, while helping bile to flow more freely through a stagnant liver and gallbladder, important for liver problems. Barberry helps clean out bronchial mucous clogs, and is a recuperative tonic for bronchitis and the early stages of tuberculosis. Barberry dilates the blood vessels, so it's good for high blood pressure. It is a specific for diseases like cholera and its malicious side effects like scabs, itch, tetters, and ringworm.

Safety Precautions: Use only root and berries - small doses for best effects. (Leaves and seeds contain methylcysticine a poisonous purgative in large doses.) Do not take if there is digestive weakness. Avoid use as a single herb during pregnancy. A high dose may slow down the heart muscle and respiratory system, constricting the bronchial tubes. Discontinue if the tincture causes nosebleeds or dizziness.

Synergy With Other Herbs: With *turmeric* to regulate liver function. With *cayenne, golden seal and lobelia* is a specific for jaundice and hepatitis. Equal parts with *wild yam root* helps eliminate gas. With *goldenseal, burdock, yellow dock, fringe tree* and *wild cherry* as a body cleanser.

• **Barley Grass,** *Hordeum Vulgare*; Family: *Gramineae*

Common Names: kung mai nieh, no mai (China), barley (Egypt), cebada (Spain), orzo (Italian).

Traditional Use: One of the most ancient grains in human food, the use of barley for medicinal purposes dates back all the way to 7000 BC. Barley seeds have been found in tombs in Asia Minor dating back to 3500 B.C. As a grain, it was used to strengthen and soothe and mainly recommended for people who are recovering from illness. In ancient Rome, gladiators ate barley for strength and stamina.

Medicinal Parts: stem and juice

Preparation Forms: drink, capsules, powder and extract. Dosage: 2-3 capsules 3x daily, or one to two tsp. daily. For recovery: 6-8 capsules daily. For weight loss: take before meals with an 8-oz. glass of water.

Nutrition Profile: Barley has a broad spectrum of concentrated vitamins, minerals, enzymes, proteins, chlorophyllins and antioxidants. Considered a "superfood," and an exceptional source of protein and essential amino acids, barley has eleven times the calcium of cow's milk, five times the iron of spinach, and seven times the vitamin C and bioflavonoids as orange juice. One of its most important contributions is to the vegetarian diet with 80mcg of vitamin B_{12} per hundred grams of powdered juice. Barley also contains glucan, the same fiber found in oat bran to reduce cholesterol levels. Barley (along with alfalfa) is one of the few foods that contains enough nutrition to sustain life from birth to old age.

Herbal Healing Actions: a digestive, diuretic, expectorant, stomachic, emollient, and nutritive, bar-

ley is especially effective for the bladder, kidneys, reproductive and lung areas.

Cleansing Properties & Detox Activity: Barley, rich in chlorophyll, normalizes metabolism and neutralizes heavy metals like mercury in the body that precipitate disease. Its small molecular proteins are absorbed directly through the cell membranes to purify and rebuild blood, and promote anti-aging. A compound in barley grass, 2-0-GIV, has antioxidant properties similar to vitamin E, that cleanse the cell membranes. Mega antioxidant enzymes in barley (including SOD, *super-oxide dismutase*) stop free radical attacks, destroy nitro-compounds, (environmental pollutants which build up in the body) and stimulate healing. Barley eliminates fecal matter and toxins in the colon.

A green drink with barley is a tonic, regenerating drink – a chlorophyll-containing aid to the digestive system, an ideal anti-inflammatory food for healing stomach and duodenal ulcers and hemorrhoids. It's a specific for blood sugar balance, particularly in cases of hypoglycemia and diabetes. Barley grass acts directly on DNA to repair cellular damage, and boosts the cells' ability to fight diseases like cancer.

Safety Precautions: None in common use.

Synergy With Other Herbs: with *spirulina, bee pollen* and *alfalfa* to restore strength after exhaustion or illness. with *vitamin c* and *sea vegetables,* to neutralize and cleanse the body of heavy metals.

• **Bayberry,** *Myrica cerifera,* Family: *Myricaceae*

Common Names: wax myrtle, sweet bay, tallow shrub, candleberry, vegetable tallow, waxberry, mirika (Tu), American bayberry, candleberry, American vegetable wax.

Traditional Use: Bayberry is considered a true reviving herb, one of the most useful in medical herbal practice because it helps insure that vital nutrients are absorbed into the blood. Chinese tradition treats it as a yang tonic of the highest caliber. Nineteenth century Eclectic physicians prescribed bayberry bark with cayenne to treat hepatitis.

Medicinal Parts: bark of the root

Preparation Forms: Bayberry tea is a superior astringent for a sore, infected throat or bleeding gums; and a natural tooth powder. Use bayberry extract to stimulate a healing sweat. Bayberry douche is effective for treating a prolapsed uterus, excessive menstrual bleeding and some vaginal infections. Small doses treat chronic gastritis, enteritis, diarrhea, leucorrhea and dysentery. Dosage: Small doses improve circulation; large doses act as an emetic. Capsules: 2 -4 as needed; tincture: 15-30 drops; tea: I cup.

Nutrition Profile: Has highly active tannins and flavonoids. Tannins are tissue tightening, useful for inflamed mouth sores and digestive tract; flavonoids are antibacterial, useful for treating infections. Very high in selenium, high in calcium, chromium, iron, sodium and vitamin C.

Herbal Healing Actions: Astringent, tonic, blood balancing, diuretic, laxative, stomachic, dissolves and removes obstructions, increases perspiration, vermifuge, insecticide and wound healing.

Cleansing Properties & Detox Activity: Bayberry bark is a strong circulatory stimulant that also enhances the sympathetic nervous system. Its most effective influence is in diseased mucous accumulation of the alimentary canal, directly, as in mucous colitis, or indirectly, against incubating broncho-pulmonary organisms, like colds, flu or scarlet fever. Bayberry is a stimulant to the mucous membranes without overheating. It is an aid for digestion, and blood building. Bayberry is effective in all hemorrhage conditions — stomach, lungs, uterus or bowels.

Safety Precautions: Don't use during acute inflammation. Large doses cause nausea.

Synergy With Other Herbs: With *cayenne* to increase the body's ability to resist infection. With *comfrey root and agrimony* as a digestive astringent. In a poultice with *slippery elm.*

• **Bee Pollen**

Medicinal Parts: High quality, unsprayed, dried granules.

Preparation Forms: Use as it comes from the hive. Do not cook. Dosage: Pollen granules, 2 teasp.

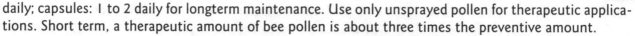

daily; capsules: 1 to 2 daily for longterm maintenance. Use only unsprayed pollen for therapeutic applications. Short term, a therapeutic amount of bee pollen is about three times the preventive amount.

Traditional Use: Pollen has been called the world's first health food, because its healing powers are described in very ancient writings. (Some think bee pollen and royal jelly were the secret "ambrosia" eaten by the gods for eternal youth.) A pollen grain is so physically indestructible that identifiable grains of the first pollen bearing plants are found in the earth's early geological strata. Ancient Greeks used honey and pollen to warm the body against chills and to cleanse open sores and carbuncles.

Nutrition Profile: A highly bio-active, complete food, bee pollen is completely balanced for all 105 of the known nutritional ingredients. No other food contains as many enzymes... an estimated 5000, with 22 amino acids, 27 minerals and all known vitamins, in fact every nutrient needed to maintain life. Bee pollen has 35% protein, about half of which is in the form of free amino acids (excellent for healing). It contains 5 to 7 times more amino acids than beef, eggs or cheese of equal weight. Bee Pollen is rich in chromium, vitamin A, B-complex vitamins (especially B$_{12}$) and vitamins C, D and E. It has one of the highest food amounts of rutin, for tissue strength. Bee pollen is a low-calorie food with 15% lecithin that helps burn away body fat. It is also 40 to 80 percent free-form glutamic acid, which can cross the blood/brain barrier, accounting for its ability to curb cravings for alcohol and increase powers of concentration.

Herbal Healing Actions: Bee pollen has antibacterial properties and antiviral properties. It offers substantial protection from many common pollutants and the toxic side effects of many drugs. It contains an antibiotic effective against *salmonella* and some strains of *E. coli bacillus.*

Cleansing Properties & Detox Activity: Bee pollen enhances a feeling of youthful vitality and provides energy. It is valuable for weight control because it helps correct metabolic chemical imbalance.

Well-documented evidence shows pollen counteracts the effects of severe toxins like radiation and environmental chemicals. More importantly, bee pollen antioxidants are clinically proven to strengthen immune response. Recent clinical tests on women with inoperable uterine cancer, show that pollen significantly reduces the side effects of both radium and cobalt-60 radiotherapy at a level of 2 TBS. a day. Red and white blood cell counts and serum protein levels both increase. The women reported notably better health, with stronger immune responses than those who did not take pollen. Pollen is regularly used in Russia to improve the immune status of patients with M.S. Pollen effectively helps chronic diarrhea and constipation, rheumatism with heart complications, kidney and liver disease, anemia (increases amount of hemoglobin), intestinal infection, fatigue, circulatory disorders, depression, colitis and prostatitis.

Bee pollen's main use is as a tree pollen and spore antidote during allergy season for control and neutralization of seasonal allergy symptoms. It relieves respiratory problems like bronchitis and sinusitis.

Safety Precautions: Pesticides used on the plants where bees gather pollen affect an extremely small number of people. Discontinue if itching, dizziness or difficulty swallowing occurs. Start with small doses.

Synergy With Other Herbs: With *panax ginseng, Siberian ginseng* and "green superfoods" such as *chlorella, alfalfa* and *spirulina;* and with CoQ$_{10}$ for immune enhancement.

• **Beets,** *Beta vulgaris,* Family: *Chenopodiaceae*

Common Names: spinach beet, sea beet, garden beet, white beet, mangel wurzel, betterave — bettarouge (Haiti), acelga (Chile & Spain), tien tsai (China), cruenta.

Medicinal Parts: leaves and root

Preparation Forms: finely grated, capsules and juice. To use the juice in a detox program, mix beets with other cleansing vegetables like carrots and spinach. No fresh beets? Open 6 capsules and mix into the cleansing juice of your choice. Dosage: Four capsules 3x daily with water at mealtime.

Traditional Use: Beets were so appreciated by the ancient Greeks that they were offered on a silver platter to Apollo at Delphi. Ayurvedic tradition recommends that the juice be sniffed up the nose for headache and toothache. For liver disease, constipation and hemorrhoids, a small tumblerful at bedtime or an hour before breakfast is recommended. Medieval medicos used beet juice for a wide variety of health

needs, from uterine diseases to skin itch and dandruff, and for ulcerous and running sores.

Nutrition Profile: Beets owe their medicinal benefits to the active ingredient betaine, a substance that helps vitalize the blood. Betaine is an essential hepatotropic, a lipotropic amino acid similar to methionine. Betaine acts on the methylation cycle of liver cells and the conversion of triglycerides for fat transport. It is a good source of vitamin A, specifically indicated for fatty degeneration of the liver.

Herbal Healing Actions: laxative, diuretic, stimulant and tonic properties. Effective kidney scourer.

Cleansing Properties & Detox Activity: Beet juice is a blood detoxifying, blood builder that cleanses eliminative, digestive and lymphatic systems, then enlivens with rich minerals and natural sugars. Beet juice is an anti-inflammatory, scouring medicinal, especially effective for the kidneys, making beet juice a good choice for a cancer program. Beet juice also aids liver and spleen function to cleanse toxic waste. It can help restore organs damaged from alcohol abuse.

Safety Precautions: none in common use.

Synergy With Other Herbs: A tea with vinegar heals itching, cleanses dandruff and dry scabs and relieves running sores and ulcers.

• **Bilberry,** *Vaccinium Myrtillus*, Family: *Ericaceae*

Common Names: black whortleberry, bleaberry, huckleberry, hurtleberry, whinberry, wineberry, dyeberry, hockelberries, blueberry, black whortles, shinberry.

Medicinal Parts: fruit and leaves

Preparation Forms: A tea, capsule or extract. Apply a strong tea for skin, mouth and throat sores. (Do not sweeten bilberry tea; it renders it therapeutically worthless.) The gel significantly increases wound healing, may also provide protection from sunburn, and results in clearer, fresher skin because of its astringent effect. Dosage: For diarrhea, boil 3 TBS. for 10 minutes in $\frac{1}{2}$ liter of water. Extract: 15 drops 2x daily; capsules: 180 mg. per day for preventive purposes, 300 mg per day for therapeutic purposes.

Traditional Use: Bilberry has a long history as a therapeutic herb, well known by ancient Greek physicians. Both Europeans and Native Americans chewed the dried berries for intestinal infections, and used bilberry wine for digestive complaints. During the second world war, pilots in England's Royal Air Force ate bilberry jam before night flying missions to dramatically improve their vision. Russian healers used bilberry as an astringent for gastric colitis. European herbalists used it to treat scurvy, urinary infections and stones, diarrhea, dysentery, diabetes, discharges and as a local application for ulcers. Bilberry grows in cool areas of North America and Eurasia, under canopies of old growth trees.

Nutrition Profile: Bilberry is rich in vitamin C, bioflavonoids, manganese, phosphorus, iron and zinc. The fruit has as much as 13% protein and 31% EFAs. Bilberries contain important medicinal compounds called anthocyanosides, bioflavonoids that provide a wide range of benefits.

Herbal Healing Actions: an antiseptic, astringent, diuretic, blood tonic and antibacterial. Bilberry has an insulin-similar effects on sugar diabetes (but is not a substitute for insulin or a good diet).

Cleansing Properties & Detox Activity: Bilberry extract is well documented for reducing and reversing damage caused by blood vessel deterioration or inflammation. It supports, strengthens and protects collagen structures, inhibits bacteria growth, and produces anti-carcinogenic benefits. It clears toxins and restrains infection. Its anthocyanodins are active free radical scavengers to boost immunity. Anthocyanodins also have cardiac protective, anti-aging activity for impressive effects on the circulatory system. Regular use of bilberry reduces hardening of the arteries by preventing oxidative damage, thus limiting calcium plaque deposits, and maintaining flexible blood vessels. Research shows impressive effects on circulation, restoring normal blood flow in patients ranging from 18 to 75 years old.

Bilberry promotes kidney cleansing and urination, to help prevent urinary tract infections. Bilberries help heal inflammation of the intestinal mucosa that accompanies chronic constipation. Flavonoids increase mucous secretion that protects the stomach lining. Also used to treat intestinal parasites, diarrhea and vaginal disharge.

Externally, bilberry extract ointment helps dermatitis, eczema, dandruff, burns and inflammations, and speeds recovery from grazes, bruises and swelling. Bilberry helps promote a clearer fresher complexion due to its astringent effect, lessening the marks of cellulite, strengthening collagen structures.

Safety Precautions: Bilberry leaf contains hydroquinone; if used for diabetes or bladder infections, it should not be taken continuously. Use for 3 weeks, then take a break for a week.

Synergy With Other Herbs: An energizing tea: equal parts of *bilberry, thyme* and *strawberry leaves.*

• **Black Cohosh,** *Cimicifuga Racemosa,* Family: *Ranunculaceae*

Common Names: black snake root, rattle root, rattleweed, squawroot, bugwort, rattlesnake's root, rich weed, American baneberry, sauco (Sp), sheng ma jou (Ch).

Traditional Use: Widely used by American Indians, especially to treat snake bites and scorpion stings. American Indians used black cohosh for kidney aliments and malaria. Records of American settlers show use from 1696. During the 19th century, hospitals used black cohosh in the treatment of rheumatism, and this use still continues in some U.S. mountain areas. The nineteenth century introduced black cohosh to the medical world as a cardiac tonic in fatty heart diseases, scarlet fever, bronchitis, rheumatism, neuralgia, hysteria, tuberculosis, dyspepsia, menstrual irregularities, measles and smallpox. Black cohosh is used in traditional Chinese medicine as a cooling diaphoretic to relieve toxicity.

Medicinal Parts: root

Preparation Forms: Root tea is effective for sore throat and rheumatism, but an alcohol extract enhances the root properties better than a tea. Capsules also effective. Dosage: capsules: 2 daily, do not exceed 4 a day (overdose can cause nervous irritation); extract: $^1/_2$ to 2 tsp.; tincture: 10 to 60 drops.

Nutrition Profile: Contains remarkable hormone-like substances. High in chromium and vitamin A.

Herbal Healing Actions: hormone balancing activity, blood cleansing, diuretic, cardiostimulant, diaphoretic, tonic, astringent, a bitter that increases gastric secretions, stimulates uterine contractions in childbirth, antispasmodic, nerve sedative. One of the best herbs for whooping cough and rheumatic pain.

Safety Precautions: Large doses may cause vertigo, tremors, reduced pulse, nausea, vomiting and prostration. Not for during early pregnancy; may irritate the uterus. Avoid during fully erupted measles.

Cleansing Properties & Detox Activity: Stimulates liver, kidneys and lymph secretions. Loosens and expels bronchial mucous; an anti-spasmodic for lung conditions, like asthma and bronchitis. Helps clear uric acid and toxic wastes from the bloodstream. A specific for female toning to relieve menstrual cramps and uterine disorders, encourage estrogen balance, and during the last weeks of pregnancy, to facilitate childbirth. Confirmed hypotensive ability to inhibit vasomotor centers (hot flashes) in the central nervous system. A specific for clearing ringing in the ears. Equalizes circulation in high blood pressure. A primary nerve and smooth muscle relaxant for irritated nerves, thus effective for arthritic, neurological, and rheumatic pain. Neutralizes some snake bites and scorpion stings.

Synergy With Other Herbs: With parturient herbs like *squaw vine* and *raspberry,* during the last two weeks of pregnancy to facilitate childbirth. In a syrup with *wild cherry bark, coltsfoot, yerba santa* and *elecampane* for whooping cough, bronchitis and asthma. For nervousness and insomnia: equal parts *black cohosh, skullcap, wood betony, passionflower, valerian* and half part *capsicum.* For menstrual pain: with *blue cohosh, red raspberry, chamomile* and *ginger.* For arthritis pain: with equal parts *angelica root, prickly ash* and *guaiacum.* For asthma spasms: with *wild cherry bark, elecampane* and *mullein.*

• **Black Walnut,** *Juglans nigra,* Family: *Juglandaceae*

Common Names: black walnut, European walnut, jupiter's nuts, carya.

Medicinal Parts: fruit, leaves and bark, green nut, rind, hulls and root.

Preparation Forms: tincture: bark and leaves. Capsules: oil, nut, nut hulls. A strong tea to gargle for sore throat and mouth infections. Tea may be used externally as well as internally, applying it as a fomen-

tation for skin conditions. Dosage: leaves are used for skin conditions as a tea or 1-3 capsules, two times daily; hull extract: 10-30 drops three times a day.

Traditional Use: Black walnut has been a food source medicine for centuries. Native Americans used the bark tea as a purging cathartic, the hull tea for ringworm, and applied the sap on inflammations. The juice of the husks boiled with honey was used as a gargle for sore mouths and throats. It was as a dependable remedy for bad blood diseases such as syphilis and diphtheria. Russians made a walnut jam so that 90 percent of the vitamins remained intact, then used it as a sweet, rich supply of vitamin C, carotene and minerals for body repair. Seventeenth century Russian hospitals used black walnut hulls as a cleansing, quick healer. Today, Russian physicians use it clinically for skin diseases and tuberculosis.

Nutrition Profile: Black walnuts are rich in oil and high in food energy, with almost as much protein as sirloin steak! The nut is rich in linolenic, linoleic and oleic fatty acids, (important for nerves, brain and cartilage), juglone (believed to have antifungal properties), in Vitamin B_{15}, and manganese. The hulls are especially high in tannins, vitamins A, B, C and E and organic iodine, useful in anti-parasite cleansing.

Herbal Healing Actions: hulls are anthelmintic (vermifuge), antifungal and antiparasitic purgative, a bitters herb; bark is a laxative and antidiarrheal with astringent properties. Helps balance sugar levels.

Cleansing Properties & Detox Activity: Black walnut hulls are useful in cleansing programs for the organs, lungs, kidneys and brain. The bark helps chronic constipation (a cleansing purgative), and liver congestion. The bark and leaves are astringent, antiseptic cleansers useful as a douche for leucorrhea, as a vermifuge for amoebic dysentery and as a mouthwash for mouth sores or sore tonsils. One study finds that several constituents of black walnut even have anti-cancer activity. Black walnut oxygenates the blood to rid the body of excessive toxins and fatty material, and is especially effective in expelling parasites. The extract of the hulls is good internally and externally for skin diseases, eczema, genital herpes, psoriasis and skin parasites. Chinese medics use black walnut to kill tapeworm with excellent success.

Safety precautions: **Avoid during pregnancy.**

Synergy With Other Herbs: For giardia (amoebic dysentery): equal parts: *black walnut, goldenseal root, mugwort* or *wormwood, chaparral* and *licorice root.* For cold sores: equal parts with *licorice root.*

• **Boneset,** *Eupatorium Perfoliatum,* Family: *Compositae*

Common Names: boneset, thoroughwort, teasel, joe pye, ague-weed, fever wort, thorough stem, cross wort, wood boneset, vegetable antimony, sweating plant, Indian sage.

Traditional Use: Boneset tea was a common home remedies in the last century, a role now enjoyed by hot lemon tea in the treatment of coughs, colds and flu. It is certainly more effective. The hot tea produces therapeutic sweating, a benefit shown to early settlers by the Native Americans. Native tribes all over the continent used boneset as an antimalarial tonic, (works better than quinine in persistent cases of malaria), as an emetic in bilious disorders, for ague, colds, fever, chills, flu and sore throat, for menstrual problems, in steam baths for body aches, gallstones and typhoid, for epilepsy, intestinal parasites, even snakebites. Appalachians did and do treat coughs and constipation with boneset tea.

Medicinal Parts: **tops and leaves**

Preparation Forms: capsules, tincture, extract and tea. Use the tea very hot for profuse perspiration and rapid bowel evacuation. Boneset has dual action depending on how it is administered: when cold— tonic, when warm—emetic and diaphoretic. Dosage: tea: 3-oz three times daily. Drink 4 to 5 cups while in bed to encourage sweating; capsules: $^1/_2$ to 1 gram; extract: $^1/_2$ to 1 tsp. three times daily; tincture: 10 to 40 drops three times daily; 2 TBS tincture added to hot water can be used for sweating to break fevers.

Nutrition Profile: Boneset contains vitamin C, calcium, some PABA, magnesium and potassium.

Herbal Healing Actions: **an expectorant, laxative, stimulant, digestive, diuretic, purgative and tonic.** Boneset contains diaphoretic compounds that promote sweating, are antiseptic and decrease mucous thickness while increasing mucosal fluid.

Cleansing Properties & Detox Activity: **Boneset is closely related to gravel root and has similar**

cleansing constituents. As a hot tea, boneset is widely used and practically unequalled in its effectiveness as a reliable diaphoretic, providing slow, gentle perspiration to clear flu and cold infections. As a cold tea, it works as a soothing tonic on the stomach, liver, bowels and uterus, relaxing the muscular structures, and clearing areas of waste buildup and congestion. Liver detoxification helps clear the skin, bilious fevers, and other inflammation (like that associated with arthritis and rheumatism.)

Safety Precautions: **Large doses may result in severe flu like symptoms.**

Synergy With Other Herbs: **To treat flu, combine with** *yarrow, elder flowers, cayenne* **or** *ginger.* **Use with** *ginger* **and** *anise* **for coughs for children. Use as a fomentation with** *hops* **for tumors.**

• **Borage,** *Borage officinalis,* Family: *Boraginceae*
Common Names: **burrage, bugloss, common bugloss, beebread, bee plant.**

Traditional Use: **Indigenous to Great Britain and northern Europe, borage is a wildflower that has been used as a food for a thousand years. In Roman times, Pliny extolled the plant's virtues for a feeling of well-being. In the sixteenth century, a weak tea was considered valuable for eye inflammations.**

Medicinal Parts: **the whole plant and the oil**

Preparation Forms: **Borage seed oil capsules: for eczema, rheumatoid arthritis, menstrual irregularity, irritable bowel syndrome and first aid for hangovers; lotion: use equal parts juice and water for dry skin and rashes; liquid extract drops: for depression or anxiety; poultice: for inflammatory swelling; flower syrup made from strong tea: an expectorant for coughs; leaf tea: for early stages of colds, and fevers, tincture: for drug toxin removal.** Dosage: **extract: 2-10 ml three times a day; powder: 12 to 20 grains; tea: 2 teaspoons dry herb steeped 10-15 minutes, three times daily; oil: 500mg daily.**

Nutrition Profile: **the most potent natural, currently known source of GLA (22% gamma-linolenic acid) which shows promise in the treatment of alcholism and diabetes, Contains vitamin C, and large amount of salts of potassium and calcium salts. The fresh juice has almost 30 percent potassium. The stems and leaves supply rich saline mucilage, responsible the invigorating properties of borage.**

Herbal Healing Actions: **diuretic and diaphoretic, adrenal stimulant and expectorant; mucilaginous properties make it a superior soothing demulcent and emollient. A good cleansing eyewash.**

Cleansing Properties & Detox Activity: **Borage purifies the blood by promoting kidney activity. It is anti-inflammatory against pleurisy and pneumonia. It may be used as a tonic for exhausted adrenals as a restorative agent for the adrenal cortex, especially after cortisone or steroid drugs. It is a remedy for jaundice and ringworm. Borage is used for heart and lung congestion. Its demulcent properties make it effective against ulcers, both internal and external. The leaf tea can be a poultice for external inflammations.**

Safety Precautions: **Pyrrolizide alkaloids are present in very small amounts. Though used by traditional people around the world for thousands of years, borage is not the type of nutritive tonic herb to take regularly over a period of months. It is more of an occasional acute remedy for fevers and might be considered safe to use as a sole agent for no more than three to seven days maximum.**

Synergy With Other Herbs: **With** *marshmallow or mullein* **as an expectorant.**

• **Buchu,** *Barosma Betulina,* Family: *Rutaceae*
Common Names: **bucco (Dutch), buchu (French, Sp., U.S.), diosma (Italian), diosme (Fr), gotterstraunch (Ge). Buchu means "fragrant."**

Traditional Use: **Originating in the southwest region of South Africa, buchu is used by the Hottentots of South Africa under the name of Bookoo or Buku, as a brandy remedy for problems of the stomach, bowels and bladder, as a stimulant tonic, and for wounds. Buchu brandy is a stock item in bars in South Africa today. Buchu was introduced into European medicine around 1821 for bladder and kidney ailments.**

Medicinal Parts: **leaves**

Preparation Forms: **tea, fluid extract and capsules. Overnight cold water maceration, extract or long**

infusion are the best preparations to retain the active essential oil. Works best when given as a cold infusion, which may be applied to bruises and rheumatic pains. Dosage: 2 cups tea daily; 20 drops three times a day; three 200mg capsules three times a day.

Nutrition Profile: The essential oil has antiseptic properties and is highly bacteriocidal.

Herbal Healing Actions: diuretic, carminative, stimulant, diaphoretic, emollient, stomachic and tonic.

Cleansing Properties & Detox Activity: Buchu is effective for chronic cystitis, irritation of the urethra, first stage diabetes, urine retention, nephritis and cystitis. It is highly regarded for cleansing the kidney and urinary tract, increasing the quantity of urinic fluids and solids, acting at the same time as a tonic, astringent and disinfectant. Its volatile oil is excreted virtually unchanged by the kidneys, rendering the urine itself antiseptic.

Safety Precautions: too strong a diuretic to use during pregnancy. Don't use during acute inflammatory conditions or serious kidney infections. Large doses produce mouth burning, nausea, severe diarrhea, heart palpitations and sweating. Breaks of several days are advisable every two weeks.

Synergy With Other Herbs: With *uva ursi* for water retention. For urinary tract infections: with *juniper berry* and gentle, antiseptic and anti-inflammatory herbs, like *cornsilk* or *marshmallow.* With *yarrow, uva ursi* or *couchgrass* for cystitis.

• **Buckthorn,** *Rhamnus cathartica,* Family: *Rhamnaceae*

Common Names: alder buckthorn, black dogwood, black alder dogwood, frangula bark, tufty thorn (U.K.), bourdaine, bourgène, aune noir, rhubarbe des paysans (French).

Traditional Use: An old country medicine - the bark was boiled in ale for jaundice.

Medicinal Parts: the branch and young tree bark

Preparation Forms: fluid extract (used in sunscreen preparations); as a decoction: 1-oz. bark in 1-qt. water, boiled down to a pint. As a fomentation to relieve itchy skin. Dosage: Fluid extract: 15 drops per dose; decoction in teaspoon doses; syrup: 1-2 tablespoons daily for a purgative effect.

Nutrition Profile: contains anthraquinones and bitters for better digestion and elimination.

Herbal Healing Actions: a blood purifying, gentle purgative. Very similar to *rhubarb* and *cascara.*

Cleansing Properties & Detox Activity: A gentle laxative for chronic constipation — does not cause cramping, is not habit forming, relieves hemorrhoids. Buckthorn is a blood cleansing tonic remedy for gallstones, hardening of the liver and spleen, lead poisoning, clearing toxic blood, gout and rheumatism. Taken hot, diaphoretic properties cause perspiration and help lower fevers.

Safety Precautions: Bark must cure for at least one year prior to use or it acts as an irritant on the gastrointestinal tract, causing griping pains and nausea. Contraindicated for pregnancy.

Synergy With Other Herbs: For persistent constipation, combine with *senna, peppermint* and *caraway seed,* or with *chamomile* and *fennel* as a tea.

• **Bugleweed,** *Lycopus Virginicus,* Family: *Labiatae*

Common Names: sweet bugle, water bugle, gypsywort, gypsy-weed, gipsy herb, water horehound, virginian bugle, wolffoot, carpenters herb.

Traditional Use: The Cherokee used bugleweed externally for snakebites. Bugleweed first appeared as a medicine in the early 1800s with the early Eclectics who recognized it as a sedative, mild narcotic, and astringent as a remedy for diarrhea and dysentery.

Medicinal Parts: the whole fresh flowering herb

Preparation Forms: powder, infusion, tincture. Dosage: infusion: three times a day; tincture: take 1-2 ml three times a day.

Nutrition Profile: flavone glycosides, volatile oil, tannins

Herbal Healing Actions: an astringent, bitters tonic and antitussive, bugleweed is a peripheral vaso-

constrictor (for problems when capillary flow needs to be diminished, like hemorrhoids or intestinal bleeding from the lungs or bowels). Bugleweed is a cardio-active diuretic like digitalis, quieting the pulse and lessoning its frequency when treating pericarditis and endocarditis.

Cleansing Properties & Detox Activity: Treats Graves' disease (an overactive thyroid condition with tightness of breathing and nervous heart palpitations), where a thyroid-stimulating antibody is found in the blood. The antibody binds to and is inhibited by bugleweed extract. Very useful for relieving widespread pain regardless of location. It is a mild gastric tonic and a remedy for painful indigestion. One of the mildest, best narcotics in the world. As a sedative cough reliever, it eases irritating coughs. Bugleweed's cardiotonic properties aid a weak heart, especially where there is build-up of fluid retention.

Safety Precautions: Use with caution during pregnancy.

Synergy With Other Herbs: With *dong quai, honeysuckle* and *licorice root* for abscess swelling and pain. With nervines like *skullcap* or *valerian* as a natural sedative. With *motherwort* for the high thyroid condition Grave's disease. With *kelp, bladderwrack, vitamin C, astragalus, Irish moss, licorice rt., parsley* and *prickly ash* it helps neutralize and release hazardous chemicals from the blood.

• **Bupleurum,** *Bupleurum falcatum, (Chai hu),* Family: *Umbelliferae*
Common Names: Misima-saiko (Ja), Tzu Hu (Ch), Hare's Ear Root, Thorowax Root (Eng)
Medicinal Parts: **root**
Preparation Forms: **tea, capsules, extract, soup.** Dosage: 3-10 grams daily.

Traditional Use: Known from the 1st century B.C., bupleurum was primarily used by the Chinese, who considered it to strengthen the liver qi, as a liver tonic. Rediscovered in western medicine in the 1960's, bupleurum has shownspecial promise in treatment for hepatitis, a liver malfunction.

Nutrition Profile: Sakiosaponins found in bupleurum are capable of inhibiting measles, herpes simplex virus. Rich in flavonoids.

Herbal Healing Actions: Diaphoretic, antibiotic and antiviral, anti-inflammatory, analgesic, bile stimulant, liver and adrenal gland protector, blood purifier. Effective for: dysmenorrhea, lung congestion, malaria, muscle cramps, tumors, inflammatory skin conditions, angina pain, epilepsy, even depression.

Cleansing Properties & Detox Activity: An ideal herb in a detoxification program, bupleurum is a prime liver detoxifier, toner and strengthener. Its antibiotic abilities inhibit micro-organisms like influenza and polio. A tonic immune-enhancer with the ability to stimulate T, B, and phagocyte immune cells. Stabilizes the central nervous system with an antispasmodic quality, especially effective for menstrual cramping. Clears and reduces blood cholesterol levels.

Safety Precautions: May cause nausea or vomiting in large doses.

Synergy With Other Herbs: With *bee pollen, white pine bk., elecampane, scullcap, royal jelly, ephedra, acerola cherry,* and *ginger rt.* to maintain harmony during high risk seasons. Used with *ginseng* and *gotu kola* to promote strong nerves, energy and raise vitality.

• **Burdock,** *Arctium Lappa,* Family: *Compositae*
Common Names: grass burdock, burr seed, hardock, hareburr, turkey burseed, niu-pang-tzu (China), goboshi (Japan), thorny burr, beggar's or cockle buttons, love leaves, philanthropium.

Traditional Use: Burdock has been a healing remedy since ancient Greek times. In Western herbalism, it was an important blood purifier throughout the Middle Ages, an effective pain killer and rheumatism treatment. Native Americans also used burdock tea to treat rheumatism, to purify the blood, for female weakness, kidney gravel, scurvy and venereal diseases. Chippewa and Ojibwa used burdock as an anodyne and tonic. American herbalists used burdock to alleviate arthritis. The Chinese found it valuable as a healing diaphoretic and diuretic to eliminate toxins and cool the heat of infections. The Chinese consider burdock a strengthening female aphrodisiac. Used in Ayurvedic medicine for skin conditions like boils,

carbuncles and rashes. Also used for addiction detoxification.

A cancer folk remedy all over the world, burdock has been used for cancers, indurations or tumors of the breast, glands, intestine, knee, lip, liver, sinus, stomach, tongue and uterus, as well as for corns and warts. It is a primary herb of the cancer folk remedy "Essiac."

Medicinal Parts: **root, herb and seeds**

Preparation Forms: **Powder, poultice, tea, tincture. Massage oil into the scalp for dandruff. Dosage: tea: 1 cup 3x daily; tincture: 30 to 60 drops 3x daily; extract: $\frac{1}{2}$ to 1 tsp. 4x daily; capsules: 6-10 daily.**

Nutrition Profile: **abundant in iron and insulin for the blood. High in chromium, magnesium, manganese, silicon and thiamine. Also high in dietary fiber, phosphorus, potassium, vitamin A and zinc.**

Herbal Healing Actions: **Inulin, a polysaccharide (reduces cell mutation), is the source of most of burdock's curative powers. Burdock is antibacterial, tumor-protective and an inhibitor of cancer-causing agents. Antipyretic, antiseptic, strongly diaphoretic and diuretic. Also alterative, demulcent, carminative, cholagogue, tonic, bitter, fungicide, hepatic, laxative, refrigerant.**

Cleansing Properties & Detox Activity: **Burdock is one of the herb world's best blood purifiers. It helps arthritis, rheumatism and sciatica inflammations, reducing swelling around joints and ridding the body of calcification deposits. It helps cleanse the blood of toxins during a weight loss regimen. Burdock is useful for arthritis, rheumatism, gout, asthma and sciatica. It has volatile oils which make it a good diaphoretic which clears the kidneys of excess wastes and uric acid by increasing the flow of urine. Aids the pituitary gland in releasing an ample supply of protein to help adjust hormone balance. Burdock alleviates ulcerated, glandular and white tumors.**

Documented effects include treatment of venereal eruptions (particularly gonorrhea) and skin conditions, such as ringworm and eczema. Homeopaths prescribe the tincture of fresh root for acne, since most poor skin conditions result from blood toxicity. Herbal formulas for weight loss include burdock to help cleanse the body of toxins. Burdock markedly enhances liver, gallbladder and bile functions. It helps cleanse the body of toxins and wastes that accumulate during illness.

Safety Precautions: **none in common use.**

Synergy With Other Herbs: **For detoxifying the liver from addictions: equal parts** *turmeric, barberry, gotu kola* **and** *burdock.* **With** *calendula, oregon grape, gumweed, cleavers, black haw* **for herpes. With** *sheep sorrel, slippery elm* **and** *turkey rhubarb* **in the cancer-fighting "Essiac" formula.**

• **Butcher's Broom,** *Ruscus Aculeatus,* Family: *Liliaceae*

Common Names: **kneeholm, box holly, pettigree, sweet broom, Jew's myrtle, brusca (Europe).**

Traditional Use: **The branches were used by butchers to sweep their blocks, thus, the name** *butcher's broom.* **Used in the Middle Ages for its cleansing and opening qualities. Used by the ancient Greeks as a laxative and diuretic for dropsy, urinary and nephritic obstructions. Helps mend broken bones.**

Medicinal Parts: **fleshy rootstock**

Preparation Forms: **Decoction and alcohol extract for internal use. As an ointment, suppository for hemorrhoids, poultice, compress, salve, bolus and herbal tea enema. Dosage: 100mg daily.**

Nutrition Profile: **Flavonoid-rich. High in chromium, iron, silicon, manganese, niacin and zinc. Measureable in calcium, magnesium, phosphorus, selenium, sodium, vitamins A and C.**

Herbal Healing Actions: **Diaphoretic, laxative and diuretic—especially for cellulite release. The ruscogenins and neoruscogenins (similar to** *wild yam's* **steroidal constituents) exert anti-inflammatory effects and increase vein tone, reduce capillary fragility and boost circulation.**

Cleansing Properties & Detox Activity: **Butcher's broom is effective for varicose veins, leg cramps and heaviness in the legs. It is useful for arthritic, rheumatic and hemorrhoidal pain, diabetic retinopathy, atherosclerosis, thrombosis, fevers, and congestive headaches, such as migraines. Useful for post-operative recovery where there is heavy or prolonged bleeding.**

Safety Precautions: should only be used short term (1 week to 1 month), so that blood chemistry can achieve its own balance.

Synergy With Other Herbs: With *dandelion* as a diuretic. Synergistic with *centella* and *bilberry*. With *pau d' arco, kukicha, ginkgo biloba, hawthorn, sage, sassafras, ginger, calendula, yellow dock, peppermint, bilberry* and *licorice* for blood cleansing, to stimulate circulation and deter blood lipid stickiness.

• **Butternut,** *Juglans Cinerea,* Family: *Juglandaceae*

Common Names: noyer (France), nogal (Chile), noguiera (Portugal), noce commune (Italy).

Traditional Use: Used in the Revolutionary War to staunch bleeding. In Appalachia, the bark tea is still used as a laxative. Native Americans used the bark tea to check the bowels but also as a cathartic. They applied the bark to the temples for headaches and to teeth for toothaches. The Delaware Indians boiled butternut to the consistency of soap, and used it as a hemostatic, even for a ruptured artery. Also used on fresh wounds to prevent swelling and speed healing.

Medicinal Parts: inner bark of young stems and roots, leaves and nut

Preparation Forms: Alcohol tincture, tea and decoction. Dosage: decoction: 1-2 teaspoons 3x daily; tincture: up to 5ml a day for skin ailments, liver health or slow digestion; infusion: 1-oz. bark in 1C. water.

Nutrition Profile: contains juglandic acid, juglandin and juglone and tannins.

Herbal Healing Actions: laxative, purgative, alterative, astringent, ferbrifuge, cholagogue, vermifuge. For dysentery, cancer (stomach), constipation, eczema, liver congestion, parasites, tumors, warts.

Cleansing Properties & Detox Activity: Used for constipation, sluggish digestion, as a liver cleanser and stimulant, and for skin diseases and fevers. Especially helps skin ailments resulting from incomplete cleansing of the body via the bowels. It has been used as a vermifuge and is recommended for syphilis and old ulcers. The expressed oil of the fruit removes tapeworms.

Safety Precautions: As a purgative, it should not be used on fragile invalids.

Synergy With Other Herbs: To combat infections, fevers and colds, some part of the treatment should be laxative to help the body rid itself of bacteria-laden wastes. With *barberry, rhubarb, psyllium husk, fennel seed, licorice, ginger, Irish moss* and *capsicum* for evacuation of the bowels.

• **Calendula,** *Calendula Officinalis,* Family: *Compositae*

Common Names: bull's eyes, goldes, holigold, marsh marigold, marigolde, oculis christi, souci (Fr), fiore d'ogni mese (It), chin chan hua (Ch), maravilla (Spain), mercadela (Mex).

Traditional Use: In the Middle Ages, calendula flowers were used for bright, clean eyesight, for intestinal troubles, for liver obstructions, for snake bites and to strengthen the heart. It was used in 1700s as a remedy for headache, jaundice, red eyes and ague. Employed in the Civil War to treat wounds and as a remedy for measles, smallpox and jaundice. In World War 1: for dressing wounds.

Medicinal Parts: The flowers, leaves and root

Preparation Forms: tea, lotion, tincture, ointment, mouth wash (for mouth ulcers and gum diseases). Dosage: Infusion: 1 TBS. each hour or one cup daily for skin eruptions, hemorrhage, small pox and measles, fevers; tincture: 15 to 30 drops three times daily for bleeding hemorrhoids, cramps, skin eruptions; extract: $^1/_2$ to 1 tsp. three times daily for bleeding hemorrhoids, cramps, hemorrhage, skin eruptions.

Nutrition Profile: Flavonoids, bitters, and steroidal compounds. Essential flower oil contains carotene and lycopene. High in phosphorus, manganese, carotenes and vitamins A and C.

Herbal Healing Actions: a blood purifying tonic, analgesic, astringent for skin and wound healing, anti-bacterial, carminative, cholagogue, diaphoretic and diuretic, laxative, stimulant and tonic.

Cleansing Properties & Detox Activity: Internally, effective for stimulating lymphatic drainage and decreasing inflammation of the lymph nodes. Blood cleansing activity helps stomach ache, digestive sluggishness and stagnant liver. For external application, calendula is effective in treating burns, wounds and

skin irritations like shingles, eczema, athlete's foot, sunburns, warts, corns and boils. May be taken internally and applied topically for hemorrhoids and anal fissures, and for varicose veins.

Safety Precautions: **Don't apply to infected, draining wounds or acne pustules; they may close prior to proper drainage. Contra-indicated during pregnancy or if excessive menstrual bleeding.**

Synergy With Other Herbs: **Topically with** *plantain leaves, wormwood* **and** *chickweed* **to relieve eczema; with** *chamomile* **and** *St. John's wort* **for ear infections; with** *tea tree oil* **as a suppository for vaginal yeast infections; with** *goldenseal* **and** *myrrh* **as an antiseptic lotion; with** *marshmallow* **and** *cranesbill* **for digestive problems; with** *senna, fennel, ginger, papaya, hibiscus, lemon balm, peppermint* **and** *parsley* **as a simple laxative tea; with** *mullein, pleurisy rt., marshmallow, rose hips, ephedra, licorice, boneset, ginger, peppermint* **and** *fennel* **as an expectorant tea to clear mucous congestion.**

• **Capsicum,** *Capsicum annuum, Capsicum Frutescens,* Family: *Solanaceae*
Common Names: **cayenne pepper, bird pepper, chili (Mezoaztec), guinea pepper, pi po (China).**
Traditional Use: **An American spice, used as a folk medicine for weak digestion and loss of appetite, especially if accompanied by flatulence and sluggish elimination. It also found use as a stimulant for circulation and to stave off colds and flus and was said to be an aphrodisiac. In the 1800s, it was popular in the U.S. for expelling the contagion of serious infectious diseases.**
Medicinal Parts: **fruit and seeds**
Preparation Forms: **tinctures, ointments, liniments, salves and dried powder.** Dosage: **One to 2 capsules with meals or $\frac{1}{4}$ tsp. extract 3x daily. Apply powder externally to stop bleeding.**
Nutrition Profile: **Capsaicin, a main constituent of capsicum is rich in carotenoid, iron and zinc. High in Vitamins A, B complex, and C; lower in calcium potassium and magnesium, to allow the stimulant effects to work at maximum potential.**
Herbal Healing Actions: **Capsicum is like an express train for herbal transportation. Cayenne is best when combined with other herbs to speed circulation, acting as a catalyst or carrier to convey herbal agents to the sites needed. May be used alone as a dilute extract or with honey to regulate cardiac activity and stop angina. Cayenne is a specific for breaking up mucous congestion during colds and flu. Cayenne is anti-inflammatory, antiseptic, antispasmodic, a blood thinner and cardiovascular tonic, a carminative and stomachic for digestion, a diaphoretic for cleansing, and a hemostat and vulnerary for wound healing.**
Cleansing Properties & Detox Activity: **Capsicum is a catalyst in the blood purification process, stimulating the vital organs to greater activity, promoting cardiovascular activity, lowering blood pressure. Capsicum is popular today as an ointment for relief of arthritis pain, rheumatism, neuralgia, sprains and bruises, for skin ailments like shingles, even gangrene. It increases circulation, and is used as a stimulant for people with sluggish metabolisms. Recent studies point to capsicum's fat burning qualities with proven thermogenesis enhancement; it slows fat absorption from the small intestine. Stimulates circulation in the stomach and intestines to improve digestion. It acts directly as a diaphoretic, stimulating excretion of wastes in sweat. Also effective for fatigue, infections, tumors, and healing stomach ulcers.**
Safety Precautions: **Keep away from the eyes.**
Synergy With Other Herbs: **With herbs like** *ginger* **and** *garlic* **protects against colds and flu.**

• **Cascara Bark,** *Rhamnus purshiana,* Family: *Rhamnaceae*
Common Names: **cascara sagrada, chittem bark, Christ's thorn, holy bark, persian bark.**
Traditional Use: **As a Native American folk medicine, cascara extract was used in laxative combinations. Early pioneers processed a cold infusion by soaking the bark overnight which they used as a body cleansing tonic, especially for intestinal worms. Adopted into medical use in 1877and is still used in OTC laxative formulas. Grows in the Rocky Mountains west to the Pacific Coast.**
Medicinal Parts: **aged, dry bark. The bark must be aged for at least one year prior to use.**

Preparation Forms: extract, capsules and decoction. Dosage: dried powdered bark: 2-4 tsp. at bedtime; extract: 2-5 ml at bedtime.

Nutrition Profile: high in calcium, cobalt, and vitamin A.

Herbal Healing Actions: laxative, bitter tonic, nervine, emetic, promotes peristaltic action in the intestinal canal. Anti-leukemic activity due to the presence of aloe-emodin.

Cleansing Properties & Detox Activity: Cascara is a cleansing laxative for stagnant conditions and general toxicity and non-habit forming for chronic constipation. A bitters tonic that stimulates digestive secretions for the liver, gallbladder, stomach and pancreas. It is a proven remedy for colitis, ridding the body of gallstones, indigestion, intestinal mucous congestion, gout, hemorrhoids, and liver disorders, especially an enlarged liver. A specific for chronic constipation and flatulence from gas. Useful for hemorrhoids because of poor, flaccid bowel structure or constipation. There is evidence of anti-tumor activity.

Safety Precautions: Pregnant and nursing mothers should avoid - transfers in milk. Large doses of the bark may cause inflammation; habitual use can result in diarrhea.

Synergy With Other Herbs: With *dandelion, licorice, celery seed, cayenne* and *wild yam* for liver disorders. With *butternut bark, rhubarb, ginger, licorice rt., Irish moss* and *cayenne* as a laxative. With *red clover, chaparral, licorice rt., Oregon grape, stillingia, burdock, sarsaparilla, prickly ash, buckthorn* and *kelp* for detoxification and toning. With *butternut, barberry, rhubarb, psyllium husk, fennel seed, licorice, ginger, Irish moss* and *capsicum* for evacuation of the bowels by normal peristalsis.

• **Chaparral,** *Larrea Tridentata*, Family: *Zygophyllaceae*

Common Names: creosote bush, greasewood.

Traditional Use: Used by Native Americans as a remedy for colds, rheumatism, bowel cramps, as an emetic, for STDs, as a diuretic for menstrual cramps, and for tuberculosis. Used externally as a poultice for sores and bruises. Used externally in Mexico and central America for insect bites, rheumatism, skin ulcers, wounds, bruises and swellings; internally for stomach and intestinal problems, for kidney problems as a urinary antiseptic, and for uterine and gallbladder pain.

Medicinal Parts: leaves and stems

Preparation Forms: tea, tincture and powder, poultice, fomentation and liniment. Dosage: tea $\frac{1}{2}$ oz. infused in a pint of water; tincture: 10-30 drops, 3 times daily.

Nutrition Profile: Famous for its primary constituent NDGA, a significant antioxidant, antitumor and anticancer element. Its amino acid content is rich: arginine, tryptophane, phenylalanine, glycine, glutamic acid, aspartic acid, cystine and tyrosine. Also contains carotenes, vitamin C, potassium, calcium, magnesium, iron, chlorine, natural salts, and sulfur.

Herbal Healing Actions: a bitters tonic and cleanser that is diuretic, antiseptic and astringent. Diuretic, expectorant, antibiotic, antioxidant, blood purifier and parasitcide with vasodepressant effects.

Cleansing Properties & Detox Activity: Chaparral's blood purifying, antioxidant value is legendary. Effective blood purifying uses include kidney infections, respiratory infections, allergies, auto-immune diseases and several types of cancers. It often works for difficult toxic blood conditions when other herbs are ineffective. Chaparral is a specific analgesic to relieve arthritis and rheumatic pain. It is a system toner to rebuild tissue strength. It is one of the best herbal antibiotics, effective internally and externally against bacteria, viruses and parasites. It is used for colds and flu, TB, diarrhea, urinary tract infections, venereal disease, leukemia, acne, eczema, some STD's and tetanus. It is effective externally as a poultice for sores and bruises. I have seen it used successfully in reduced dosage for dogs with certain cancers.

Safety Precautions: Because of its potency and swift action, chaparral must be used with care and direction. NDGA in concentrated and overlong use can affect liver health leading to jaundice and possibly hepatitis. Longterm heavy dosages should be avoided to prevent possible formation of kidney lesions.

Synergy With Other Herbs: With *echinacea, goldenseal, garlic* and *usnea* to heighten its antibiotic, detox properties.

• **Chlorella**

Common Names: Green micro-algae

Medicinal Parts: Entire plant

Preparation Forms: Dried, liquid extract and tablets. Dosage: average nutritional level: 15 tablets per day; poor nutritional levels: 30 tablets per day; very poor nutritional level: 45 tablets per day. Children under 15 should take the number of tablets daily that corresponds to their age in years.

Origins & Traditional Use: Believed to have existed on Earth for over 2.5 billion years. Due to its extremely high protein content and nutritious profile, chlorella was used to help feed people during food shortages of World War II.

Nutrition Profile: Chlorella is 60% protein, rich in minerals and contains 12% chlorophyll, the largest amount of any plant on Earth. The richest food source of vitamin B$_{12}$, higher than liver or sea vegetables. with a protein yield greater than soy beans, corn or beef. Phytoplankton like chlorella are the most potent source of beta carotene in the world with all B vitamins, vitamin C and E, an abundance of the antioxidant superoxide dismutase (SOD), and many trace minerals high enough to be supplementary amounts. Phytoplankton are the only foods, other than mother's milk, with GLA, an essential fatty acid and precursor to the body's master hormones (GLA deficiency contributes to obesity, heart disease and PMS).

Herbal Healing Actions: a tonic, antibiotic, anti-tumor and anti-carcinogen plant. Inhibits growth and development of toxic bacteria.

Cleansing Properties & Detox Activity: The cell wall material of chlorella has a particular effect on intestinal and bowel health, detoxifying the colon, stimulating peristaltic activity, and promoting the growth of beneficial bacteria. Chlorella is effective in eliminating heavy metals, such as lead, mercury, copper and cadmium. Antitumor research shows it is an important source of beta carotene in healing. It strengthens the liver, the body's major detoxifying organ, so that it can free the system of infective agents that destroy immune defenses. It reduces arthritis stiffness, lowers blood pressure, and relieves gastritis and ulcers. Its rich nutritional content has made it effective in weight loss programs, both for cleansing ability, and in maintaining muscle tone during lower food intake. Chlorella also enhances tissue growth and repair (beneficial to hypoglycemic and diabetic people), accelerates healing, protects against radiation, prevents degenerative diseases and promotes longer life. It improves the complexion and aids in skin disorders such as eczema, recurrent cold sores, warts, atopic dermatitis and acne.

But its most important benefits come from a unique molecular composition called Controlled Growth Factor, that provides a noticeable increase in stamina and immune health when eaten on a regular basis.

Safety Precautions: none in common use.

Synergy With Other Herbs: 1) an herbal revitalizer: *American ginseng* and *chlorella*. 2) in a whole green drink with chlorophyllins, trace minerals and full spectrum amino acids: *barley and alfalfa sprouts, bee pollen, acerola fruit, Siberian ginseng, sarsaparilla rt., dandelion, quinoa and oat sprouts* and *chlorell*.

• **Cleavers,** *Galium Aparine,* Family: *Rubiaceae*

Common Names: cleever (Australia), clivers, catch-weed, bedstraw, robin-run-in-the-grass, everlasting friendship, loveman, goosebill (U.K.), chu yang yang (China); grateron (France).

Traditional Use: Extolled in England for its powers as a blood purifier and spring tonic to cleanse the liver. In the 14th century, it was used as an ointment for scalds and burns, later for colds and swellings. It was a medieval remedy for snake and spider bites.

Medicinal Parts: aerial portions

Preparation Forms: fresh juice, infusion, tincture, compress. Dosage: 3 - 9 gms. of tea infusion.

Nutrition Profile: contains chlorophyll, saponins (to prevent red blood cell destruction), tannins (useful as astringents), citric acid, coumarins, trace minerals, glycosides and a mild laxative, asperuloside.

Herbal Healing Actions: diuretic, blood cleanser, laxative, tonic, astringent, refrigerant, diaphoretic, anti-inflammatory. Helps in hepatitis, cystitis and some venereal diseases. A good cleanser for eczema,

psoriasis and other skin diseases. A good compress for tumerous growths.

Cleansing Properties & Detox Activity: Cleavers is a blood cleansing diuretic with mild laxative activity. Used to dissolve kidney stones and sediment. It eliminates excess fluid, both as a diaphoretic and as a diuretic. It counteracts inflammations, urinary infections, hepatitis and venereal disease. It is an astringent herb for the treatment of psoriasis and various skin diseases. A lymphatic cleanser for swollen or enlarged lymph glands, including prostate disorders, glandular fever and tonsillitis. Also for ailments where toxic conditions and skin problems exist as well as urinary ailments like cystitis and stones.

Safety Precautions: Care should be taken if diabetes exists.

Synergy With Other Herbs: With *juniper berry, uva ursi, goldenseal* and *marshmallow* as a diuretic and sediment dissolver. To prevent itching, scaling and skin discomfort use with *burdock rt., dandelion rt., echinacea purpurea rt., st. john's wort herb, yellow dock rt., nettle's herb, kelp* and *tumeric.* To gently relieve and relax use with *parsley, cornsilk, uva ursi, dandelion, juniper berry, ginger, marshmallow rt.* and *kelp.*

• **Comfrey Root,** *Symphytum officinalis,* Family: *Boraginaceae*

Common Names: gum plant, ass ear, slippery rt., blackwort, boneset, bruisewort, knitbone (Eng); herbe aux coupures, orielle d'ane (French); scharzwurz, schermurz (Gr.)

Traditional Use: Known since the Middle Ages, comfrey was used as a poultice for healing wounds and broken bones until the 1800s. Brought to N. America by the early settlers and introduced to the natives, the Indians were soon using it with much greater skill than the settlers.

Medicinal Parts: root and leaves

Preparation Forms: capsules, compress, douche and bolus, extract, gargle, ointment, plaster, poultice, salve, suppository, tea and tincture. Dosage: 3-9 grams, 10-30 drops tincture, 1 tsp. extract 3x daily, 30-60 grains powder 3x daily, no more than two weeks at a time.

Nutrition Profile: A main constituent, allantoin, works like calcium stimulating cell production for healing connective tissue, bone and collagen. High in sodium, calcium, cobalt, iron, manganese, potassium and vitamins A and B_2. One of the few plants that can produce vitamin B_{12} from the cobalt in the soil.

Herbal Healing Actions: Comfrey is blood purifying, anti-inflammatory, anti-spasmodic and antiviral. It is an anti-catarrhal expectorant. It is hemostatic against wounds. Its mucilaginous, yet astringent properties makes it effective for absorbing toxins, regulating intestinal flora and providing demulcent, antacid, healing action to the colon. Its nutritive content makes it useful after prolonged illness.

Cleansing Properties & Detox Activity: Comfrey leaves and root cleanse the upper respiratory system—effective for asthma, bronchitis, colds, tuberculosis and pleurisy. Helps stop lung hemorrhage accompanying severe inflammation of coughing. The richest source of mucilage, soothing and stimulating mucous membranes, it is also an expectorant, removing toxic material from the lungs. Comfrey is a blood cleansing tonic that treats cystitis, colitis, bladder and prostate infections. It works both internally and externally to promote healing of sores, bones, muscles and tissues. It works well for anemia, arthritis and rheumatism, and for boils, bruises, burns, diarrhea, eczema and other skin infections.

Safety Precautions: Although used for thousands of years safely and effectively, recent investigation shows comfrey contains hepatotoxic pyrrolizidine alkaloids (PA's), such as echimidine. Whether this is from environmental toxins or is naturally present in the plant, *but neutralized by other plant substances, has not been determined.* Until a safe source can be guaranteed, comfrey should not be used during pregnancy and nursing or for children. I recommend using an organically grown source for a short limited time, or using comfrey externally until more information on these alkaloids is known. Not for use when on dietary potassium restrictions.

Synergy With Other Herbs: With *goldenseal, slippery elm* and *aloe vera* as a laxative to detoxify and heal inflamed tissues in the digestive system. With *peppermint, marshmallow, slippery elm, pau d'arco, ginger, aloe vera, wild yam* and *lobelia* as a gentle bowel cleanser when there is irritable bowel disease.

- **Cornsilk,** *Zea Mays,* Family: *Gramineae*

Traditional Use: **Native north and central American Indians used the silk tea for intestinal gravel. Folk medicine history lists cornsilk to stop bleeding and bed-wetting, to lower blood pressure and cholesterol and to treat arteriosclerosis.**

Medicinal Parts: **silk hair surrounding ears of corn.**

Preparation Forms: **infusion, tincture, extract and powder.** Dosage: **tincture: 5 to 20 drops 3x daily; extract: $^1/_2$ tsp. 3x daily; infusion: $^1/_2$ cup as needed; powder: 1 to 5 caps 3x daily.**

Nutrition Profile: **Very high in silicon, high in iron, significant in zinc, magnesium, Vitamin B$_1$, chromium, cobalt, phosphorus and potassium.**

Herbal Healing Actions: **Soothing diuretic to remove stones and sediment, cholagogue to help boost bile production, a lithotropic for relieving fluid retention and for urinary stones and sediment.**

Cleansing Properties & Detox Activity: **Cornsilk is effective for cleansing when there is inflammation of the urethra, bladder, prostate or kidneys. Helps conditions such as cystitis, urinary stones and painful urination, prostatitis, edema from hypertension, and inflamed kidneys. Helps lower high blood pressure and high cholesterol and clear arteriosclerosis.**

Safety Precautions: **None in common use.**

Synergy With Other Herbs: **To relieve fluid retention, with** *uva ursi, juniper bry., parsley, dandelion lf., plantain, marshmallow rt., ginger* **and** *cleavers.* **Or with** *juniper bry., uva ursi, dandelion, marshmallow rt., goldenseal rt., ginger, parsley* **and** *honey.*

- **Cranberry,** *Vaccinium macrocarpon,* Family: *Ericaceae*

Common Names: **New England bogberry; bogberry**

Traditional Use: **Folklore history used the juice for combating urinary tract infections. Native Americans steeped the tea for pleurisy; a leaf tea was used for nausea and for tumors, dysentery and wounds.**

Medicinal Parts: **berries**

Preparation Forms: **juice, powder and douche.** Dosage: **16-oz. per day of juice.**

Nutrition Profile: **high in phosphorus, potassium, and calcium; contains significant amounts of iron, magnesium, manganese, sodium and B-complex vitamins.**

Herbal Healing Actions: **Antibacterial compounds in cranberries inhibit urinary infecting bacteria from adhering to tract walls so that they are flushed from the system. It is a good source of bioflavonoids and vitamin C for tissue tone. Has anti-cancer, blood purifying and immuno-stimulant effects.**

Cleansing Properties & Detox Activity: **A specific for cystitis and other urinary tract infections because it helps neutralize acids and dissolve sediment. New research shows excellent results in clearing kidney stones. Now used successfully in the prevention of asthma attacks, dilating bronchial passages during an attack. A good antidote for reducing ammonia urinary odors in the elderly. Inactivates polio virus type 1. A natural benzoyl peroxide which is a preventative of acne. It prevents the acne-causing bacteria from penetrating the skin so breakouts are less frequent and less severe.**

Safety Precautions: **none in common use**

Synergy With Other Herbs: **In a balancing, cleansing combination rich in bioflavonoids with** *pau d'arco, cranberry, rose hips, burdock, damiana, echinacea rt., myrrh, lemon balm, cinnamon, hibiscus.*

- **Dandelion,** *Taraxacum officinalis* Family, *Compositae*

Common Names: **jin yin hua, pu kung ying, (China), diente de leon (Sp), dente de lion, pissenlit (Fr).**

Medicinal Parts: **The root, roasted or raw, and the leaves**

Preparation Forms: **extract, tea, herbal wine, and capsules.** Dosage: **tincture: 10-15 drops 3x daily; capsules: 1-2 capsules with each meal; tea: 1 cup in the morning and the evening for 4-6 weeks.**

Traditional Use: **Early Medieval medicinal use was for liver congestion, skin problems, fevers and**

boils. It was used in China for cancer, liver diseases and digestive ailments.

Nutrition Profile: Dandelion is very high in Vitamin A, with balanced mineral content.

Herbal Healing Actions: a powerful diuretic; stimulates the liver to release blood toxins.

Cleansing Properties & Detox Activity: Because of its high potassium level, dandelion is an excellent diuretic choice over pharmaceutical diuretics. It can even maintain potassium in the body often leached by over-ambitious pharmaceutical formulas. It is a mucilaginous, blood purifying herb that soothes the digestive tract while absorbing toxins, inhibiting unfriendly bacteria, and allowing friendly fauna to thrive. It scours the liver and kidneys, softens deposits, encourages urination and removes intestinal congestion. As a bitters tonic, dandelion helps the liver and gall bladder produuce bile for better assimilation.

Dandelion is beneficial for a wide variety of ailments including arthritis, rheumatism, gout, skin eruptions, eczema, herpes, acne, abscesses, ulcers, bladder irritation, kidney infections and stones, jaundice, hepatitis, anemia, edema, high blood pressure, tumors, constipation, and heartburn.

Safety Precautions: Large amounts may cause heartburn.

Synergy With Other Herbs: Use with *red clover, licorice rt., chaparral, burdock, pau d'arco, echinacea rt., ascorbate vitamin C, goldenseal rt., garlic, kelp, alfalfa, poria mushroom, American ginseng, sarsaparilla, astragalus, yellow dock, butternut, milk thistle seed, ginger, prickly ash* and *buckthorn bk.* for a strong detoxification formula. With *watercress, yellow dock, pau d' arco, hyssop, parsley, Oregon grape rt., red sage, licorice rt., milk thistle seed* and *hibiscus* for a liver flush. Use with *bancha lf., kukicha* and *chicory* as a cleansing coffee substitute.

• **Echinacea,** *Echinacea Angustifolia and E. Purpurea,* Family: *Compositae*

Common Names: snakeroot, Kansas snakeroot, purple coneflower, comb flower, black sampson, hedgehog, scurvy root, indianhead (Am), kegelblume, kupherblume (Gr).

Traditional Use: The North American Indian pharmacopeia valued echinacea much the same as the Chinese valued ginseng - widely. For snakebites, insect stings, and infective conditions like syphilis, other STDs and respiratory complaints. Introduced into Western culture and medicine in the late 1700s.

Medicinal Parts: root and whole plant

Preparation Forms: tincture, extract, capsules, gargle, douches, washes, compress and tea. Dosage: 10-50 drops of extract or tincture; 2 to 3 capsules every two hours for acute conditions – three times a day for chronic conditions.

Nutrition Profile: high in cobalt, silicon and zinc, chromium, iron, manganese, selenium and in vitamins C, B-3 and riboflavin.

Herbal Healing Actions: a blood cleanser, antiseptic, diaphoretic, stimulant, antibiotic, antiviral, immunostimulant, tonic and antitoxin. Echinacea increases phagocytic activity of leukocytes (antibodies), stabilizes red blood cell count and stimulates T-Cell formation by inhibiting hyaluronidase enzymes. A panacea that activates immunity, restrains infection and clears toxins; reduces inflammation, antidotes poison, promotes tissue repair and arrests discharge, dredges the kidneys, enlivens the lymph, promotes skin cleansing, resolves fever and pushes out eruptions.

Cleansing Properties & Detox Activity: Echinacea is indicated whenever reinforcement for resistance is needed and to stimulate body defense mechanisms — for the onset of colds, flus and other respiratory infections, or for any acute inflammatory condition, like mumps, measles, scarlet fever, rheumatic fevers, urinary infections, venereal infections, herb, food borne infections, bites, stings, Also used for skin conditions: acne, eczema, psoriasis; for congested lymph gland diseases, like chicken pox, ulcers, goiter, strep throat, even cancer and tumors.

Safety Precautions: none known in common use

Synergy With Other Herbs: With *ginsengs, goldenseal* and other tonifying herbs for rebuilding and restoring health. With *red clover, licorice root, chaparral, burdock root* for blood purifying.

• **Elder Bark, Berries & Flowers,** *Sambucus Nigra,* **Family:** *Caprifoliaceae*

Common Names: boretree, scot tree, pipe tree, devil's wood and winlin berries (Eng), parsley elder (Am), hautbois (Fr), kisseke (Ge); American, black or common elder (Am).

Traditional Use: A medicine chest for country people in times past both in Europe (for inflammations of all kinds) and in America. All parts of the tree were useful for everything from a toothache to the plague. Native Americans used all parts of the tree for ailments like rheumatism, fevers, infections, blood disorders, jaundice, children's colic, bronchitis and sore throats.

Medicinal Parts: flowers, berries, inner bark, roots, twigs and leaves.

Preparation Forms: infusion, tincture, decoction, syrup, cream, eyewash, gargle. Dosage: Cream: apply freely. Flowering tops tea: I cup 3x daily. Flowering tops extract: I tsp. with water 3-4 times daily. Decoction of berries: 100 ml. 3x daily.

Nutrition Profile: Elder flowers contain quercetin and rutin, noted for their anti-inflammatory and anti-allergic actions. The berries are high in both vitamin A, B-complex and C. Contains the amino acids: alanine, arginine, aspartic acid, choline, cystine, glutamic acid, histadine, iron, lysine, methionine, phenylalanine, threonine, tryptophan and tyrosine and the minerals: calcium, phosphorus and potassium.

Herbal Healing Actions: Elder flowers are expectorant, diaphoretic, diuretic, and anti-inflammatory in topical applications. Elder berries are diaphoretic, diuretic, laxative and respiratory cleansers. Mild bitter properties accompanied with mucilage activity work as a good detoxifier. The bark is a purgative, emetic (in large doses), diuretic, soothing emollient (topically), bitter and detoxicant.

Cleansing Properties & Detox Activity: Elder reduces inflammation and clears toxins. It acts as an expectorant to remove phlegm and normalize lung function. It is a diuretic to relieve edema and fluid congestion, and is diaphoretic to reduce fevers. Use for the onset of colds and flu with fever, respiratory infections including sinusitis, chest congestion, bronchial asthma, tonsillitis and laryngitis. It may be used for pneumonia with pleurisy, boils, abscesses, burns, rashes, bruises and sprains, arthritis and rheumatism. Effective for childhood diseases—rheumatic fever, measles, chickenpox, even food poisoning. Apply topically to relieve boils, abscesses, rashes, bruises and sprains.

Safety Precautions: Bark must be aged at least one year prior to use or it can be toxic. Recommended for occasional use only. Do not use when pregnant or while nursing.

Synergy With Other Herbs: The juice of the berries with honey for an effective cough syrup. Topically with equal parts *elder* and *chamomile* for inflammations, stiff joints and muscles. Flowers with equal parts *sassafras* in a tea for acne; with equal parts *mint* and *yarrow blossoms* for colds.

• **Fennel Seed,** *Foeniculum vulgare,* **Family:** *Umbelliferae*

Common Names: sweet fennel, roman fennel, wild fennel, large fennel; fenouil (Fr); fenchel and brotanis (Ge); hsiao hui hsiang, shih lo and tzu mo lo (China); uikyo (Japan).

Traditional Use: Romans used fennel to stimulate digestion and for better vision. Its ancient name, marathoron, meant to grow thin, for weight reduction. In Renaissance Europe, fennel was used in broths "for those that are grown fat." It also helped open obstructions of the liver, spleen and gallbladder, to relieve painful swellings there. Native Americans used it for colds, colic and labor as a tonic.

Medicinal Parts: seeds

Preparation Forms: tincture, decoction, infusion, fluid extract, powder, syrup. Dosage: Infusion: 6-oz. 3x daily; fluid extract: 5 to 60 drops 3x daily.

Nutrition Profile: Fennel seeds are high in calcium, magnesium, phosphorus, selenium, sodium and vitamin B_1, and contain significant amounts of iron, manganese, potassium, zinc and vitamins B_2 and B_3.

Herbal Healing Actions: carminative for digestive stimulation, antispasmodic, tonic, and diaphoretic. Stimulates gastrointestinal mucous membranes for food assimilation. Promotes urination, menstruation and lactation due to its phytoestrogens. Tonifying for the kidneys and spleen and the immune system.

Cleansing Properties & Detox Activity: In a cleansing compound, fennel is helpful for indigestion,

gas and flatulence, abdominal cramping, urinary incontinence and bladder irritation, urinary stones, nausea and PMS. As an expectorant, it relieves coughs, hoarsness, loss of voice, bronchial asthma. For nausea and vomiting; for inflammation of the eyes and floaters in the vision; and externally for healing snake bites.

Safety Precautions: **Because they have a stimulating effect on the uterus, fennel seeds are contraindicated during pregnancy. Fennel oil may cause pulmonary edema, respiratory problems and seizures.**

Synergy With Other Herbs: **With** *rhubarb root* **for digestive disorders. To calm and soothe coughs: with** *wild cherry bk., slippery elm bk.* **and** *licorice rt.* **For digestion in kids: with** *peppermint, chamomile, papaya, ginger* **and** *orange peel.*

• **Fenugreek,** *Foenum-graceum,* Family: *Leguminosae*
Common Names: **hu lu pa, ku tou (China), alholva (Spain), bird's foot (English).**
Medicinal Parts: **seeds**
Preparation Forms: **poultice, tincture, powder, capsules.** Dosage: **tincture: 1-2ml 3x daily; powder: 1-2 tsp. daily or 1-2 capsules with meals.**
Traditional Use: **Both the ancient Egyptians and used fenugreek seeds for medicinal purposes, as a poultice drawing treatment for boils, styes and gastrointestinal problems, even roasted them as a coffee. Benedictine monks introduced foenugreek to Europe in the 9th century for diabetes and tuberculosis. By the 16th century, it was popular in England as a sprouting seed and vegetable in their diet. Foenugreek was used in India as a spice for curries and a source for yellow cloth dye.**
Nutrition Profile: **The seed is 30% galactomannan-like mucilage with lecithin, making an excellent choice for a poultice; 20% protein and high in fiber, making the seed a good choice for a cleansing fiber.**
Herbal Healing Actions: **Antiseptic properties make fenugreek a topical specific for boils, gout and abscesses. Reduces intestinal inflammation and normalizes bowel activity to relieve diarrhea and constipation. Also an antiviral, expectorant, diuretic, and emollient.**
Cleansing Properties & Detox Activity: **Fenugreek helps reduce total and LDL (bad) cholesterol without altering levels of HDL (good) cholesterol, makings it helpful in preventing atherosclerosis. It reduces blood glucose, plasma glucagon, and somatostatin levels including sugar-induced hyperglycemia allowing less insulin doses in diabetics. Fenugreek can reduce the amount of calcium oxalate deposited in the kidneys. It helps relieve excess mucous and respiratory congestion and lower blood pressure.**
Safety Precautions: **Large doses may result in hypoglycemia.**
Synergy With Other Herbs: **To help breakdown toxic buildup use with** *gotu kola, garlic, red sage, black cohosh, lecithin, goldenseal rt., quassia wood, bilberry, poria mushroom, fennel sd., milk thistle sd., tumeric, kola nut* **and** *kelp.* **For a cleansing combination use with** *flax sd., gotu kola, fennel sd., parsley, uva ursi, senna, bancha, burdock rt., gymnema sylvestre, red clover, lemon peel, hibiscus* **and** *bladderwrack.* **With** *cranberry juice ext., echinacea ang. rt., coriander, wild yam rt., dandelion, marshmallow, juniper bry., uva ursi* **and** *kava kava* **for a tissue toning formula. For respiratory ailments use with** *marshmallow, mullein, ma huang, rosemary, ginkgo biloba, passionflowers, wild cherry bk., angelica, lobelia, cinnamon.*

• **Fo-Ti-Tieng Root,** *Polygonum multiflorum* (See Ho-Shou-Wu)

• **Garlic,** *Allium sativum,* Family: *Liliaceae*
Common Names: **cropleek, poor man's treacle (UK); hsiao suan (China), ail (Fr.), ajo (Spain).**
Traditional Use: **Garlic has been known for medicinal use dating back to the early dynasties of China, to Egypt and the Pharoahs. The Roman Pliny extolled its detoxifying properties, as a remedy for snakebites and for neutralizing the effects of poisonous plants like henbane. It was used against gangrene and infections. In Chinese folk medicine, it was a stomachic, detoxifier and antiparasitic.**
Medicinal Parts: **bulb**

Preparation Forms: Fresh: either topical or juice; capsule, tincture, tea, oil, poultice, enema, implant. Dosage: **One clove 3x daily; Garlic oil capsules: 3 a day or 3 capsules 3x daily when infection occurs.**

Nutrition Profile: **Loaded in fiber, garlic is high in calcium, iron, magnesium, phosphorus, potassium, vitamin A and C, and B-complex vitamins. It contains 33 sulphur compounds. Garlic's primary benefit comes from its rich antioxidant compounds (at least 15 different), including germanium, chromium, selenium, zinc, vitamins A and C and 17 amino acids.**

Herbal Healing Actions: **a proven antiseptic, antibacterial, and antiviral, garlic helps overcome infections by boosting immune response and attacking the microorganism. A diaphoretic and diuretic to enhance kidney activity. A specific in controlling arteriosclerosis and high blood pressure, raising good HDL cholesterol while lowering bad LDL. It is a vermifuge to rid the body of parasites. It is a liver stimulant and stomachic for bile production, and important in re-establishing beneficial flora in the digestive tract.**

Cleansing Properties & Detox Activity: **Garlic's list of cleansing and detox benefits is wide ranging. It is a blood purifying tonic that helps restore good body chemistry against pollutants and allergens. Garlic is a part of almost every kind of detoxification compound, especially those involving digestive waste elimination. It is a specific for removing candida albicans yeast overgrowth. It is effective for almost every type of respiratory congestion problem, from colds, coughs and flu to chronic bronchitis and asthma. Recent tests show that garlic has anti-cancer (especially stomach cancer) and antitumor effects. Garlic is good as an enema for detoxification and to expel worms as a liver stimulant for bile production and as part of a compound to re-establish friendly, beneficial flora in the digestive tract. It is effective as part of a compound for arthritis and rheumatism.**

Safety Precautions: **stomach irritating if taken raw; not for use in medicinal doses during pregnancy.**

Synergy With Other Herbs: **With** *echinacea angustifolia, siberian ginseng, rosehips, goldenseal rt., hawthorn, guggul, pau d' arco, astragalus, elecampane, peppermint* **for herbal defense in high risk seasons.**

• **Gentian,** *Gentiana Lutea,* Family: *Gentiaceae*

Common Names: **yellow gentian, felwort, bitterwort and baldmoney (Eng), gentiane, quinquina du pauvre (Fr), magenwurzel, bitterwurz, kreuzwurz, and gänzene (Ge).**

Traditional Use: **Used in medieval times as a strengthener to prevent fainting and against poisoning from mad dog bites. As a pain reliever from griping and bruises. Used for ailing livers and bad stomach.**

Medicinal Parts: **root**

Preparation Forms: **decoction, tincture, infusion, powder, extract.** Dosage: **Large doses to drain wastes; small doses for restoring. Tincture: 10-30 drops $1/_2$ hour before meals to help digestion.**

Nutrition Profile: **Gentian is high in magnesium, phosphorus, selenium, zinc and vitamins B_1 and B_3. It contains significant amounts of calcium, chromium, iron and vitamins A, C and B_2.**

Herbal Healing Actions: **As a primary bitters tonic, gentian is a good addition to any liver cleansing program. The bitter properties stimulate the mucous membranes of the stomach and gallbladder, increasing the flow of bile, helping absorption of nutrients and speeding elimination of wastes. Gentian calms the liver and gall bladder, relieving irritability, promoting bile flow and bowel movement, and clearing toxins. It is anti-inflammatory, blood cleansing, and a cholagogue to lower cholesterol.**

Cleansing Properties & Detox Activity: **Gentian restores strength to the liver, spleen and stomach. It stimulates the upper digestive tract and helps to maintain proper digestive function. It is helpful even in severe liver-related problems, such as jaundice and hepatitis. It is also beneficial for almost all digestive-related problems, such as chronic diarrhea, constipation, gastritis, heartburn, ulcers, Crohn's disease, poor appetite and anorexia. It is a primary herb to help clear vaginal yeast infections.**

Safety Precautions: **Not recommended when emaciated or if weak digestion is a problem. Use caution with a sensitive stomach. May aggravate hyperacidity of the stomach. May also cause nervousness and muscle spasms. Do not use if hypoglycemic.**

Synergy With Other Herbs: **With** *ginger, capsicum* **and** *wormwood* **for indigestion and heartburn. A good addition to any liver cleansing formula.**

• **Ginger Root,** *Zingiber Officinalis,* Family: *Zingiberraceae*
Common Names: **gingembre (Fr), ingwer (Ge),jiang or chiang (Ch).**
Origin & Traditional Use: **Ginger's known use dates back over 4000 years in India and China; it is listed in Chinese texts from 2000 years ago for its medicinal properties. Traditionally used to promote perspiration during colds, to aid in digestion, for headaches and as a cough remedy. Native of Asia, it is now cultivated in the West Indies, Jamaica, India and Africa.**
Medicinal Parts: **root**
Preparation Forms: **fresh and dried, essential oil, decoction and tincture, tea, capsules.** Dosage: **tea: 2-oz. 3x daily; tincture: 15 to 30 drops 3x daily; extract: 5-20 drops 3x daily; caps: 2 to 4 3x daily.**
Nutrition Profile: **Ginger is very high in aluminum, manganese and silicon; contains high amounts of magnesium and potassium, and vitamins C, B$_2$ and B$_3$. Contains a wealth of amino acids.**
Herbal Healing Actions: **Ginger is a digestive stimulant and carminative to help food assimilation, settle the stomach, increase amylase in saliva and tone intestinal muscles. It acts as a diaphoretic to increase perspiration for removal of toxic wastes and promotes expectoration to release congestion from the respiratory system. It works as an immune stimulant and helps fight infections. It is a circulatory tonic and reduces serum cholesterol levels in the blood. It is an effective anti-inflammatory to reduce pain and swelling of both rheumatoid arthritis and osteoarthritis.**
Cleansing Properties & Detox Activity: **Use ginger for colds and flu, fever, bacterial and viral infections, bronchitis, tonsilitis, laryngitis, stomach upset, ulcers, flatulence and bloating, motion and morning sickness, food poisoning, and PMS congestion. Promotes toxin cleansing through the skin by opening pores and stimulating perspiration. Helps cleanse the bowels and kidneys, and stimulates digestion. It is effective for nausea, gas, heartburn, flatulence, diarrhea and dizziness.**
Safety Precautions: **Use carefully in early stages of pregnancy (low doses for morning sickness-1 gm).**
Synergy With Other Herbs: **With** *capsicum, wormwood* **and** *gentian* **for indigestion and heartburn. With** *mullein, pleurisy rt, marshmallow, rose hips, ephedra, licorice, calendula, boneset, peppermint* **and** *fennel seed* **to clear mucous congestion.**

• **Ginkgo Biloba,** *Ginkgo biloba* **(Bai guo)** Family: *coniferales*
Common Names: **gingold, maidenhair tree, icho (Ja), pai-kuo, yin hsing (Ch), living fossil (Eng).**
Medicinal Parts: **leaves**
Preparation Forms: **Best results from extract, also capsules, tea.** Dosage: **1 tablet 3x daily.**
Traditional Use: **In existence over 200 million years, ginkgo is believed to be one of the oldest trees in the world. But we can see a recent example of its amazing survival ability in modern times. In 1945, Ginkgo was the only tree that survived the A-bomb blast of Hiroshima. Ginkgo is mentioned in 2800 B.C. in a medicinal materia medica of China, where was used to treat asthma, allergies and coughs, to relieve wheezing and to lessen phlegm, and to treat incontinence. It was not until the 1950's that ginkgo began to be researched in modern pharmacology in the west. Today, wild ginkgo trees have become extinct except those cultivated in the Far Eastern temple gardens.**
Nutrition Profile: **The leaves contain flavone glycosides, bioflavones, sitosterol and anthocyanin.**
Herbal Healing Actions: **Antioxidant, anti-inflammatory, antiallergenic, antispasmodic, antiasthmatic, circulatory stimulant and tonic. A primary brain and mental energy stimulant, it increases both peripheral and cerebral circulation through vasodilation. Ginkgo has the ability to protect against nerve damage from neurotoxic material. Effective against vertigo, dizziness and ringing in the ears. As an anti-oxidant, it protects the cells against damage from free radicals, reduces blood cell clumping which can lead to con-**

201

gestive heart disease, and reduces lung inflammation leading to asthmatic attacks. It also helps return elasticity to cholesterol-hardened blood vessels.

Cleansing Properties & Detox Activity: **Stimulates circulation and supplies oxygen to the brain,** specifically to brain-damaged areas. Ginkgo protects and nourishes brain cells, enhances mental alertness and defends against disorders that cause senility or Alzheimer's. It increases circulation in people with hardening of the arteries, helping to return elasticity to cholesterol-hardened blood vessels. Provides specific cardiac protection against stroke and atherosclerosis. Because Ginkgo inhibits PAF (platelet activating factor), it can prevent blood clotting in congestive heart disease, asthma, skin problems and hearing problems. Ginkgo boosts acetylcholine levels - thus the ability to better transmit body electrical impulses.

Safety Precautions: **In extremely large, high doses, ginkgo may cause irritability, restlessness and diarrhea. The fruit pulp and raw seed are toxic. Direct contact with the pulp may cause contact dermatitis. Swallowing the seeds may cause stomach ache, nausea, diarrhea, convulsions, difficulty in breathing and shock. Not recommended for pregnant or lactating women. Do not use ginkgo if taking anticoagulants.**

Synergy With Other Herbs: **It is a specific in anti-aging and regenerative compounds. For relief of** respiratory and circulatory conditions, with *mullein, wild cherry bk., pleurisy rt., plantain.* **and** *horehound.* **For asthma, with** *marshmallow rt., fenugreek sd., mullein, ma huang* **and** *rosemary.* **For mental clarity, with** *gotu kola* **and** *panax ginseng.*

• **Ginseng, Panax,** *Ren-shen (Ch),* Am Panax Ginseng, (*Quinquefolium*), Family: *Araliaceae*
Common Names: man root (Eng), kraftwurzel (Ge), ren shen (Che), five fingers, tartar root, cherokee root, red berry, sang/santa root, seed of the earth, panacea, jinshard, garantoquen (Native Am), ninsin.

Traditional Use: **Ginseng has been known for all of man's known history — at least 7,000 years; it** has been valued for its remarkable therapeutic benefits for centuries. Ginsengs have been used for over 5,000 years to keep natives of different cultures well. Wars have been fought for control of the forests where it grew. There are even references to "Pannag," the all-healing ginseng, being used for trade in the marketplace of Israel in The Old Testament. During the 9th century, the Arabs brought ginseng to Europe for its ability to improve stamina and resistance to stress.

In traditional Chinese belief, ginseng is the crystallization of the essence of Earth in the shape of man. Considering it the best tonic for old age, the Chinese used ginseng so heavily over the centuries (it takes 6 to 10 years to mature) that Asian ginseng is now extremely hard to get and very expensive. American panax ginseng was one of the most important medicines used by Native Americans, highly esteemed by every native culture with access to it. For the elderly, ginseng was a special tonic that strengthened mental power. Some tribes used it for women to increase fertility and to induce child birth without suffering; others to cure nosebleeds, treat shortness of breath or for men as a "woman catcher." Finally, in the 18th century the West learned of its stimulating and healing qualities.

Medicinal Parts: **root - dried or fresh**

Preparation Forms: **capsules, tablets, tea, extract.** Dosage: **about 500 mg daily or** $^1/_2$ **tsp. powdered** root 3x a day. Ginseng benefits are cumulative in the body. Taking ginseng as a tonic for several months to a year is more effective than short term doses.

Nutrition Profile: **Ginseng has measurable amounts of germanium for tissue healing. Ginseng's** saponins retard plaque formation on the aorta to help prevent stroke. Ginseng's polysaccharides protect against alcohol induced ulcers and increase the protective cells in the gastrointestinal lining.

Herbal Healing Actions: **adaptogenic, tonic, immuno-stimulant, anti-ulcer and hypoglycemic. The** most effective adaptogen of all tonic herbs, capable of stimulating both long and short term energy. A premier brain and memory center stimulant.

Cleansing Properties & Detox Activity: **Ginseng is a strong tonic for boosting energy and rejuvena-**tion during detoxing. As an adaptogen, ginseng provides energy to all body systems, promotes regeneration from stress and fatigue, and rebuilds foundation strength. Ginseng increases the body's ability to

fight disease. Ginseng is an effective stimulant to the central nervous system, but in a gentler, calmer way than stimulant drugs like caffeine and nicotine, so it also improves sleep and relieves pain. Ginseng can improve memory, concentration, alertness, visual motor control and reaction time. It reduces the risk of heart attacks by thinning the blood, suppresses arrythmias, and helps regulate blood pressure by regulating cholesterol levels in the blood. Ginseng influences carbohydrate metabolism and has the ability to stimulate the removal of sugar from the blood, preventing hypoglycemic blood sugar swings.

Safety Precautions: In large amounts, may cause insomnia or high blood pressure. Avoid while consuming caffeine. Do not take during pregnancy or during acute diseases, high fever or severe inflammation.

Synergy With Other Herbs: With *licorice rt.* to regulate blood sugar swings. With *prince ginseng, kirin ginseng, suma, echinacea angustifolia* and *purpurea rt., pau d' arco, astragalus, St, John's wort, ashwagandha* and *aralia* to energize and restore body defenses. With *bee pollen, Siberian ginseng rt., gotu kola, fo ti rt., kirin ginseng, prince ginseng., suma, aralia rt., alfalfa, dong quai* to revitalize the system.

• **Ginseng, Siberian, (Eleuthero),** *Eleutherococcus Senticosus (Wujiashen)*
Common Names: eleuthero, wujiashen, prince of tonics, ciwujia, devil's shrub, touch-me-not, ussurian thorny pepper bush.

Medicinal Parts: root

Preparation Forms: tea, liquid and powdered extract, capsules, herbal wine. Dosage: Take 2 capsules dried herb 2-3 times daily; or take 1 dropperful of tincture two to three times daily.

Traditional Use: Originally used in China for over 4,000 years as a general tonic for vitality, mental clarity and virility. Its greatest tradition comes from Russian history. It was the Soviet Union in modern times who brought world wide attention to Siberian ginseng for clinical use. A 15 year Russian study with over 20,000 people chronicled Siberian ginseng's ability to boost energy, relieve fatigue, reduce PMS irritability and menopause symptoms. Russian scientists also gave it to their athletes to increase their performance during Olympic games. In 1986 following the nuclear disaster at Chernobyl, it was given to the people to aid in exposure to radiation and toxic chemicals.

Nutrition Profile: Assists carbohydrate metabolism to normalize blood sugar levels in diabetics. Effective in lowering blood pressure and cholesterol. A highly complex herb - contains ginsenoids, polysaccharides, triterpenoids, saponins, lignans, sterols, B complex vitamins, vitamins A, D and E, selenium, amino acids, minerals and enzymes. Its glycosides provide antioxidant influence and overall resistance to chemical factors. Its generous amount of germanium preserves oxygen and stimulates immunity.

Herbal Healing Actions: A prime adaptogen and tonic, Siberian ginseng helps prevent infection and maintain well-being making highly useful for avoiding disease and recovering from illness. It was used by Russian astronauts to help their transition into weightlessness in space. Immuno-stimulant, antispasmodic, antirheumatic. Eleuthero accelerates body recovery after intense activity, decreases lactic acid build-up and increases resistance to developing injury. Siberian ginseng increases oxygen uptake, a highly desired quality for those who suffer from respiratory disorders. Traditional Chinese medicine uses Siberian ginseng is a primary herb for insomnia.

Cleansing Properties & Detox Activity: Siberian ginseng exhibits many of the rejuvenative, adaptogen properties of its cousin panax ginseng in terms of energy and endurance and raising sexual potency. It is an all-body tonic and an energizer which combats depression and fatigue, and helps the body rebuild system strength after mental or physical exhaustion. It should be a prime part of any immune rebuilding herbal combination to increase body resistance to disease, especially heart disease. In fact, Siberian ginseng promotes an enormous increase in the number of immune cells (particularly natural killer cells) to support the immune system against infections of all types. It is an excellent nutritive tonic for both the adrenal and circulatory systems, helping the body withstand heat, cold, infection and radiation.

Safety Precautions: Not recommended for persons with hypertension. Avoid caffeine while using. Some people may experience insomnia when consuming large doses.

Synergy With Other Herbs: **With** *kava kava, kirin ginseng, American ginseng, prince ginseng, dong quai, fo-ti rt., suma, kola nut* and *gotu kola* **for mental inner energy. With** *American ginseng, Chinese kirin ginseng, prince ginseng, fo-ti rt., suma, gotu kola, wild oat tops* **and** *sarsaparilla* **for active physical energy.**

• **Goldenseal,** *Hydrastis canadensis,* Family: *Ranunculacaea*

Common Names: yellow root, Indian dye, tumeric root, yellow puccoon, eye balm root, ground raspberry (Am), racine d' or, racine orange (Fr), wasserblatt and gelbwurzel (Ge).

Traditional Use: First used by Native Americans as a stomachic and tonic applied for ailments like hepatitis, cancers, inflammations, fevers, indigestion, catarrh, eye infections, mouth ulcers, gonorrhea and dyspepsia. Introduced to European culture in 1760 and made popular by 19th century Eclectics.

Medicinal Parts: root

Preparation Forms: tincture, powder, douche, skin wash, gargle, ear drops. Dosage: capsules: 2 to 4 caps 3x daily; tincture: small doses for liver restoration; medium doses for astringent, decongestant, disinfectant and anti-inflammatory actions; large doses for laxative and stimulating actions.

Nutrition Profile: Very high in cobalt and silicon; high in iron, magnesium, zinc and vitamin C; significant amounts of chromium, phosphorus, potassium, selenium, and vitamins A, B_1, B_2, and B_3.

Herbal Healing Actions: Two main compounds in goldenseal, the alkaloids berberine and hydrastine, have strong antibiotic action, and help scour the liver and gall bladder through bile secretion. Goldenseal has tonic, astringent and anti-inflammatory effects on mucous membranes, making it helpful in resolving mucous obstructions, arresting infections and clearing toxins. It strengthens the body through its tonifying action on the intestines, liver, stomach, veins and skin. It is antiseptic, astringent and hemostat making it a good choice for skin rashes, acne, measles, dermatitis, open sores, ulcers and varicose veins. It is effective both internally and externally.

Cleansing Properties & Detox Activity: Goldenseal is a broad spectrum medicinal with a wide range of detoxification benefits. Its properties include effective blood cleansing by removing circulatory congestion to restore veins and enliven the blood. It stimulates blood supply to the spleen, increasing spleen activity to release immune potentiators. It is a bitter tonic with laxative, bowel regulating effects against constipation diarrhea and hemorrhoids. It helps resolve infectious tumors of the breast, uterus and stomach and skin. It is effective in cleansing and healing formulas for cystitis, gonorrhea, candida albicans, eye inflammations, head and sinus congestion, bronchitis, gallstones, gastric ulcers and chronic gastritis, fevers, flu, tonsillitis and malaria.

Safety Precautions: Not for use during pregnancy - a uterine stimulant; not for use with high blood pressure. Extended use can weaken good intestinal flora.

Synergy With Other Herbs: **With** *echinacea, garlic* **and antibiotic herbs for immune stimulation. With** *chaste-tree berry* **for PMS. With** *licorice rt., chaparral, burdock, pau d' arco, echinacea, ascorbate vit. C, goldenseal rt., garlic, kelp, alfalfa, dandelion, poria mushroom, American ginseng, sarsaparilla, astragalus, yellow dock, butternut, milk thistle seed, ginger, prickly ash* **and** *buckthorn bark* **in a detox formula.**

• **Gravel Root,** *Eupatorium purpureum,* Family: *Compositae*

Common Names: trumpet-weed, gravelweed, joe pye weed, jopi weed, purple boneset, feverweed, kidney root, queen-of-the-meadow root (Am).

Traditional Use: Used medicinally by native Americans as a blood and kidney remedy, for typhus, colds and coughs, wounds, burns, irregular menstruation and nephrosis. Gravel root got its name Joe Pye weed from a New England Indian of that name who used it to cure typhus among the settlers.

Medicinal Parts: root

Preparation Forms: tincture, infusion, decoction. Dosage: tincture: $1/2$ to 1 tsp. 3x daily; or 10-30 drops 3x daily; infusion: 1-oz. root to 1pt. water.

Nutrition Profile: **A flavonoid-rich, high tannin herb with strong bitters principles for digestion.**

Herbal Healing Actions: **Gravel root promotes urination, removes fluid congestion and relieves bloating. It helps clean out toxins by dissolving sediment and stones. It also helps to dissolve the systemic inorganic crystalline deposits of gout, rheumatism and arthritis. Actions are tonic, nervine, stimulant, blood cleansing, diaphoretic and digestive.**

Cleansing Properties & Detox Activity: **Gravel root is a diuretic for the urinary and reproductive systems that also reduces inflammation and fever, with disinfecting action. It clears excess uric acid, and strengthens the tissues against urinary incontinence. Especially effective for urinary infections, stones and irritation, excess uric acid, urinary incontinence, edema, gout, rheumatism and arthritis.**

Safety Precautions: **none in common use**

Synergy With Other Herbs: **To aid in elimination of sediment, with** *dandelion rt., parsley rt., hydrangea rt., wild yam rt., marshamallow rt., licorice rt., lecithin, lemon balm herb, ginger rt., and milk thistle sd.* **With** *devil's claw rt., red clover blsm., Oregon grape rt., ginkgo biloba, licorice rt., horsetail, slippery elm, elm bk., prickly ash bk., ginger rt., flax sd.* **for a soothing and relaxing formula.**

• **Green Tea,** *Thea sinensis*

Common Names: **Bancha leaf, kukicha twig, Cha (China)**

Medicinal Parts: **leaves (unfermented), leaf buds.**

Preparation Forms: **tea, capsules, extract.** Dosage: **1 cup green tea daily or 1 capsule (5-15 mg) daily.**

Origins & Traditional Use: **Green tea was discovered by a Chinese emperor in 2700 B.C. We have written information about its use from the third century B.C. Cultivated from the 6th century A.D. to satisfy demand. Traditionally, a beneficial fasting tea providing energy and mental clarity during cleansing. The Chinese regard green tea as a stimulant, an astringent for clearing phlegm and a digestive remedy.**

Nutritional Profile: **rich in flavonoids with antioxidant and anti-allergen activity; contains potent polyphenols like catechins, that act as antioxidants, yet do not interfere with iron or protein absorption.**

Herbal Healing Properties: **antioxidant, vasodilator, anticancer, antitumor, antibacterial, antiviral. During detoxification green tea's polyphenols are remarkably valuable at lessening the production of uremic toxicity to protect the kidneys.**

Cleansing Properties & Detox Activity: **Traditionally a good fasting tea, providing energy support and clearer thinking during cleansing. Combats free radical damage to protect against degenerative disease. Boosts enzyme production in the body. Green tea is fully enzyme-active for weight loss and cleansing. Green tea is a vasodilator and smooth muscle relaxant in cases of bronchial asthma. Highly valued as a cancer preventive. Recent research in Japan shows that several cups of green tea on a regular daily basis are effective in reducing lung cancer death rates, even in men who smoked two packs of cigarettes a day. Other studies in Tokyo indicate the same success with stomach and liver cancers. It shows definite evidence of tumor and skin cancer prevention in animals, even when exposed to ultraviolet radiation.**

Green tea is equally valuable as a heart protector, especially against atherosclerosis. Prevents LDL cholesterol development and PAF (platelet aggregation factor), blood stickiness. Green tea has antibiotic qualities, amazingly even combatting antibiotic-resistant microorganisms. It can lower iron levels in the body, having a direct anti-viral effect on abnormal types of hepatitis viruses.

Safety Precautions: **none in common use.**

Synergy With Other Herbs: **With** *burdock rt., gotu kola herb, kukicha twig, fo ti rt., hawthorn bry., cinnamon bk.,* **and** *hisbiscus flowers* **for a cleansing, energizing antioxidant tea.**

• **Hawthorn,** *Cratageus oxyacantha,* Family: *Rosaceae*

Common Names: **hedgethorn, whitethorn, red haw, hagthorn, quickthorn; aubépine, epine blanche, pain d' oiseau (Fr), weissdorn, hagendorn, hühnerbeere, mehlbeerstaude, vogelbeer (Ge).**

Traditional Use: **Mediterranean cultures used hawthorn against urinary stones and dropsy. During the Renaissance, it was used for digestive complaints and urinary tract ailments. TCM used the berries to improve digestion and eliminate stagnant blood and food, and as a remedy for dyspepsia and bloating.**

Medicinal Parts: **berries, flowers and leaves**

Preparation Forms: **extract, tea, tincture, capsules. Dosage: Cumulative effects over a lengthy period for best effects. Tincture: 15-30 drops 3x daily; extract: 10-15 drops 3x daily; infusion: 1 cup 3x daily.**

Nutrition Profile: **high in chromium and selenium and contains significant amounts of calcium, cobalt, magnesium, phosphorus, potassium, sodium and vitamins A and C with bioflavonoids.**

Herbal Healing Actions: **Hawthorn is one of the top three cardiovascular tonics in the world. It has a dilating action on the coronary arteries to improve the blood supply to the heart and limit cholesterol build-up on artery walls. It is a calming stimulant for the entire circulatory system, toning the heart muscle, regulating its beat and calming cardio-pulmonary restlessness. It has collagen stabilizing properties that help maintain muscle and joint integrity and prevents free radical damage.**

Cleansing Properties & Detox Activity: **Hawthorn is a specific for a wide range of circulatory conditions: congestive heart failure, angina, arrhythmias, arteriosclerosis, high blood pressure, difficult breathing, hypertension and insomnia from cardio-pulmonary problems. It relieves edema and fluid congestion, and promotes hormone balance. It acts quickly as well as longterm, to offer a feeling of well-being.**

Safety Precautions: **None in common use**

Synergy With Other Herbs: **With** *red clover, pau d' arco, nettles, sage, alfalfa, horsetail herb, milk thistle seed, gotu kola, echinacea, blue malva, yerba santa* **and** *lemon grass* **for a blood cleansing and purifying tea. With** *spirulina, bee pollen, rose hips, barley grass, Siberian ginseng, alfalfa, sarsaparilla, raspberry, kelp, parsley, carrots, golden seal, mullein* **to rebuild the body.**

• **Hibiscus,** *Hibiscus sabdariffa,* Family: *Malvaceae*

Common Names: **Jamaica sorrel, roselle, rozelle; karkadé (Fr); hibiscusblüten.**

Traditional Use: **In African folk medicine, used as a diuretic, liver and bile aid, antibacterial, antispasmodic and antiparasitic. The leaves were used as an emollient, as a poultice for abscesses, and for coughs.**

Medicinal Parts: **flowers and leaves**

Preparation Forms: **tea, extract, decoction. Dosage: 2 cups 3x daily as a tea; extract: as needed.**

Nutrition Profile: **Leaves and flowers are rich in chromium, manganese and selenium; high in calcium, iron, potassium and silicon and contain significant amounts of magnesium, phosphorus, sodium and vitamins A, C, and B$_3$. Flavonoids may used for tissue tightening (in cellulite), and weight control.**

Herbal Healing Actions: **A diuretic, tonic, demulcent, emollient, antiseptic, astringent, digestive, mild laxative, anti-inflammatory and bile stimulant.**

Cleansing Properties & Detox Activity: **The flowers decrease the viscosity of the blood helping to reduce blood pressure and stimulate intestinal peristalsis. Hibiscus flowers are used to dissolve phlegm, for catarrh of the upper respiratory passages, as a gentle laxative and diuretic, and for circulation disorders. Helps to clear the body of alcohol after a "hard night."**

Safety Precautions: **none in common use**

Synergy With Other Herbs: **Works with almost any herbal combination to counteract bitterness of other herbs. With** *senna, fennel seed, ginger, papaya, lemon balm, peppermint, parsley* **and** *calendula* **for a simple laxative tea. With** *dandelion, watercress, yellow dock, pau d'arco, hyssop, parsley, Oregon grape, red sage, licorice* **and** *milk thistle seed* **for a liver flush tea.**

• **Ho-Shou-Wu, Fo-Ti-Tieng Root,** *Polygonium multiflorum,* Family: *Polygonaceae*

Common Names: **fo-ti, fo-ti-tieng (Eng), she chien tsao (Ch), fleeceflower, hill-brother, hill-father**

Traditional Use: **In legend, Ho-Shou-Wu was the grandchild of a man who at age 58 had not been**

able to father a child. A monk told him to eat a certain herb (Ho-Shou-Wu). Not only did he father a child but his hair turned black again. His son lived to be 130 and he himself lived to be 160 years old.

Medicinal Part: **root.**

Preparation Forms: **tea, extract, capsules.** Dosage: **capsules: 2 capsules with meals 2x daily.**

Nutrition Profile: **A source of beta-carotene, calcium, carbohydrates, chromium, fiber, iron, lecithin, potassium, selenium, vitamin C, thiamin and zinc. Also contains leucoanthrocyanidins (LAC), a bioflavnoid-like compound, which have anti-inflammatory, cardiotonic, hypotensive and vasodilating action. Currently being studied for one of its compounds, LAC, effective in reducing inflammatory conditions such as ulcers and arthritis.**

Herbal Healing Actions: **An effective liver tonic, an anti-toxic blood cleanser, gentle diuretic and laxative. A potent antibacterial and antiviral, it has anti-cancer activity. An astringent, it helps stop leakage of nocturnal emission, spermatorrhea, even vaginal discharge. Cardiotonic for the cirdulatory system, ho-shou-wu is vasodilating in normalizing blood pressure. A mild sedative, used in Chinese traditional medicine for poor sleep.**

Cleansing Properties & Detox Activity: **Ho-shou-wu rejuvenates, restores energy, increases fertility. For the elderly, it helps maintain strength and vigor. Strengthens and tonifies the liver, kidneys and blood. A good choice for hypoglycemia and diabetes because of hypoglycemic blood-glucose-lowering activity. Lowers blood cholesterol levels and inhibits atherosclerosis by decreasing blood coagulation. Reduces hypertension and coronary disease. It moistens the intestines and unblocks bowel movements.**

Safety Precautions: **Use caution in cases of spleen deficiency, phlegm and diarrhea. Do not use while taking or using onion, chives or garlic.**

Synergy With Other Herbs: **With** *bancha lf., burdock, gotu kola, kukicha twig, hawthorn bry., cinnamon, orange peel* **for a cleansing, energizing tea with antioxidants. For calm energy use with** *St. John's wort, kava kava, American ginseng rt., ashwagandha, gotu kola, scullcap, Siberian ginseng rt., rosemary, wood betony* **and** *ginger.* **To boost vigor use with** *American ginseng rt., Chinese ginseng rt., Siberian ginseng, suma, gotu kola, prince ginseng rt., dong quai, sarsaparilla* **and** *ginkgo biloba.*

- **Horseradish,** *Cochlearia armoracia or Armoracia rusticana,* Family: *Cruciferae*

Common Names: **mountain radish, radcole and raifort (Eng), moutarde des allemandes or des capucins, ravenelle and cranson de bretagne (Fr), meerrettich, kren, märek (Ge).**

Traditional Use: **Used in medieval times as a plaster for sciatica, gout, joint-aches and hard swellings of the spleen and liver.**

Medicinal Parts: **root**

Preparation Forms: **syrup, extract, gargle, tincture, tea, plaster, wash, poultice.** Dosage: **grated root: 2-4 grams; tincture: 1 to 1 $^1/_2$ teaspoons or 6-12 drops.**

Nutrition Profile: **high in potassium and vitamin C, with significant amounts of calcium, iron, phosphorus, potassium, sulphur, protease, selenium and vitamin B.**

Herbal Healing Actions: **diuretic, stimulant, digestive, expectorant, laxative, stomachic, diaphoretic and blood cleansing. Stimulates circulation, reduces infections promoting tissue repair and benefits the skin. Aids in digestion. Acts as a powerful expectorant to remove phlegm and lymph congestion. Stimulates urination helping to clear kidney congestion, infections and edema.**

Cleansing Properties & Detox Activity: **A cold and flu herb that warms the body, relieves sinus ache, and releases excess mucous. Particularly good for asthma. An herb to relieve urinary infections and stones. Helps rheumatism, gout, colitis, asthma, chronic bronchitis, sore throat and coughing, intestinal parasites, skin ulcers and acne.**

Safety Precautions: **Very strong. Don't use if there is acute inflammation, during pregnancy or thyroid imbalance. Overdose can irritate the kidneys or gastric mucosa. Discontinue if diarrhea or nightsweats occur.**

Synergy With Other Herbs: With *honey* and *apple cider vinegar* for rheumatism. With *mustard seed* for water retention. With *water* and *honey* for a sore throat gargle.

• Horsetail, *Equisetum Arvense*, Family: *Equisetaceae*

Common Names: shave grass, joint weed, bull pipes and tad broom (Am); Dutch rushes, paddock pipes and pewterwort (Eng); prêle, equisette, queue de chat/de cheval (Fr), schaftheu (Ge).

Traditional Use: Native Americans used horsetail for constipation, kidney ailments, dropsy and lumbago. In the Middle Ages, it was used to stop bleeding, both internally (ulcers) and externally (wounds). The decoction taken in wine helped remove urinary stones. It strengthened the intestines and helped sinus congestion and coughs. The warm fomentation was used to take down inflammations and skin breakouts (still effective today for this).

Medicinal Parts: above ground portions

Preparation Forms: capsule, tea, ointment, gargle, wash, poultice. Dosage: Extract: 30 drops 3x daily.

Nutrition Profile: very high in chromium, iron and silicon; high in calcium, magnesium, manganese, potassium and vitamin A; significant amounts of cobalt, phosphorus, selenium, and vitamins C, B_2 and B_3.

Herbal Healing Actions: diuretic, astringent, hemostatic, carminative, anti-inflammatory, antibiotic, bitter tonic and antiseptic. Effective in treating urinary and venereal infections, kidney ailments, dysentery, sores, boils, cancerous lesions, heavy metal poisoning, and ear, nose and throat infections, TB, asthma, emphysema, arteriosclerosis, urinary stones, eczema, acne, chronic ulcers, gout and arthritis.

Cleansing Properties & Detox Activity: Horsetail herb is useful as a diuretic and tonic for a "spring cleaning" detox. It nourishes and strengthens the kidneys, lungs, bones and connective tissue. Recent tests show that it helps build strong blood. It is anti-inflammatory, restraining infection and clearing toxins through antiseptic activity. It promotes urination, scours the kidneys and softens sediment deposits. It is rich in silica which benefits the skin, hair and nails by assisting tissue and collagen repair.

Safety Precautions: Use extract or tea ONLY.... not just ground up powder. Caution during pregnancy. Horsetail breaks down B vitamins; take with nutritional or brewer's yeast for B vitamins.

Synergy With Other Herbs: With *nettles* or *sage* or *Irish moss* for chronic lung conditions; with *parsley* or *cornsilk* for bladder conditions. With *dandelion* for connective tissue ailments.

• Lemon Balm, *Melissa officinalis*, Family: *Labiatae*

Common Names: melissa, balm, sweet balm, mélise, herbe au citron (Fr), melisse, königsblume, bienenkraut and herzkraut (Ge).

Traditional Use: Known in Medieval times as an elixir of youth; in the 17th century as a remedy for melancholy, and a strengthener for memory and the brain. Well known among warriors for staunching the bleeding of wounds. Melissa refers to the honey bee — lemon balm is considered an equal to royal jelly and bee pollen. Native to southern Europe, naturalized in the U.S.

Medicinal Parts: leaf

Preparation Forms: infusion, compress, tincture, extract, essential oil; douche, ointment. Dosage: tincture: 5-10 drops; essential oil 1-2 drops in water; infusion: 1-2 cups daily. Its gentle properties and mild bitters provide a pleasant flavor for children who find it difficult to consume strong bitter herbs.

Nutrition Profile: Lemon balm citronella terpene has sedative-like effects. High in antispasmodic and antibacterial volatile oil that acts on the digestive tract and central nervous system. Polyphenols and tannin give lemon balm its anti-viral properties and are, perhaps, responsible for its success and effectiveness in inhibiting the herpes simplex virus and mumps.

Herbal Healing Actions: Lemon balm is a diaphoretic-febrifuge to sweat out toxins and reduce fever. It is a carminative for flatulence and gastritis. It is a nervine for a nervous stomach and easy digestion.

Cleansing Properties & Detox Activity: Lemon balm restores the nervous system and has relaxing

tonic action upon the heart (especially palpitations) and circulatory system. It helps calm coughing spasms and asthma spells and expels phlegm. It resolves fever and expels phlegm, expels heat and helps to dissipate tumors. Lemon balm is a good choice for insomnia, tension headaches and depression. It is an effective compress for herpes and cold sores; a good wash for eye inflammations.

Safety Precautions: **none in common use.**

Synergy With Other Herbs: **With** *elecampane* **and** *sage* **as a restorative from depression and exhaustion. With** *senna, fennel seed, ginger, papaya, hibiscus, peppermint, parsley* **and** *calendula* **for a laxative**.

• **Licorice Root,** *Glycyrrhiza Glabra,* Family: *Papilionaceae*

Common Names: **réglisse, herbe-aux-tanneurs and bois doux (Fr), süssholz (Ge).**

Traditional Use: **First recorded on Assyrian tablets nearly 3000 years ago. Ancient use was for dry coughs, asthma and respiratory diseases, colds, sore throats, gastrointestinal complaints and as a tonic. TCM use includes clearing heat, removing toxins, as a tonic for the spleen and for harmonizing the actions of other herbs. Native to Mediterranean region and parts of Asia.**

Medicinal Parts: **root**

Preparation Forms: **tincture, extract, tea, capsules, syrup, wash.** Dosage: Extract: 1-1.5 tsp. 3x daily.

Nutrition Profile: **very high in magnesium, silicon and sodium; high in chromium, cobalt, iron and vitamin B$_3$; significant amounts of calcium, manganese, potassium and vitamins C and B$_1$.**

Herbal Healing Actions: **Licorice is a blood-purifying tonic herb. It stimulates the immune system, helps to protect the liver, fights infection and inflammations, stimulates digestion, regulates the nervous system and supports gland balance. It is a demulcent and expectorant for chest congestion and throat problems. Recently, its phytohormone properties have been recognized for many male and female hormone problems, from change-of-life symptoms to certain types of cancers.**

Cleansing Properties & Detox Activity: **Both antibacterial and antiviral, licorice is effective against many infections, including hepatitis, herpes, dermatitis, eczema and most respiratory infections. It cleanses the blood of toxic pollutants, making it effective for allergies, asthma, candida albicans and arthritis. It restores exhausted adrenals, making it a good choice for fatigue and weakness, including serious adrenal conditions, such as Addison's disease. It is as specific for sore throat, laryngitis and vocal strain.**

Licorice is a good remedy for flu, colds and all lung problems; it is a good expectorant for coughs and bronchial congestion. Its action is complex in normalizing vital blood salt concentrations to stimulate and sustain proper adrenal function. Licorice enhances blood purity by protecting the body's blood detoxification plant- the liver.

Safety Precautions: **Not when high blood pressure is a problem.**

Synergy With Other Herbs: **With** *mullein, pleurisy, marshmallow, rose hips, ephedra, calendula, boneset, ginger, peppermint* **and** *fennel seed* **for a tea to clear mucous congestion. In a capsule with** *sarsaparilla, bladderwrack, Irish moss, uva ursi, rose hips, ginger, capsicum* **for an adrenal activator.**

• **Lobelia,** *Lobelia inflata,* Family: *Lobeliaceae*

Common Names: **indian tobacco, bladderpod, puke weed, asthma root, eyebright, lobélie enflée (Fr), aufgeblasene lobelie (Ge).**

Traditional Use: **Native Americans used it for aches, asthma, boils, colic, croup, coughs, sore throat and stiff necks. Later made popular by the 19th century Eclectics -one of the most frequent herbs used.**

Medicinal Parts: **The whole plant**

Preparation Forms: **tincture, extract, tea, capsules.** Dosage: capsules 2-4; tincture: 5-15 drops.

Nutrition Profile: **high in manganese and vitamins A and C; significant amounts of calcium, iron, magnesium, phosphorus, potassium and vitamins B$_1$ and B$_3$.**

Herbal Healing Actions: **a bitters tonic, diuretic, laxative, diaphoretic and sedative. Lobelia is a**

powerful herb with non-addictive action similar to nicotine— relaxing and stimulating depending on the amount used (a stimulant in small doses, a decongestant and relaxant in large doses). A specific in "stop smoking" combinations to decrease desire for tobacco. As a muscle relaxant, it is used in combinations for spasmodic lung and respiratory problems and to liquefy viscous phlegm. Lobelia relaxes and restores the nerves. It is cardiotonic for circulation. Lobelia causes sweating to resolve fever, push out eruptions and reduce inflammation. It stimulates the adrenals by releasing adrenaline. It helps activate immunity.

Cleansing Properties & Detox Activity: Lobelia is a specific for bronchial asthma, both to calm spasms and open passages and as an emetic to throw out mucous obstruction. Lobelia extract may be used as an emergency measure to revive a person who has overdosed on a narcotic or is in convulsions from epilepsy. It cleanses in cases of blood poisoning, both food and heavy metal. Lobelia antidotes poison though emesis. It works for several childhood diseases including colds, fevers, chicken pox, mumps, measles, scarlet fever, croup and allergies. It helps clear both lung and lymphatic congestion. It is a specific in formulas to relieve the pain and swelling of insect bites and stings and poison ivy or oak.

Safety Precautions: There is a long standing debate over whether lobelia is poisonous or not - allopathic doctors and FDA say yes; alternative medicine says no.

Synergy With Other Herbs: With *capsicum, grindelia* and *ephedra* for asthma. With *peppermint/ peppermint oil, comfrey, marshmallow, slippery elm, pau d'arco, ginger, aloe vera powder* and *wild yam* for gentle cleansing of the bowel for irritable bowel, colitis inflammation or diverticular disease.

• **Ma Huang,** *Ephedra sinica,* Family: *Ephedraceae*
Common Names: ephedra, Mormon tea, Brigham tea, ma huang gen (Ch),desert tea, joint fir.
Medicinal Parts: aerial parts
Preparation Forms: tea, capsules. Dosage: 2 to 6 grams in tea daily; 2 -4 capsules daily.
Traditional Use: A primeval herb, ma huang has been found in middle Eastern neolithic graves indicating probable use and existence 60,000 years ago. Ma huang is mentioned as a medicinal plant in the Vedas, India's most ancient scriptures. The Chinese too, have used it for over 5,000 years to treat asthmatic conditions. Both Native American and Chinese varieties of ephedra have been used in treatment of arthritic and rheumatic ailments. The bodyguards of Genghis Khan used ma huang tea to stay alert because they were threatened with beheading if they fell asleep. Zen monks used ephedra to enhance calm concentration during meditation.

Nutrition Profile: ephedrine, alkaloids and pseudo-ephedrine are responsible for bronchial dilating effects and central nervous stimulation.

Herbal Healing Actions: diaphoretic, stimulant, treats water retention, antirheumatic and astringent. A strong, natural bronchodilator and decongestant for respiratory problems.

Cleansing Properties & Detox Activity: Ephedra works similarly to ma huang, but is not as strong. Both are long lasting CNS stimulants that calm the mind as they stimulate the body. Excellent for mental energy during a long test or meditation. Helps relieve congestive conditions almost immediately from allergies and bronchitis and sinusitis. Beneficial in balancing combinations for circulatory stimulation, strengthening and restoring the body's vitality. Ma huang is thermogenic and can raise metabolism, making it a primary herb in weight loss programs. It is extremely effective without being overly strong in its actions, but only when properly utilized. Topically, may be used as an eyewash.

Safety Precautions: For best results, use in combination with other herbs. Not for those suffering from hypertension, not for long-term use, and not for people who are using MAO inhibitors for depression. Should also be avoided in severe cases of glaucoma and coronary thrombosis. A cardiac stimulant that should be used with caution by anyone with high blood pressure. Other precautions may include heart palpitations, nervousness, insomnia, headaches and perhaps dizziness.

Synergy With Other Herbs: With *marshmallow rt., bee pollen, goldenseal rt., white pine bk., burdock, juniper bry., parsley, acerola cherry, mullein, rosemary, lobelia* and *capsicum* as a breathing formula. An

asthmatic aid, with *marshmallow rt., fenugreek sd., mullelin lf., rosemary lf., ginkgo biloba, passionflowers, wild cherry bk., angelica, lobelia* **and** *cinnamon.* **For a cleansing combination, with** *licorice rt., mullein, pleurisy rt., rose hips, marshmallow, boneset, calendula, ginger, fennel sd., peppermint* **and** *stevia.*

• **Marshmallow,** *Althea Officionalis,* Family: *Malvaceae*
Common Names: **mallards, mauls, schloss tea, mortification root, mallowwild.**
Traditional Use: **Its botanical name,** *Althea* **is derived from the Greek 'altho' meaning 'to cure'; the family name Malvaceae comes from the Greek** *'malake'* **meaning** *'soft,'* **(thus softening and healing). The Roman used marshmallow to boost immunity to be free from all diseases, and as a poultice to draw out thorns and reduce inflammation.**
Medicinal Parts: **leaves, roots and flowers**
Preparation Forms: **root, tincture, decoction, capsule, poultice, ointment.** Dosage: **tincture: 30-60 drops 3x daily; extract: 1-2 tsp. 3x daily; capsules: 2 to 4 daily.**
Nutrition Profile: **very high in aluminum, iron, magnesium and selenium; high in chromium, sodium and vitamin C; significant amounts of calcium, cobalt, manganese, potassium, silicon and vitamin B$_3$.**
Herbal Healing Actions: **actions include emollient, demulcent, expectorant, blood cleanser, bitter, diuretic and wound healing. It has mild immuno-stimulating activity.**
Cleansing Properties & Detox Activity: **Marshmallow is used to reduce inflammation for arthritis, respiratory infections including allergies and asthma, urinary tract infections, kidney stones and venereal diseases. It is effective for diarrhea, hemorrhoids and ulcers. It is a soothing to insect and for any skin sore or inflammation. Marshmallow's mucilaginous properties help bind and eliminate toxins regulating bowel activity and increasing colonic flora to allow the body to cleanse itself. It soothes and heals the mucous membranes to lubricate the lungs, intestines and kidneys.**
Safety Precautions: **none in common use.**
Synergy With Other Herbs: **With** *spearmint* **for urinary ailments. With** *mullein, pleurisy, rose hips, ephedra, licorice, calendula, boneset, ginger, peppermint* **and** *fennel seed* **as an expectorant tea. With** *peppermint/peppermint oil, comfrey, slippery elm, pau d'arco, ginger, aloe vera powder, wild yam* **and** *lobelia* **for a mild, gentle cleansing of the bowel.**

MEDICINAL MUSHROOMS
• **Kombucha,** *Fungus Japonicus*
Common Name: **Csinii Grib (Russian), Chamboucho (Romanian), Champignon De Longe Vie (Fr), Combucha (Japanese), Hongo (Spanish), Tea Mold (Java), Theezwam Komboecha (Dutch).**
Medicinal Parts: **fungus cap**
Preparation Forms: **tea.** Dosage: Use only as directed.
Traditional Use: **First recorded in the Chinese Tsing Dynasty in 221 B.C. kombucha was a tea-like beverage thought to have magical powers to heal. Traditionally, and to the present, used for acne, arterioclerosis, arthritis, constipation, dizziness, dysentery, fatigue, gout, chronic headaches, hemorrhoids, low energy, multiple sclerosis, nervous tension, old age, rheumatism and tonsilitis.**
Nutrition Profile: **An enzyme-rich, immune boosting detoxification agent effective in cleansing the liver, eliminating toxic deposits and promoting optimal digestion and absorption.**
Herbal Healing Actions: **Kombucha stimulates T-cell activity helping to combat HIV replication. Its usnic acid gives it anti-cancer properties. As a powerful liver cleanser and detoxifier, kombucha helps eliminate rheumatic and arthritic conditions. As a colon aid, it helps eliminate constipation and promotes healthy intestinal activity. It has adaptogen qualities to balance body functions—especially lowering blood pressure, restoring blood sugar balance.**
Cleansing Properties & Detox Activity: **Kombucha is especially effective as a blood and liver cleanser.**

As a detoxifier, kombucha is considered a good source of Glucuronic Acid, a substance that can interact with body toxins, make them easier to excrete, and prevent them from being absorbed by the intestines.

Safety Precautions: Avoid using kombucha if you drink large amounts of alcohol; it may cause adverse effects, such as jaundice, dizziness, nausea even liver damage. I believe there is high risk of contamination with dangerous pathogens if the mold is not managed correctly. Immune suppression and antibiotic resistant bacteria may occur. Drinking large amounts of the mold tea is not recommended. Persons with HIV are not recommended for kombucha treatment.

Synergy With Other Herbs: Use alone, or with *green tea* and *echinacea* for immune strengthening.

• **Maitake Mushroom,** *Grifola frondosa,*
Common Names: hen of the woods, sheep's head, king of mushrooms.
Traditional Use: Discovered by people in the deep mountains of northeastern Japan, where it was used to promote longevity and long term health. Its health benefits were so impressive it could be exchanged for its weight in silver. In fact, it was so precious that those who knew where to find it did not tell even members of their family. Only years ago did modern cultivation of Maitake begin.
Medicinal Parts: fungus cap
Preparation Forms: capsules, tea, and tincture Dosage: As a preventative: 2-3 caplets per day. For hypertension: 6 caplets daily then 2-4 caplets per day to maintain lowered blood pressure. For HIV: 4-10 caplets per day. For diabetics: 10 caplets per day, then 3-6 caplets once blood sugar balanced. For AIDS: 8-10 caplets per day. For tumors: 4-10 caplets daily. For cancer: 8-10 caplets daily.
Nutrition Profile: contains amino acids, enzymes, lectins, triglycerides, EFAs, vitamins, nucleotides, amino acids. Orally taking maitake is more effective than taking reishi or shiitake; its polysaccharide beta-glucan is more readily than other mushroom immune-stimulating polysaccharides.
Herbal Healing Actions: immuno-stimulating, detoxifying, anti-tumor, anti-cancer, adaptogen. Helps lower high blood pressure. A superior adaptogen that helps regulate endocrine functions.
Cleansing Properties & Detox Activity: Maitake is a specific in formulas to combat cancers (especially leukemias, prostate cancer, fibroid and breast cancers, ovarian and uterine cancers). Many healers use it as an option to chemotherapy drugs. Maitake have strong immuno-stimulating properties for diseases like chronic fatigue syndrome and rheumatoid arthritis. They inhibit replication of HIV by increasing T-cell counts. In one test, maitake inhibited tumor growth 86% after 31 days. Four of ten animals showed complete tumor resolution. Another study reports maitake activates various immune effector cells (macrophages, natural killer cells, T-cells) to attack tumor cells, including lymphkines and interleuken-1.
Safety Precautions: None in common use.
Synergy With Other Herbs: *Maitake* and *Echinacea* are a good immune boosting compound. Use with *reishi* and *shiitake* for a medicinal mushroom superfood. Use as a specific in a weight control formula with thermogenic herbs like *garcinia, sida cordifolia* and *ephedra.*

• **Reishi Mushroom,** *Ganoderma lucidum (Ling zhi)*
Common names: Ling Zhi (Ch), Shi Rh -plant of immortality (Ch), phantom mushroom.
Medicinal Parts: fungus cap
Preparation Forms: capsules, extract, tea. Dosage: tincture: 10ml 3x day; tablets: 1g. tablets 3x day.
Traditional Use: Reishi has been used as a healing method for at least 4,000 years in China and Japan. Traditionally used for normalizing blood pressure, preventing blood clotting, strengthening and cleansing the heart, regenerating the liver and reviving the immune system. The Japanese and Chinese with cancer or other degenerative diseases traveled great distances to obtain it. We in the West, we did not know or utilize reishi until the late 1970s.
Nutrition Profile: contains protein, lipids, minerals, fiber, carbohydrates, high levels of germanium,

and ergosterol, a provitamin which converts into vitamin D with the presence of sunlight.

Herbal Healing Actions: immunostimulating, anti-inflammatory, antihistamine, anti-tumor. Vitamin D activity is a specific for osteoporosis prevention. An adaptogen for blood sugar regulation.

Cleansing Properties & Detox Activity: Promotes longevity and health. Increases vitality and immunity during a cleansing program. Has special effectiveness against wasting, and degenerative diseases like cancer and AIDS. Stimulates T-cell activity and inhibits the replication of the HIV virus and demonstrates anti-tumor activity. In 1977, an extract of reishi (PSK) was approved in Japan as a treatment for cancer. (After five years, 62 percent of PSK treated cancer patients were disease-free, compared with 35 percent treated with surgery alone.) Helps reduce the side effects of chemotherapy for cancer. In several Chinese hospitals, a reishi formula tested on 2,000 cases of chronic bronchitis, one of the hardest-to-handle allergic reactions, is proven effective in up to 91% of cases. After several months of treatment with reishi, patients showed an increase in their immunoglobulin A (Ig A), the major immune system defender in the respiratory tract. Reishi is also a powerful antioxidant, used therapeutically for a wide range of serious conditions like hepatitis and Chronic Fatigue Syndrome. Detoxifies and regenerates the liver. Lowers cholesterol and triglycerides. Reduces coronary symptoms and high blood pressure. Calms the nervous system and relieves insomnia. Helps strengthen recovery from longterm illness. Excellent even for children.

Safety Precautions: Use only when needed, not continuously. Do not use during pregnancy. Do not mix with aspirin. Take with food. If overused, reishi may cause diarrhea and skin rash.

Synergy With Other Herbs: Works well with *ginseng or chlorella* to rebuild the system after illness.

• **Shiitake Mushroom,** *Lentinus edodes (Hsiang-ku)*

Common Names: Snake butter, Pansia Fungus, Forest Mushroom, Hua Gu (China)

Traditional Use: Has centuries-old tradition as a general tonic and invigorating stimulant to the body's natural defenses. It has been used with steamed vegetables in soups as medicine to reduce cholesterol, promote urination and ease stomach irritation by the Japanese since 199 A.D.

Medicinal Parts: fungus cap

Preparation Forms: fresh and dried, capsules, tincture, extract. Dosage: 1-2 capsules a day before breakfast. The dried or fresh mushroom may be added to soups.

Nutrition Profile: contains LEM, vitamins, minerals, amino acids, polysaccharides and abundant in nutrients such as potassium, phosphorus, silicium, magnesium, calcium, sulphur.

Herbal Healing Actions: Antitumor, anti-inflammatory, shiitakes help shrink existing tumors, lower blood cholesterol levels, and fight colds and flu. At least two different extracts from shiitakes act as immune system stimulators and possess antiviral activities: LEM, and lentinan, an extract from the mushroom's fruit. Anti-viral tests show shiitake can even combat the HIV virus infection, and boost the immune system against chronic fatigue syndrome and lupus. Shiitakes are linked to cures for cancers and tumors for centuries in Oriental medicine. Chinese traditional doctors regularly use them to prevent high blood pressure and heart disease and to reduce cholesterol. Shiitake, eritadenine, lowers serum cholesterol by as much as 45 percent.

Cleansing & Detox Activity: Shiitakes work in a complex way - apparently producing a virus that stimulates interferon production in the human body. Shiitake mushrooms are a tonic mushroom useful for maintaining immune defenses after a cleanse. Shiitakes have precise activity on immune response: they stimulate the immune system powerhouses, the macrophages and NK (natural killer) cells to act more quickly and aggressively against invading pathogens; they combat existing infections; and they increase antibody production and interferon for greater disease resistance. Shiitakes are now used all over the world to fight cancer, Candida infections and environmental allergies.

Safety Precautions: None in common use

Synergy With Other Herbs: With *chlorella* as a superfood immune booster for anti-cancer activity. In miso soup and brown rice for strengthening immunity.

• **Milk Thistle,** *Silybum Marianum,* Family: *Compositae*

Common Names: marian thistle, holy thistle, our lady's thistle, variegated thistle.

Traditional Use And History: The Romans used milk thistle with honey to remove excess bile. In the 17th century, it was known as an effective friend to the liver and blood and against all melancholy diseases. It was prescribed for agues, for preventing and curing plague infections and for removal of obstructions of the liver and spleen. In 18th century Europe, it was used as a great remedy for hepatitis and jaundice. Native in southern Europe, Asia Minor and North Africa.

Medicinal Parts: seed and herb

Preparation Forms: tincture, extract, powder, tea. Dosage: tincture or extract: 20 drops 3-4x daily.

Nutrition Profile: Very high in chromium, iron, manganese, phosphorus and selenium; high in magnesium and zinc; contains significant amounts of calcium, cobalt, potassium and vitamin A.

Herbal Healing Actions: Milk thistle is a tonifying, detoxifier for the liver, and is a specific for the gallbladder, with high antioxidant properties to prevent free radical damage. The active constituent silymarin has a triple action mechanism which helps stabilize liver structure, stimulate protein synthesis to accelerate regeneration of damaged liver tissue and acts as a liver-specific antioxidant. Active flavonoids are strong antioxidants that inhibit uncontrolled free-radical activity and protect the liver from environmental toxins. A bile stimulant, blood cleanser, tonic and demulcent.

Cleansing Properties & Detox Activity: Milk thistle is a specific for all liver, spleen and gallbladder conditions including jaundice, hepatitis (chronic and viral), liver cirrhosis and fatty liver. It is also effective for asthma and allergy attacks and anaphylactic shock. Extensive clinical trials substantiate the ability of milk thistle to reverse the symptoms of liver disorders, like hepatitis and cirrhosis, and to stimulate liver cells to replace tissue that which has been damaged or destroyed by disease.

Safety Precautions: None in common use

Synergy With Other Herbs: With *beet, Oregon grape, dandelion, wild yam, yellow dock, licorice, ginkgo biloba, barberry bark, gotu cola, ginger, wild cherry bark* for liver cleansing and support.

• **Mullein,** *Verbascum thapsus,* Family: *Scrophulariaceae*

Common Names: great or white mullein, torches, our lady's flannel, velvet dock, candlewick, wild ice, Aaron's, Jacob's or Peter's staff, golden rod, beggar's blanket, cuddy's lungs, feltwort.

Traditional Use: The ancient Greeks used mullein for coughs, insect stings, sore throats, tonsilitis and eye infections.

Medicinal Parts: flowers and leaves

Preparation Forms: tincture, infusion, syrup, gargle, oil, suppository, powder. Dosage: tincture: 30 - 60 drops, often; oil: 2 -3 drops 3X daily.

Nutrition Profile: Very high in iron; high in calcium, chromium, cobalt, magnesium, manganese, phosphorus, silicon and in vitamins A , C and B_3; contains significant amounts of potassium.

Herbal Healing Actions: Mullein is an antispasmodic, astringent herb, effective for a wide range of respiratory problems acting as an expectorant to loosen and remove mucous. It helps reduce swollen membrane conditions, especially in the glands and joints. It is an expectorant, demulcent, anti-inflammatory healing herb. Mullein acts both as mucilage and expectorant for the respiratory organs. It is a mild diuretic, a wound healer, nervine and blood balancer.

Cleansing Properties & Detox Activity: Mullein is an anti-spasmodic and astringent herb, a specific for all types of respiratory problems asthma, bronchitis, swollen glands, whooping and hacking coughs, sinus congestion and hay fever. Mullein is particularly good in treating atrophied lung tissue of emphysema. It is a main ingredient for ear infections, especially for children, and is also effective for other childhood diseases - mumps, fevers, toothaches, diarrhea and constipation. Topically, the oil is used for bruises, skin ailments, warts and swellings.

Safety Precautions: **none in common use.**

Synergy With Other Herbs: **With** *horehound, lobelia* **and** *coltsfoot* **for use against bronchitis. With** *pleurisy, marshmallow, rose hips, ephedra, licorice, calendula, boneset, ginger, peppermint* **and** *fennel seed* **for a tea to clear mucous congestion.**

• **Nettles,** *Urtica dioica,* Family: *Urticaceae*

Common Names: **stinging nettle, scaddie, ortie piquante (fr), brennessel and donnernessel (Ge).**

Traditional Use: **Nettle beer is a folk remedy made with** *nettles, dandelion, ginger* **and** *cleavers* **for gout and rheumatic pains. Nettle tea is a long-standing spring medicine used to purify the blood, for gouty gravel, for chronic rheumatism and loss of muscle tone. The seeds were a recommended remedy for the bites and stings from venomous creatures and mad dogs, and for counteracting the poisons of hemlock, henbane and nightshade. Native Americans used nettle for ague, dyspepsia, diarrhea complaints, arthritis, backaches, stomach aches, colds and flus, pneumonia and for fatigue.**

Medicinal Parts: **leaves**

Preparation Forms: **tea, tincture, powder, extract, juice, syrup, gargles, compresses, washes, ointment.** Dosage: **tincture: 5 - 15 drops as needed; juice: 1 tsp. as needed, infusion: as needed.**

Nutrition Profile: **Nettles is very high in calcium, chlorophyll and magnesium; high in chromium, cobalt, iron, phosphorous, potassium, zinc, and in vitamins A, C, and B$_1$, and contains significant amounts of manganese, selenium, silicon and vitamins B$_2$ and B$_3$ and vitamin K.**

Herbal Healing Actions: **Nettles' chlorophyll makes it a good detoxifier for dissolving deposits and stones, draining fluid congestion and edema, and mucous. It stimulates blood building and circulation by enriching the liver. Nettles is a powerful blood-purifying herb, driving toxins and metabolic waste products out of the body by stimulating the kidneys to excrete more water. It stimulates thyroid function for better metabolism. Nettles is rich in balanced minerals for boosting skin, hair and nails. Nettles is diuretic, blood cleansing, tonic, astringent, expectorant, stimulant, vermifuge and hemostatic.**

Cleansing Properties & Detox Activity: **Nettles is effective for arthritis, sciatic pain, and all types of respiratory conditions, including asthma, chronic bronchitis, hacking coughs and excess mucous. Nettles has a draining action, clearing mucous through expectoration. It has a role against cancer and tumors. Its diuretic qualities make it effective for cardiac edema and eczema. Used in cleansing formulas for hives, hepatitis, kidney stones, kidney and bladder infections, diarrhea and constipation. Its tonic qualities make it a favorite for fatigue and loss of energy, anemia and thyroid conditions. Its chlorophyll and mineral content make it a good choice for digestive problems such as gastric acidity and allergies.**

Safety Precautions: **none in common use.**

Synergy With Other Herbs: **With** *marigold, burdock and figwort* **for an ointment for skin conditions. With** *beets, alfalfa, dandelion, Siberian ginseng, yellow dock, parsley, burdock, dulse, bilberry* **and** *capsicum* **as a hemoglobin builder. With** *alfalfa, Irish moss, yellow dock, watercress, parsley, borage seed, dulse and barley grass* **for an effective mineral formula.**

• **Oats,** *Avena sativa,* Family: *Graminae*

Common Names: **groats, avoine (Fr), hafer, gäbelshaber and hoven (Ge).**

Traditional Use: **A stabilizing, high mineral food staple for centuries. Middle Ages used oats for the removal of freckles and spots from the skin by boiling oatmeal with vinegar and applying.**

Medicinal Parts: **The beard**

Preparation Forms: **tincture, decoction, extract, tea, powder, poultice, wash, soap.** Dosage: **tincture: 20 drops, frequently, at the first sign of a cold or flu.**

Nutrition Profile: **Oat grain is one of the richest sources of zinc in the plant kingdom. Other important minerals include boron, calcium, chlorine, chromium, copper, iodine, iron, magnesium, manganese,**

phosphorous, potassium, selenium, silicon, sodium, sulfur; vitamins A, B-complex, choline, folic acid, D and E, and many amino acids including, lysine, methionine, phenylalanine, tryptophan and tyrosine.

Herbal Healing Actions: As a calcium-magnesium nutrient, oats actions are nourishing and restorative. They stimulate the immune system and enhance immunity. Its active constituents are some of the most extensive of all herbs benefiting skin, blood, nerves, brain, musculoskeletal, endocrine, immunity and regulating the entire metabolism. Actions include nervine, antispasmodic, diaphoretic and reportedly aphrodisiac (he's feeling his oats!).

Cleansing Properties & Detox Activity: Oats can combat withdrawal symptoms from drug addictions and toxic conditions. They tonify the blood, nerves, and endrocrine systems providing increased vitality. Particularly helpful for thyroid deficient conditions, depression, diabetes, insomnia, anti-inflammation for eczema, shingles and herpes, PMS, headaches, rheumatism, gout, sciatica and ulcers.

Safety Precautions: People sensitive to gluten should be careful of dosage.

Synergy With Other Herbs: With *nettles* and *sea buckthorn* for libido. With *flax seed, psyllium husk, vegetable acidophilus, guar gum, apple pectin, organic fennel seed* for a fiber food to regulate and maintain peristalsis. With *barley grass, bee pollen, Siberian ginseng, alfalfa, apple pectin, dulse, acerola cherry, sarsaparilla, licorice, dandelion, gotu kola, lemon juice* and *rice protein* to normalize body chemistry.

• **Oregon Grape,** *Mahonia Aquifolium,* Family: *Berberidaceae*
Common Names: mountain grape, holly grape, trailing mahonia, California barberry.
Traditional Use: West Coast Native Americans used it for appetite stimulation, cancer and arthritis. Native to Pacific Northwest America.
Medicinal Parts: root bark
Preparation Forms: tincture, decoction, infusion, fluid extract, powder, wash. Dosage: tincture: 10-30 drops 3x daily; fluid extract: $1/_2$ tsp. 3x daily; capsules: 2 to 4 3x daily.
Nutrition Profile: Contains measureable calcium, chromium, iron, cobalt, magnesium, phosphorus, potassium, selenium, silicon, sodium and vitamins B_1, B_2 and B_3.
Herbal Healing Actions: A strong blood purifier, liver, and organ cleanser that helps release stored iron into the bloodstream for stronger blood and immune defense. A specific in a liver, gallbladder or overall waste cleansing formula. Improves poor digestion, stimulates bile secretion and thyroid activity. It is an astringent and antibiotic. Its actions include alterative, blood cleansing, diuretic, expectorant, laxative, purgative, tonic, antiseptic, bile stimulating, hepatic, bitter and stomachic. Oregon Grape root is similar to Barberry, but more restorative and liver-centered. (See Barberry)
Cleansing Properties & Detox Activity: Oregon grape is effective liver support against jaundice and lymphatic congestion, enhancing the flow of bile through the liver and gallbladder to purify the blood. It may be used for all liver diseases including hepatitis and gallstones. Its blood cleansing properties are strong against arthritis, acne, herpes, psoriasis, eczema, syphilis, vaginitis, bronchitis, anemia and even some cancers. Also used for skin diseases, bronchial congestion, arthritis, cancers and tumors.
Safety Precautions: Not when pregnant or when hyperthyroid. Overdosing can cause fatal poisoning.
Synergy With Other Herbs: With *dandelion root* for a tea for hepatitis and jaundice. With *dandelion, watercress, yellow dock, pau d'arco, hyssop, red sage, licorice, milk thistle seed* and *hibiscus* for a liver flush tea. With *beet, milk thistle seed, dandelion, wild yam, yellow dock, licorice, ginkgo biloba, barberry bark, gotu kola, ginger, wild cherry bark,* for a liver cleansing and support formula.

• **Parsley,** *Petroselinum Crispum,* Family: *Umbelliferae*
Common Names: petersylinge, persil, petersilie, garteneppich and bittersilche (Ge).
Traditional Use: The Greeks used parsley to adorn their champion warriors and to purify the dead. Greek physicians recommended it for dropsy. People in the Middle Ages found that it "made the stomach

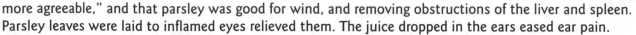

more agreeable," and that parsley was good for wind, and removing obstructions of the liver and spleen. Parsley leaves were laid to inflamed eyes relieved them. The juice dropped in the ears eased ear pain.

Medicinal Parts: **leaf and root**

Preparation Forms: **tincture, decoction, fluid extract, tea, capsules, chlorophyll drink. Dosage: tincture: 20-40 drops 3x daily, fluid extract: $1/2$ to $3/4$ tsp. 3x daily; capsules: 2-4, 3x daily.**

Nutrition Profile: **Parsley is rich in chlorophyll, potassium, and vitamin A, making it a strengthening diuretic to relieve fluid congestion. It is a specific for liver, kidney and bladder problems. It is a nutritive digestive aid that stimulates secretion of stomach acids. It enhances the immune system, acts as a tonic on the blood and is a chlorophyll source to clean up toxic blood.**

Herbal Healing Actions: **Parsley is a key diuretic herb with balancing potassium to relieve fluid congestion. It contains constituents that work as natural calcium channel blocking agents. Its actions include diuretic, carminative, emmenagogue, blood cleanser, stomachic, expectorant, tonic and bitter.**

Cleansing Properties & Detox Activity: **Useful for all kidney and bladder problems, including kidney and gall stones, bladder infections and bloating, jaundice, hepatitis and anemia. Helps indigestion, gas, flatulence and ulcers. Effective in formulas for arthritis, PMS, asthma, hay fever and swollen glands.**

Safety Precautions: **Not during pregnancy in high doses.**

Synergy With Other Herbs: **With** *kelp, dulse, barley grass, spirulina, dandelion, watercress, alfalfa* **to revitalize metabolic activity. With** *beets, alfalfa, dandelion, Siberian ginseng, yellow dock, nettles, burdock, dulse, bilberry* **and** *capsicum* **for a hemoglobin builder. With** *dandelion, watercress, yellow dock, pau d'arco, hyssop, Oregon grape, red sage, licorice, milk thistle seed* **and** *hibiscus* **for a liver flush tea.**

- **Pau d' Arco Bark,** *Tabebuia Impetiginosa,* Family: *Bignoniaceae*

Common Names: **la pacho, taheebo, ipe roxo, trumpet bush.**

Medicinal Parts: **inner bark**

Preparation Forms: **tea, extract, capsules, ointment, cream. Dosage: 2-5 capsules 3x daily.**

Traditional Use: **An Amazon rainforest herb and 1000-year-old folk remedy. Wide-range uses for boils, colitis, dysentery, bedwetting, fever, sore throat, snake bites, wounds, and cancers of the esophagus, head, intestine, lung, prostate, and tongue. Used all over South America to treat skin cancers, flus, colds, infections, gonorrhea, syphilis and malaria. Used by the Indians of Brazil - primarily for skin cancer treatment. Rediscovered in the 1960's from major Brazil experiments with cancer patients.**

Nutrition Profile: **Rich in quinones, mainly lapachol. In fact, pau d' arco contains 18 different quinones including naphthoquinones and anthraquinones which are rarely found together in a plant. High in iron, iodine and the bioflavonoid quercetin. A good source of natural COQ10. Considered ozoniferous which means fresh, pure and free from pollution, smog, exhaust, smoke and pesticides. Pau d' arco gets most of its chemical and mineral substances from the soil in which the tree grows and not the bark itself.**

Herbal Healing Actions: **antibiotic, a valuable treatment for allergies and asthma; antifungal, for overcoming candida, athlete's foot, thrush, nail fungus and ringworm. Anti-bacterial qualities (externally and internally), heal cold sores and lesions.**

Cleansing Properties & Detox Activity: **A primary blood cleanser and immune stimulant, especially purifying blood toxicity against dermatitis and psoriasis. Anticancer against leukemia. Anti-viral qualities boost the immune system against viruses such as HPV, flu, herpes and hepatitis, and, amazingly, against AIDS. Effective against warts, diabetes, ulcers, rheumatism and liver disease.**

Safety Precautions: **May produce nausea and loose bowels; anti-coagulant blood effects in high doses.**

Synergy With Other Herbs: **With** *dandelion, gentian, myrrh, goldenseal rt., witch hazel, lomatium, grapefruit sd., propolis, vitamin D gel* **to provide relief for itchy skin conditions. For serious cleansing, with** *red clover, licorice rt., burdock, ascorbate vitamin C, sarsparilla, alfalfa, kelp, echinacea rt., garlic, butternut, panax ginseng, goldenseal rt., astragalus, poria mushroom, yellow dock, buckthorn bk, prickly ash, dandelion,* **and** *milk thistle sd.*

• **Peppermint,** *Mentha Piperita,* Family: *Labiatae*

Common Names: brandy mint, curled mint, lamb mint, menthe poivrée (Fr), pfefferminze, edelminze, hausminze (Ge), po ho (Ch).

Traditional Use: Egyptians, Greeks and Romans recognized peppermint for medicinal use. Icelanders used it by the 1200s. It became popular as a medicine in Europe during the 1700s, as a stimulant and aid for digestion, vomiting and for hiccups.

Medicinal Parts: leaf and oil

Preparation Forms: tincture, oil, tea, fluid extract, powder, compress, wash, inhalant. Dosage: tincture: 20-40 drops 3x daily; oil: 5-10 drops 3x daily; tea: 1 cup 3x daily.

Nutrition Profile: Peppermint is very high in magnesium, phosphorus and in vitamins A, B_1 and B_2; high in calcium, iron, potassium, sodium and in vitamin B_3, and contains significant amounts of cobalt, manganese, selenium and vitamin C.

Herbal Healing Actions: Peppermint is a stimulant and tonic herb. Its bitter properties stimulate digestion. It energizes the liver to help blood cleansing activity and circulation. Its diaphoretic qualities encourage sweating to expel toxins and lower fever for body comfort. Its nervine properties help neuralgia, nervousness, and headaches of all kinds. It is an antiseptic and antispasmodic -helpful for aches and pains. Its carminative properties help nausea, indigestion, gas and heartburn.

Cleansing Properties & Detox Activity: Peppermint is an effective body cleanser and toner. It reduces inflammations and expels phlegm to benefit the skin and lungs. Peppermint is good enzyme therapy herb to stimulate the liver and gall bladder, promote the flow of bile, cleanse the colon and improve digestion. Peppermint is a good choice for the onset of colds, flu, cough and fever, bronchitis and asthma.

Safety Precautions: Don't use while breast feeding (reduces the flow of milk); use sparingly with very young children; oil may cause contact dermatitis on the skin. Keep oil away from eyes.

Synergy With Other Herbs: With *comfrey, marshmallow, slippery elm, pau d'arco, ginger, aloe vera, wild yam* and *lobelia* for a mild gentle cleanser for the bowel when there is irritable bowel soreness, colitis, or diverticular disease. With *senna, fennel seed, ginger, papaya, hibiscus, lemon balm, parsley and calendula* for a simple herbal laxative. With *mullein, pleurisy rt., marshmallow, rose hips, ephedra, licorice, calendula, boneset, ginger* and *fennel* for an herbal expectorant tea.

• **Plantain,** *Plantago lanceolata,* Family: *Plantaginaceae*

Common Names: ribwort, lamb's tongue, dog's ribs, bent, leechwort, snake plantain, black plantain, ribble grass, black jack, jackstraw, hen plant, plantain lancéolé (Fr), lungenkraut (Ge).

Traditional Use: Ancient Greeks used plantain to arrest bleeding, clear inflammations and heal ulcers. Medieval Europeans used plantain for yellow jaundice and dropsy.

Medicinal Parts: leaves

Preparation Forms: juice, extract, tea, capsules, ointment. Dosage: juice: 2 tsp. 3x daily; tincture: 2-60 drops 3-4x daily; extract: $^1/_2$ to 1 tsp. 3-4x daily.

Nutrition Profile: contains vitamins A, C, K, B_2, B_3; also calcium, iron, zinc and tyrosine.

Herbal Healing Actions: a soothing astringent, plantain reduces inflammations, fights fevers and infections. It is an expectorant to expel phlegm and remove congestion in the lungs, intestines and lymph glands. It is a specific for kidney and bladder cleansing. Plantain staunches bleeding, encourages tissue repair and promotes healthy skin. Other actions include diuretic, blood purifier, emollient and laxative.

Cleansing Properties & Detox Activity: A cleanser in cases of chronic diarrhea, dysentery, leucorrhea, kidney and bladder infections and inflammations, lymphatic infections, edema, lung and throat inflammations and infections, bronchitis, allergic asthma, hayfever, rhinitis, venereal infections, wounds, burns, boils, abscesses, bug bites and stings, snakebites, rashes, poison oak, blood poisoning, skin infections, dry skin, ulcers, eye, mouth and ear inflammations and hemorrhoids.

Safety Precautions: **None in common use.**

Synergy With Other Herbs: **For respiratory aid with** *mullein, wild cherry bk., horehound, ginkgo biloba, slippery elm bk., marshmallow rt., chickweed, licorice rt., kelp, acerola cherry, cinnamon, ma huang* **and** *capsicum.*

• **Pleurisy Root,** *Asclepias tuberosa,* Family: *Asclepiadaceae*

Common Names: **butterfly weed, yellow milkweed, archangel, tuber root, colic root, orange swallow-wort, flux root and chiggerflower; asclépiade tubereuse (Fr); seidenpflanze (Ge).**

Traditional Use: **Native Americans have used pleurisy root for centuries for pneumonia with pleurisy, diarrhea and dysentery, rheumatism, heart trouble, fevers, flu, dog and snake bites, bruises, wounds, swellings and to induce vomiting.**

Medicinal Parts: **root**

Preparation Forms: **tincture, decoction, tea, capsules.** Dosage: **tincture: 30-60 drops every three hours; tea: 2-3 oz. as needed; powder: 20-40 grains 4x daily.**

Nutrition Profile: **contains flavonoids like rutin and quercertin; glycosides (including cardioactive glycosides), bitters and tannic acids.**

Herbal Healing Actions: **Actions include diaphoretic, carminative, diuretic, digestive bitter tonic and antispasmodic. Pleurisy root is one of the best herbal expectorants. It clears phlegm from the lungs with good diaphoretic activity to induce sweating and break fevers. It stimulates urination to clear toxins, and acts as an antiviral that reduces discharges in colds and flu.**

Cleansing Properties & Detox Activity: **Pleurisy root is as specific for pleurisy, pneumonia, bronchitis, asthma and all respiratory infections. Helps in formulas for headaches, fevers, colds and flu, cramps and diarrhea. A digestive aid for flatulence and intestinal inflammation. For childhood diseases such as chicken pox and measles.**

Safety Precautions: **Not during pregnancy (a uterine stimulant). An emetic in large doses.**

Synergy With Other Herbs: **With** *angelica* **and** *sassafras* **for perspiration in fevers and pleurisy. With** *mullein, marshmallow, rose hips, ephedra, licorice, calendula, boneset, ginger, peppermint* **and** *fennel seed* **for an expectorant tea.**

• **Psyllium Husk,** *Plantago psyllium,* Family: *Plantaginaceae*

Common Names: **psyllium seeds, fleaseed, psyllion, psyllios barguthi.**

Traditional Use: **Native to the Mediterranean region, India and the U.S.**

Medicinal Parts: **The seed husk**

Preparation Forms: **The husk is powdered and added to bulk laxative formulas.** Dosage: **powder: 1-2 tsp. in warm water or juice 3x daily.**

Nutrition Profile: **husk contains measureable calcium, iron, phosphorus and vitamin A.**

Herbal Healing Actions: **When ingested, psyllium husk absorbs water and expands into a jelly-like mass stretching along the intestinal walls. Since it is indigestible material, the expanded jelly-like mass acts as a brush or sweeper absorbing and removing toxins that are entrapped in the colon. It also acts as a balancer and regulant for digestive and colon bacteria. Externally, a poultice of the husk can draw out infections from wounds and sores. Other actions are laxative and demulcent.**

Cleansing Properties & Detox Activity: **Widely used as a laxative for chronic constipation and detoxifying bowels and colon. For inflammatory diverticulitis and colitis, a lubricant for ulcerous intestinal tract tissue, for dysentery, gastritis, hemorrhoids and ulcers. Psyllium also decreases LDL cholesterol.**

Safety Precautions: **May cause allergic response in a small number of people.**

Synergy With Other Herbs: **With** *oat bran, flax seed, vegetable acidophilus, guar gum, apple pectin* **and** *fennel seed* **as an effective fiber mix to regulate peristalsis and provide a cleansing action.**

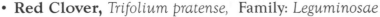

• **Red Clover,** *Trifolium pratense,* Family: *Leguminosae*

Common Names: purple clover, field clover, suckles, meadow trefoil, trèfle rose and trèfle des prés (Fr), wiesenklee, rotklee and fleischblume (Ge).

Traditional Use: Long known as a blood purifier and spring tonic, European gypsy cultures have used it as a medicinal herb for centuries. Native Americans used it as a remedy for whooping cough, fevers, kidney ailments and as a blood purifier. Famous in the U.S. as part of the Hoxsey cancer formula.

Medicinal Parts: flower head.

Preparation Forms: tincture, tea, capsules, fluid extract. Dosage: tincture: 5-30 drops, as needed; powder: 30-60 grains; infusion: 4-6 cups daily.

Nutrition Profile: high in chromium, calcium, magnesium, phosphorus, potassium, and vitamins C, B_1 and B_3; contains significant amounts of manganese, selenium and vitamins A and B_2.

Herbal Healing Actions: Red clover acts as a restorative for the blood and relieves nerve spasms. Other actions include antispasmodic, deobstruent, antibiotic, depurative, nutritive and tonic.

Cleansing Properties & Detox Activity: Red clover is a definitive blood purifying herb with mild antibiotic and anti-inflammatory properties. It promotes cleansing and the elimination of toxins and deposits through urination and expectorant actions. It improves skin conditions through cleansing.

Red clover cleanses are used for cancer and tumors, arthritis, gout and rheumatism, heavy metal poisoning, all types of skin ailments, including eczema, all types of respiratory infections, including bronchitis, spasmodic coughing, asthma, swollen glands, and tuberculosis, and all kinds of elimination system problems including constipation, urinary tract infections and diverticulitis.

Safety Precautions: Dilute doses for older children.

Synergy With Other Herbs: **With** *hawthorn lf.* and *flwr., pau d' arco, nettles, sage, alfalfa, horsetail, milk thistle seed, gotu kola, echinacea purpurea, blue malva, yerba santa* **and** *lemongrass* **for a blood purifying tea. With** *licorice rt., chaparral, burdock, pau d' arco, echinacea, ascorbate vit. C, goldenseal rt., garlic, kelp, alfalfa, dandelion, poria mushroom, American ginseng rt., sarsaparilla, astragalus, yellow dock, butternut, milk thistle seed, ginger, prickly ash* **and** *buckthorn bark* **for a detox formula.**

• **Rhubarb Root,** *Rheum palmatum,* Family: *Polygonaceae*

Common Names: Turkey or China rhubarb, East India rhubarb, Rhubarbe (Fr), da huang (Ch).

Traditional Use: An Asian herb, rhubarb was used as a detoxifier for over 2000 years in the Chinese materia medica, especially for eliminating inflammation in the lower intestine. In Europe, around the 1st century A.D., where its reputation as a medicinal was famous, expeditions began to the East in search of its source. In 17th century Europe it was known for liver cleansing and as an amazing purgative.

Medicinal Parts: root only

Preparation Forms: tincture, capsules. Dosage: Small dose: (astringing) tincture, 6-12 drops; Medium dose: (mild stimulating, laxative) tincture, 15 drops; Large dose: (purgative) tincture, 50-100 drops.

Nutrition Profile: High in minerals like calcium, copper, iodine, iron, magnesium, manganese, phosphorus, potassium, silicon, sulphur and zinc, as well as vitamins A, C and B-complex. Oxalic and other acids help oxygen transport in the blood. Has an inhibiting effect on both cancerous tumors and bacteria, due to an antibiotic, antimicrobial and antitumor anthraquinone in the root.

Herbal Healing Actions: Rhubarb acts as a stimulating tonic on the liver, gall ducts and mucous membranes promoting the removal of toxic substances from the bowels and blood. It reduces liver congestion. In large doses, it gives a purgative action and in small doses, an astringing and calming effect.

Cleansing Properties & Detox Activity: Rhubarb root is effective for elimination problems: constipation, diarrhea and dysentery; for digestive problems: acute gastritis, food poisoning, swollen painful abdomen, duodenal and stomach ulcers, and gallstones; for skin conditions: jaundice, dermatitis, eczema, herpes, and boils, and for cleansing the body of parasites. Rhubarb root acts as a stimulating tonic

on the liver, gall ducts and mucous membranes to promote removal of toxic substances from the bowels and blood. It reduces liver congestion, infections and tumors. In large doses, it is a purgative.

Safety Precautions: **Not during pregnancy or with arthritis or gout. The leaves are poisonous.**

Synergy With Other Herbs: **With** *sheep sorrel, slippery elm* **and** *burdock rt.* **for the cancer fighting formula Essiac. With** *butternut, barberry, cascara, psyllium, fennel seed, licorice, ginger, Irish moss* **and** *capsicum* **to normalize bowels.**

- **Royal Jelly,** *Apis mellifea L.*
Common Names: **mother's milk**
Medicinal Part: **jelly**
Preparation Forms: **Jelly, jelly/honey mix, capsules. Dosage: 1-2 capsules daily; 1 teasp. daily.**
Traditional Use: **Royal jelly has been used by royal beauties from ancient Asia and Egypt through the French Empire as a skin-enhancing cosmetic ingredient. It has been so in modern times, beginning with our Hollywood "royalty" and Charles of the Ritz and Alexandra de Markoff cosmetics after World War II. Although still an important and expensive cosmetic ingredient, royal jelly has been known since the 1960's for its success against fatigue, depression, revitalization activity and preventing senility.**
Nutrition Profile: **Contains every nutrient necessary to support life. A powerhouse of B vitamins, the minerals calcium, iron, potassium and silicon, enzyme precursors, pure acetylcholine, sex hormones and the eight essential amino acids. A rich source of pantothenic acid to combat stress, fatigue and insomnia; nourishing for proper digestion and healthy, stronger skin and hair.**
Herbal Healing Activity: **antibiotic, antibacterial, emollient. A prime skin and scar healer.**
Cleansing Properties & Detox Activity: **Royal jelly supplies key nutrients for energy, mental alertness and general well-being. Antibiotic properties stimulate the immune system, deep cellular health, and longevity. Effective for gland and hormone imbalances that reflect in menstrual and prostate problems. It helps the endocrine glands, genital organs, multiplication of cells, the immune system, and increases better replication of DNA. Aids in liver disease, pancreatitis, insomnia, stomach ulcers, kidney disease, bone fractures and skin disorders such as acne.**
Safety Precautions: **For those allergic to bees, it may cause asthma attacks and severe allergy reactions.**
Synergy With Other Herbs: **A phyto-therapy skin gel, especially for blemishes, with** *extracts of licorice rt., burdock rt., rosemary, rose hips, sarsparilla, sage, chamomile, parsley, fennel sd., thyme, dandelion, propolis, bee pollen* **and** *Korean ginseng rt.*

- **Sage,** *Salvia offficinalis,* **Family:** *Labiatae*
Common Names: **garden sage, broad-leaved white sage, narrow-leaved white sage.**
Traditional Use: **Used in the Middle Ages for better memory and also for palsy. Culpepper's Herbal recommends it for liver diseases and as a hemostat for bleeding wounds, ulcers and sores. Used by Native Americans for purification ceremonies as a smudger.**
Medicinal Parts: **leaves and whole herb**
Preparation Forms: **tea, tincture, gargle, compress, poultice, smudge stick. Dosage: tea: 1-2 cups daily; tincture: 20 to 60 drops 3x daily; powder: 10-30 grains 3x daily.**
Nutrition Profile: **Sage is high in zinc, calcium, magnesium, potassium, and vitamins A and B-1; contains significant iron, manganese, silicon and vitamins C, B$_2$ and B$_3$.**
Cleansing Properties & Detox Activity: **A good cleansing herb for colds, flu, fevers, sore throat, gas, indigestion, nerves, vertigo, trembling, depression and menopausal problems. Sage is a good memory aid.**
Herbal Healing Actions: **A "spring cleaning," high mineral tonic herb, effective in improving digestion and drying up chronic winter mucous excess. Has a vasodilating effect helping to improve peripheral circulation, and works to calm and support nerves. A stimulant, astringent, carminative, antispasmodic, antibiotic and antidiaphoretic. An antibacterial with toning action.**

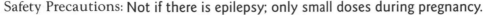

Safety Precautions: Not if there is epilepsy; only small doses during pregnancy.

Synergy With Other Herbs: With *pau d' arco, kukicha, ginkgo biloba, hawthorn, sassafras, ginger, calendula, yellow dock, peppermint, butcher's broom, bilberry* and *licorice rt.* to stimulate circulation and to deter cholesterol. With *red clover, hawthorn, pau d' arco, nettles, alfalfa, horsetail, milk thistle seed, gotu kola, echinacea, blue malva, yerba santa* and *lemongrass* for a cleansing and purifying tea. With *peppermint, rosemary* and *wood betony* for a headache remedy.

- **Sarsaparilla,** *Smilax officinalis*, Family: *Liliacea*

Common Names: Jamaica or red sarsaparilla, salsepareille (Fr), sarsaparille, klimme (Ge).

Medicinal Parts: root

Preparation Forms: extract, tea, capsules, oil. Dosage: tea: 2 cups daily; capsules: 2 to 6 daily with water at mealtime; extract: 2-4 tsp. daily or 20-40 drops 4x daily.

Traditional Use: Sarsaparilla was introduced from Jamaica into European medicine in the middle of the 16th century as a cure for syphilis. It was used for conditions that required sweating as part of the cure. The Chinese also used it as a remedy for syphilis.

Nutrition Profile: high in selenium, chromium, cobalt, iron, silicon and zinc; contains significant amounts of calcium, magnesium, manganese, phosphorus and potassium.

Cleansing Properties & Detox Activity: Sarsaparilla is an anti-inflammatory, cleansing herb that stimulates the kidneys to flush deposits and clear toxins, and promotes sweating to resolve fevers and release harmful pathogens. It binds to toxins in the gut and stops them from entering the bloodstream, it is a liver and blood restorer. Certain constituents act as natural hormone precursors, activating immunity, fighting infections, and benefiting the skin, muscle performance and female harmony.

Sarsaparilla is a primary herb for jaundice, hepatitis, gout, arthritis, rheumatism, psoriasis, herpes, acne, abcesses, boils, warts, burns, skin inflammations, venereal diseases, fevers, fatigue, anemia, impotence, sterility, bacterial infections, edema, poisons and other toxic blood conditions.

Synergy With Other Herbs: With *yellow dock* and *sassafras* for a spring tonic. With *licorice, bladderwrack* and *Irish moss* to stimulate and nourish exhausted adrenals. With *Siberian ginseng, fo-ti, licorice, Irish moss, barley grass, black cohosh, saw palmetto, dong quai, gotu kola, kelp, alfalfa,* and *ginger* as a gland balancing compound.

- **Saw Palmetto,** *Serenoa serrulata*, Family: *Palmaceae*

Common Names: dwarf palm, sabal berries, cabbage palm, fan palm.

Traditional Use: Used by natives in the southern U.S. for inner body strength and tone.

Medicinal Parts: berries

Preparation Forms: tincture, tea, extract, decoction, capsules. Dosage: tincture: 15 - 60 drops 2-3x daily; tea: 6-oz. 2-3x daily; extract: 10 drops 2-3x daily; powder: 10-20 grains 2-3x daily.

Nutrition Profile: berries contain vitamin A and lipase.

Herbal Healing Actions: diuretic, stimulant, expectorant, aphrodisiac, tonic and sedative.

Cleansing Properties & Detox Activity: Saw palmetto is a primary tissue building and gland stimulating herb for toning and strengthening the male reproductive system — hence its aphrodisiac reputation. It increases blood flow to the sexual organs, helps stimulate "good" testosterone production, reduces prostate swelling and inflammation and stimulates immunity. It increases nutrient absorption and assimilation, and helps to restore and relax nerves.

For women, it is used mainly for thyroid deficiency, ovary enlargement, infertility and bladder irritation. For men, it is used for impotence, prostate enlargement, kidney stones, and congestion. It is a strengthener against fatigue, the onset of colds and flus, and bronchitis for both sexes.

Safety Precautions: Not during pregnancy.

Synergy With Other Herbs: With *dandelion, juniper, parsley* and *anise* to flush kidney stones. With *damiana and echinacea* for enlarged and debilitated prostate. With *sarsparilla, Siberian ginseng, fo-ti, licorice, Irish moss, barley grass, black cohosh, dong quai, gotu kola, kelp, alfalfa* and *ginger* for a broad spectrum herbal gland balancing formula to nourish, regulate and extend gland and cell life.

• **Sea Vegetables,** (bladderwrack, *fucus vesiculosus*; dulse, *rhodymenia palmata*; kelp, *ascophyllum nodosum*; Irish moss: *chondrus crispus*.)

Traditional Use: Found in every ocean in the world, usually on submerged rocks near the shore, in tidepools and rocky tidal outcroppings. Traditionally, sea plants have been used as a valuable crop fertilizer, because they contain potash, (20 to 40 lbs. per ton or more when dried). Sea plants were early fodder for livestock in Mediterranean countries and food-preserving, smoking agents for drying meat and fish. Algin, a constituent of sea vegetables has been widely used for 100 years for natural gelling, emulsifying, and food stabilizing. It is also used for dental impressions and in cosmetics and lozenges. Medicinally, charcoal derived from sea plants has been used since the eighteenth century to treat goitre and scrofulous swellings. Sea plant charcoal has been used since the mid-nineteenth century for weight loss.

Medicinal Parts: entire plant - dried root, bulbs, stem and leaves.

Preparation Forms: 5-10 gm three times a day in capsules; to make an extract (70:30) using dried powdered herb: 1 part herb, 4 parts water and 2 parts alcohol. Seal and set overnight. Then, filter. Tea: pour a cup of boiling water onto 2-3 teasp. of dried plants; steep 10 minutes. Tincture: 4-8 ml three times a day for sluggish constitution. Infused oil for topical application: macerate equal parts dried sea plant and sunflower oil; heat it in warm water for two hours, then strain. As a salad or soup sprinkle, mineral drink or broth: 2 TBS. daily of dried chopped sea vegetables are a therapeutic dose.

Nutrition Profile: Sea vegetables have superior nutritional content. They transmit the energies and nutrients of the sea to us with easy absorption. They are nutritive tonics, containing over ninety elements essential to human well-being, including minerals and mineral salts, vitamins, amino acids, enzymes and trace elements. Their mineral balance is a natural tranquilizer for building sound nerve structure, and proper metabolism.

Ounce for ounce, along with herbs, they are higher in vitamins and minerals than any other food group. Some species contain over 30 minerals—rich in calcium, magnesium, iodine, manganese, potassium, selenium, chromium, silicon and zinc for human health. Sea vegetables are almost the only non-animal source of Vitamin B-12 for cell growth and nerve function. Sea plants are one of nature's richest sources of vegetable protein, and they provide full-spectrum concentrations of beta carotene, chlorophyll, enzymes and soluble fiber.

The distinctive salty taste is not just "salt," but a balanced, chelated combination of sodium, potassium, calcium, magnesium, phosphorus, iron and trace minerals. They convert inorganic ocean minerals into organic mineral usable nutrients for structural building blocks. In fact, sea vegetables contain all the necessary trace elements for life, many of which are depleted in the Earth's soil.

Herbal Healing Actions: Sea vegetables are anti-inflammatory, diuretic, immune and metabolic stimulants and thyroid restoratives. They are blood purifying, nutritive tonics, with antibiotic and detoxifying activity. Sea plants are strong antioxidants that scavenge free radicals to strengthen the body against disease. Their potent algin chelators attach to toxic metals and other wastes, removing them from the bloodstream in much the same way that water softener removes the "hardness" from tap water. As a result, less toxins enter the circulatory system. Algin lowers bowel transit time, absorbs bowel toxins for less colon putrefaction, regulates colonic flora and soothes the digestive tract.

Cleansing Properties & Detox Activity: An important part of a cleansing program, sea vegetables alkalize the body, and reduce excess stores of fluid and fat. Sea plants bind radioactive strontium, barium, and cadmium, dangerous pollutants in the gastrointestinal tract, preventing their absorption into the body. They then transform the toxic metals in the system (including radiation), into harmless salts that

the body can eliminate. They purify the blood from the acid effects of a modern diet, allowing for better absorption of nutrients. Natural iodine in sea plants stimulates the thyroid gland for help in weight control. Research indicates antiviral activity in tests against mumps and flu viruses.

Seaweed soothes irritated mucous membranes, dissolves tissue masses such as tumors, treats enlarged thyroid, lymph nodes and swollen painful testes, and reduces edema. It helps relieve rheumatism and rheumatoid arthritis when taken internally and topically applied to swollen areas. It is effective against bladder inflammation. It fights fatigue through alterative action on the glandular system.

Safety Precautions: Sea plants can contain heavy metal pollutants if gathered from areas that are polluted with high levels of mercury, cadmium and other toxins. Some experts consider sea plants unsafe for people with sensitive thyroids if taken in large doses.

Synergy With Other Herbs: With *plantain, fennel seed, licorice, marshmallow, burdock* and *hawthorn* for weight loss and bloating. With *uva ursi, dandelion, parsley, buchu, saw palmetto, bilberry* and *gentian* for a nerve tonic and normalizing blood sugar. With extracts of *alfalfa, ginger, dandelion, spearmint, capsicum, cinnamon, aloe vera gel, olive, rice bran, grapeseed oils* and *lecithin* in an herbal wrap to increase enzyme and systol/diastole action in a cleansing program. With extracts of *licorice root, sarsparilla* and *Irish moss* as a gland cleansing tonic. With *red raspberry* as part of a prenatal combination to prevent cretinism. With *wild cherry, plantain, goldenseal root, slippery elm* and *comfrey* for bronchitis to overcome inflammation. With *marshmallow, licorice* and *myrrh* as a soothing agent for gastritis and stomach ulcers. With *dong quai, damiana, sarsaparilla, wild yam, black cohosh* for female problems.

• **Senna Lf. & Pods,** *Senna alexandrina*, Family: *Leguminosae*

Common Names: Indian senna, Alexandrian senna, cassia senna and tinnevelly senna.

Traditional Use: First recorded medicinal use was in 9th century A.D. by Middle Eastern Arabs. Senna became an important trade route commodity in the late Middle Ages. By the 15th century, senna was well known by Europeans, and mainly used for constipation. Only within the last 50 years has senna has been extensively studied for its other medicinal properties and uses.

Medicinal Parts: leaf and pod.

Preparation Forms: tincture, infusion. Dosage: tincture: 10-40 drops.

Nutrition Profile: high in calcium, chromium, magnesium and vitamins A, C, B_1 and B_2; high in iron, manganese, selenium, silicon, sodium, zinc, vitamin B_3; significant phosphorus.

Cleansing Properties & Detox Activity: Senna is a bitters, purging stimulant, acting mainly on the colon to encourage peristalsis. It is a highly valued cathartic for the lower bowel, with less intestinal griping than most laxatives. It is an effective vermifuge for intestinal worms and parasites.

Herbal Healing Actions: laxative, purgative, bitter, stimulant.

Safety Precautions: Not for use when pregnant — a uterine stimulant. Not for when inflammatory conditions of the alimentary canal exist or if there are hemorrhoids. Senna is slightly habit forming, especially in its over-the-counter drug form, and should be used sparingly.

Synergy With Other Herbs: With carminatives for best results, like *ginger, cumin or fennel*. With antispasmodics like *cramp bark or lobelia* to reduce cramps. With *fennel seed, ginger, papaya, hibiscus, lemon balm, peppermint, parsley* and *calendula* for a simple herbal laxative tea.

• **Slippery Elm,** *Ulmus fulva*, Family: *Ulmaceae*

Common Names: red elm, moose elm, indian elm and sweet elm.

Traditional Use: Used by Native Americans for cancer and tumors, rheumatism, consumption, as a poultice to extract thorns, for coughs, colds, sore throat, bowel ailments, sores, wounds, eye inflammation, burns, toothache, and to ease birth. Colonists quickly integrated it into their medicines.

Medicinal Parts: inner bark

Preparation Forms: tea, extract, capsule, syrup, poultice, ointment, throat lozenge. Dosage: tincture: 15-30 drops 3x daily, powder: 30-60 grains 3x daily; tea: 6-oz. 3-4x daily, syrup: 1 TBS. as needed.

Nutrition Profile: high in vitamin B_3, calcium and vitamins B_1 and B_2, and contains significant amounts of chromium, magnesium, manganese, potassium, selenium, sodium and vitamin A.

Herbal Healing Actions: emollient, expectorant, diuretic, astringent, vulnerary.

Cleansing Properties & Detox Activity: Slippery elm soothes, nourishes, strengthens mucous membranes, especially in wasting diseases. Its mucilaginous properties aid the throat, stomach, bowels and colon helping to absorb toxins and regulate colonic bacteria. Slippery elm is a primary demulcent herb for diarrhea and constipation, colitis, irritable bowel syndrome, ulcers, indigestion, gastritis, nausea, bronchitis, congestion, coughs, asthma, croup, sore throat, inflammations, wounds, boils, burns, acne, abcesses, sores, and skin rashes. Expectorant action helps soothe respiratory ailments and discharge mucous.

Safety Precautions: None in common use.

Synergy With Other Herbs: with *peppermint/peppermint oil, comfrey rt., marshmallow rt., pau d' arco, ginger, aloe vera, wild yam* and *lobelia* in a mild gentle bowel cleanser.

• **Spirulina,** *Spirulina platensis*

Common Names: blue-green algae

Medicinal Part: dried powder

Preparation Forms: capsules, tablets, food and drink supplement. Dosage: 500-1500mg daily.

Traditional Use: The spirulina organism is said to have appeared 3.5 billion years ago. For at least five centuries it had been used by the Aztec Indians as a food and a trade item. Archeological studies conducted in Central America indicate that the Mayans used artificially constructed ponds to cultivate spirulina. In 1964, spirulina was re-discovered by modern western scientific society.

Nutrition Profile: A chlorophyll-rich "superfood," spirulina supplies 21 amino acids including the top 8 essential for health. Research shows that spirulina alone could double the protein balance of the planet! Its protein composition is 60% more by weight than any other organic whole food. Acre for acre, spirulina yields 20 times more protein than soybeans, 40 times more protein than corn, and 400 times more protein than beef. It provides amino acids, and the entire B complex of vitamins, including vitamin B_{12}, not commonly found in plants. It is rich in beta carotene, minerals, trace minerals and essential fatty acids. Extremely high in iron making it beneficial in ailments such as anemia. Digestibility is high, stimulating both immediate and long range energy.

Herbal Healing Actions: a powerful antioxidant, anti-cancer, anti-tumor, anti-viral and immune stimulant. Improves eyesight in cases of glaucoma and cataracts. A highly nutritive, blood-building micro-algae with the ability to grow in both ocean and alkaline waters. Spirulina is ecologically sound in that it can be cultivated in extreme environments which are useless for conventional agriculture.

Cleansing Properties & Detox Activity: Spirulina's chlorophyll content draws out toxins to cleanse and detoxify the body. Its alkaline properties directly help balance acidic foods like coffee, alcohol, sugar, and meat. Spirulina is easily digested providing quick energy and nourishment; helps malabsorption, especially in the elderly and the undernourished. It is a foundation nutrient for weight control and blood sugar support. Current research on spirulina identifies phytonutrients that enhance immunity. Spirulina's sulfolipids and glycolipids have amazing action on AIDS, preventing the HIV virus from attaching to or penetrating cells. Its calcium spirulan inhibits many viruses, like mumps, measles, even herpes viruses. Its anti-cancer ability is effective in stimulating an immune response that destroys malignant cells.

Safety Precautions: None in common use.

Synergy With Other Herbs: In combination with *bee pollen, alfalfa, hawthorn, chlorella, barley grass, Siberian ginseng rt., carrot rt., sarsaparilla rt., red rasberry, kelp, wild cherry bk., rose hips ext., goldenseal rt., mullein* for energy and to restore strength after exhaustion or illness. With *garcinia gambogia, sida*

cordifolia extr., bancha lf., kukicha twig, guarana sd., capsicum fruit **to balance thermogenesis. A gentle** effective herbal support program designed to re-establish friendly flora in the digestive tract combine with *pau d' arco, black walnut hulls, vegetable acidophilus, garlic, barberry, cranberry juice, burdock rt., licorice rt., echinacea angustifolia and purpurea rt., dong quai, damiana, thyme, peppermint, rosemary, rose hips.*

• **St. John's Wort,** *Hypericum perforatum,* Family: *Hypericaceae*
Common Names: hypericum, herbe de millepertius (Fr); Johanniskraut, herrgottsblut, (Ge).
Medicinal Parts: leaf, flower, buds
Preparation Forms: extract, capsules, tea, wine infusion, ointment. Dosage: tea: 1-2 tsp. herb to 1 cup hot water 3x daily; tincture: 15-30 drops 3x daily.
Traditional Use: Historically associated with devils, spirits and magic. Legend claims if hung in a window or burnt on St. John's birthday, St. John's wort will keep devils and ghosts away for a year. Medieval medics soaked it in wine for melancholy and madness, and used it to heal deep wounds. Greek healers prescribed it for sciatica, chronic fevers, and as a diuretic and emmenagogue for menstrual problems. The Romans used it for snake bites and deep wounds.
Nutrition Profile: Contains choline. Contains hypericin (its MAOI, anti-viral, and anti-cancer inhibitor ingredient), volatile oil such as carophyllene, and pseudohypericin and flavonoids.
Herbal Healing Actions: antiviral, antibiotic, antidepressive, astringent, nervine, diuretic, expectorant, serotonin-modulating.
Cleansing Properties & Detox Activity: St. John's wort is a potent antiviral, helping control viral infections of all types, including staph, strep, HPV, even HIV. It reduces congestion and tumor growth. It is immuno-modulating and lowers inflammatory reactions. It is an analgesic, anti-inflammatory, effective in compounds for colds, chest congestion, headaches, sciatica, neuralgia, rheumatism, skin sores and cancers. It is an anti-depressant for anxiety, insomnia and chronic fatigue syndrome. It acts as a nervine to curb nerve pain and rebuild strong nerve structure. It inhibits the brain chemical monamine oxidase (MAO) which triggers depression. It is a serotonin modulator that helps as an appetite suppressant.
Safety Precautions: Sun-sensitive people should avoid taking it. Very high doses may cause phototoxicity in humans, especially those with fair skin.
Synergy With Other Herbs: **With** *kirin ginseng, Chinese white ginseng, aralia, tienchi, suma, echinacea purpurea and angustifolia, pau d' arco bark, Siberian ginseng, prince ginseng, astragalus bark, reishi mushrooms, ma huang* **and** *fennel seed* **for a purifying, restorative tea.**

• **Stoneroot,** *Collinsonia canadensis,* Family: *Labiatae*
Common Names: collinsonia, pilewort, horse balm, Canadian horsemint, heal-all, richweed, knot root, knob root, hardback, oxbalm, richleaf; herbe/baume de cheval and guérit tout (Fr).
Traditional Use: Its botanical name is derived from its "discoverer," Peter Collinson. Native Americans used stoneroot for swollen breasts, as a deodorant, and for colic in horses. In the 19th century, eclectics and homeopaths used stoneroot extensively as a sediment cleanser.
Medicinal Parts: root and leaves (one of the few mint species whose root is used therapeutically.)
Preparation Forms:. tea, capsules, tincture, extract, decoction, gargle. Dosage: tincture: 15 to 30 drops 3x daily; gargle: 1 part root to 3 parts water; powder: 5-20 grains 3x daily.
Nutrition Profile: Magnesium makes it useful as a mild sedative for spasmodic pain. Tannins, a glycoside and essential oils contribute to stone root's ability to clear airways and relieve asthma.
Herbal Healing Actions: a diuretic and diaphoretic, an antispasmodic, sedative, blood and liver cleanser.
Cleansing Properties & Detox Activity: Stone root helps with all conditions that involve sediment

formation or obstruction. It is a specific for treatment and prevention of stones and sediment in the urinary system, kidney and gallbladder. It is a diuretic with tonic action on the bowels to regulate discharges and fight inflammation. The leaves are effective as a poultice for bruises, wounds, sores and cuts. The root is used for female problems such as excessive or painful menstruation. Strengthens the heart and improves circulation. For sore throats, laryngitis and bronchitis (for best results, add the tincture to a simple syrup).

It is an astringent herb that tones the venous walls and enlivens the blood, helps shrink varicose veins, hemorrhoids and prostate inflammation. It disperses mucous from the head and throat, and expels phlegm to clear congestion and inflammation from the chest.

Safety Precautions: **None in common use.**

Synergy With Other Herbs: **With honey as a gargle to relieve hoarseness. For urinary stones, with** *parsley, dandelion, gravel root* **or** *hydrangea.*

• **Uña De Gato,** *Uncaria Tomentosa,* Family: *Rubiacea*

Common Names: **cat's claw**

Medicinal Parts: **root and bark**

Preparation Forms: **tea, capsules, extract, wash.** Dosage: **tea: 2 to 3 c. daily; capsules:1- 2, 3x daily.**

Traditional Use: **A rainforest herb, Amazon Indians use una de gato as a skin treatment and a healing tea for a wide variety of ailments. In 1974, una de gato was "rediscovered" by an Austrian scientist, who introduced it to Europe. Today, una de gato is being tested in health research facilities all over the world. At the 1988 International Congress on Traditional Medicine in Lima, Peru, una de gato was presented as a serious anti-cancer herb. One doctor revealed that in his experience between 1984-1988, una de gato helped at least 700 of his patients with 14 different kinds of cancer.**

Nutrition Profile: **Contains six important oxindole alkaloids which enhance the process by which white blood cells and macrophages engulf and eliminate pathogens and cell debris. The alkaloid ryncho-phylline gives cat's claw the ability to prevent blood clotting. Rich phytochemicals like proanthocyanidins, triterpines, polyphenols, quinovic acid glycosides give it potent antioxidant properties.**

Herbal Healing Actions: **diuretic, blood cleansing, wound healing, tonic, anti-viral, anti-tumor. An powerful anti-inflammatory effective against rheumatism, arthritis, bursitis, chronic urinary tract inflammations and infections (especially in early stages) and for sores and wounds.**

Cleansing Properties & Detox Activity: **An immunostimulating herb that benefits the entire gastrointestinal system, including disorders like gastritis and peptic ulcers. Because of its ability to cleanse the colon and reduce inflammation, una de gato is especially beneficial for colon problems like Crohn's disease, diverticulitis or leaky bowel syndrome. Some patients with I.B.S. (irritable bowel syndrome) have been relieved of all symptoms after just a week of taking una de gato! Una de gato has proven effective for T-Cell enhancement against the AIDS virus. New clinical trials show it delays, even sometimes prevents, progression into full-blown AIDS. Successful against cancer, (new studies show it both reduces and normalizes the side effects of chemotherapy in cancer treatment). Halts viral infections like genital herpes.**

Safety Precautions: **Avoid during pregnancy, when undergoing skin grafts or organ transplants, if you are hemophiliac or taking fresh blood plasma, if you're being administered certain vaccines, hormone therapies, thymus extracts, or insulin. Not for children under 3 years of age. May cause diarrhea.**

Synergy With Other Herbs: **An immune restorative tonic with** *astragulus* **and** *reishi mushroom.*

• **Usnea,** *Usnea Barbata,* Family: *Usneaceae*

Common Names: **bear lichen, bearded lichen, old man's bard, larch moss, beard moss.**

Traditional Use: **Used by Native Americans from California to Washington state. Chinese medicine used usnea as an expectorant and as a poultice for external sores.**

Medicinal Parts: **lichen.**

Preparation Forms: extract (most effective), tea, raw lichen, sinus spray, gargle. Dosage: extract: 30 drops 3x daily; tea: 1 cup 3x daily.

Nutrition Profile: part fungus, part algae, with significant Vitamin C amounts. Rich in usnic acid, said to be more effective against bacterial strains than penicillin. But most medicinally effective due to the polysaccharides and mucilage found in the inner cord of the plant.

Herbal Healing Actions: powerful antibacterial, antibiotic, antifungal, alterative and aperient.

Cleansing Properties & Detox Activity: Used for sore throats, colds and flu, for strep and staph infections, sinus infections, intestinal infections, impetigo, trichomonas and urinary tract infections, fungal infections, respiratory infections and for cuts, bites and stings.

Safety Precautions: None in common use.

Synergy With Other Herbs: With *licorice and ginger* in a tea for colds and flu. *Usnea* tincture is mixed with water and used as a gargle or sinus spray.

• **Uva Ursi,** *Arctostaphylos uva ursi,* **Family:** *Ericaceae*

Common Names: rapper dandies, brawlins, cranberry (Eng); kinnikinnik, bearberry, sagackhomi, hog cranberry (Am), raison d' ours, arbre aux fraises (Fr), moosbeere, sandbeere, wolfsbeere (Ge).

Traditional Use: Used for over 1000 years as a longevity medicinal in Europe. Native Americans discovered it for urinary stones, to tone urinary organs and fight urinary infections.

Medicinal Parts: leaves

Preparation Forms: tea, tincture, extract, capsules, douche, enema. Dosage: tincture: 2ml 3x daily; tea: 3 cups daily.

Nutrition Profile: rich in iron, manganese and vitamin A; high in calcium, selenium and silicon; significant amounts of chromium, magnesium, potassium, sodium, and vitamins C, B_1 B_2 and B_3.

Herbal Healing Actions: an antiseptic, astringent to dry up mucous, a powerful diuretic, a bitter tonic, antispasmodic.

Cleansing Properties & Detox Activity: Uva ursi is a specific for bladder and kidney infections and irritations, like urethritis, acute cystitis, dysentery, mucous and blood in the urine, venereal infections, candida albicans, urinary stones and deposits, prostate irritation, hemorrhoids and bed wetting. It controls excess mucous discharge in the urine and bowels, and restores urogenital organs. It cleanses, strengthens and restores the liver, pancreas and spleen. Important as part of any cleansing formula for the skin.

Safety Precautions: Don't take when pregnant - may promote labor contractions. Not with fluid deficiency, wasting, or dryness, or with remedies which acidify the urine.

Synergy With Other Herbs: With *nettles and buchu* in a tea for bladder infections. With *couchgrass, yarrow* and *horsetail* to heal damaged mucous membranes.

• **Watercress,** *Nasturtium officinale,* **Family:** *Cruciferea*

Common Names: poor man's bread, well grass, teng tongues and billers (Eng); cresson, and santé du corps (Fr); brunnenkresse, garten/wasserkresse, quellkranke, wassersenf (Ge).

Traditional Use: The Romans thought watercress a good food for disturbed mental conditions. Used topically in the 17th century for the removal of acne, blotches, freckles and spots and also applied to the forehead with vinegar for mental alertness. Native Americans used it to dissolve kidney stones.

Medicinal Parts: leaves and root

Preparation Forms: juice, tincture, tea, capsules. Dosage: Fresh juice: 2 tsp. in water 3x daily.

Herbal Healing Actions: diuretic, stimulant, tonic, alterative, nutritive, expectorant, laxative, stomachic, depurative and cholagogue.

Nutrition Profile: One of the best herbal sources for vitamin E. Has high iron, calcium, phosphorus, potassium, iodine, magnesium, manganese, sulfur, zinc, B-complex vitamins and many amino acids.

Cleansing Properties & Detox Activity: A spring cleansing purifier, watercress is a chlorophyll-rich herb for conditions that need blood building along with cleansing, like anemia, eczema and other chronic skin eruptions. Watercress is a potassium-rich diuretic, effective as a liver and organ cleanser in a formula to stimulate better metabolic activity, increase bile production and dispel gas.

Watercress restores the endocrine, nervous and immune systems. It tonifies the blood, regulates metabolism and relieves fatigue. It stimulates digestion, removes mucous accumulations in the lymph and liver, promotes urination, and resolves blood toxins. Watercress helps remove respiratory congestion by dissolving viscous phlegm and promoting expectoration. Recent studies indicate that watercress is particularly potent against lung cancer.

Safety Precautions: Don't take if there are gastric or duodenal ulcers, or inflamed kidneys.

Synergy With Other Herbs: With *fresh nettle* and *dandelion* for blood purification. With *dandelion, yellow dock, pau d' arco, hyssop, parsley, Oregon grape, red sage, licorice, milk thistle seed* and *hibiscus* for a liver flush tea. With *kelp, dulse, barley grass, parsley* and *alfalfa,* for naturally occurring, absorbable potassium to revitalize metabolic activity. With *alfalfa, nettles, Irish moss, yellow dock, parsley, borage seed, dulse* and *barley grass* for strong bones.

• **Wheat Grass,** Family: *Gramineae*

Common Names: cereal grass

Traditional Use: People have been using wheat berries as food for at least 15,000 years. Doubtless, sprouted wheat berries and wheat grass were also valued nutrients. In the 1960s, Ann Wigmore, founder of Hippocrates Health Institute, referred to her Bible in creating her healing, organic raw foods programs. She read a verse in Daniel that instructed King Nebuchadnezzar to go into the field and "eat grass as did the oxen." Wigmore found wheatgrass was the most potent and nutritious of the grasses and began the widely popular movement in the U.S. of wheat grass juicing, enemas and implants for body cleansing.

Medicinal Parts: grass

Preparation Forms: tablets, powder, juice, poultice, rectal implants (especially effective for colon cancer). Dosage: 1 tsp. dehydrated juice to $\frac{1}{2}$ cup water; 1 TBS. whole grass powder to $\frac{1}{2}$ cup of water; tablets: up to 10 grams daily. For external use: soak cloth in fresh juice, apply locally or make a poultice of crushed grass pulp. Retention enema: 1 to 4-oz. fresh juice. Taken with water before meals, wheat grass has the ability to purge candida yeasts from the body. Builds red blood cells and can treat anemia.

Nutrition Profile: Highly nutritious - 15 lbs of wheatgrass has the nutritional value of 350 pounds of vegetables! A rich source of vitamin A, C, B$_{12}$, fiber, chlorophyll (over 70%), minerals, amino acids (including lysine, leucine, tryptophan, phenylalanine, threonine, valine and leucine. High SOD contributes to wheat grass's ability to protect against free radical damage caused by chemicalized foods, pollution, radiation (from X-rays, cancer treatment or computers) and other toxins. An excellent vegetarian source of protein, laetrile (an anti-cancer compound) and mucopolysaccharides. High nutrient content aids in appetite suppression for weight loss. High chlorophyll in wheat grass detoxifies the liver and bloodstream and helps neutralize pollutants like carbon monoxide. Note: Wheat grass is NOT a source of the gluten responsible for much of wheat grain allergy today (OK for wheat-sensitive people.)

Herbal Healing Actions: a high chlorophyll superfood for treating malignant growths; nutritive, anti-inflammatory, blood purifying, digestive, stomach, liver, pancreas and circulatory cleanser. Stimulates metabolism and enzyme activity. Wheat grass is a primary anti-cancer agent with scientific findings revealing that it can decrease the ability of mutagens to cause cancer by as much as 99%.

Cleansing Properties & Detox Activity: Wheat grass cleanses the blood and gastrointestinal tract. Abundant in alkaline minerals, wheat grass can reduce over-acidity in the blood making it useful for over-acid body conditions like arthritis, rheumatism, candida yeast overgrowth, chronic fatigue, AIDS, and allergies. Wheat grass normalizes the thyroid gland, beneficial for thyroid-related obesity, fatigue and constipation. High chlorophyll and the fraction P4D1 in wheat grass also protects against damage from

radiation exposure, and renews cellular DNA. Restores energy levels in people with chronic fatigue by improving the oxygenation of body tissues.

Wheat grass used externally can successfully treat skin ulcers, impetigo or other allergic, itchy skin conditions. It is a powerful healing tool as a colon implant for colon cancer, bowel toxicity or chronic constipation. High chlorophyll in wheat grass attributes to its action as a natural body deodorizer.

Safety Precautions: Large amounts of undiluted wheat grass juice may cause nausea and dizziness. Adding a small "shot" to other fresh vegetable juices is advised. Used therapeutically for detoxification, wheat grass juicing may induce a short "healing crisis" characterized by diarrhea or headaches and is usually a good indication that the body is beginning to detoxify. If symptoms continue, reduce dosage.

Synergy With Other Herbs: With *spirulina or chlorella* to cleanse the body of toxins.

• **White Pine Bark,** *Pinus Strobus,* Family: *Pinaceae*
Common Names: soft pine, deal pine.
Traditional Use: Frenchman Jacques Cartier in 1535, the first European to arrive in Canada, said that Quebec Indians saved the lives of he and his crew from scurvy by giving them a tea made from white pine bark. Native Americans used pine to treat bleeding gums, loose teeth, fragile bones and skin membrane bleeding. Modern rediscovery began in the 1960's, by Dr. Jack Masquelier, when large amounts of antioxidant proanthocyanidins were discovered in the bark.
Medicinal parts: bark.
Preparation forms: tea, capsules, extract. Dosage: as an antioxidant during high risk seasons, capsules: 1-2 capsules every 6 hours.
Nutrition Profile: Full of vitamin C, bioflavonoids and proanthocyanidins (PCO's).
Herbal Healing Activity: most valued for its potent antioxidant activity. Also expectorant, circulatory stimulant, astringent, demulcent, alterative and anodyne (a pain reliever).
Cleansing Properties & Detox Activity: An antioxidant and powerful circulation stimulant used in to overcome or prevent the onset of colds, flu, even rheumatism by raising circulatory action. An expectorant for respiratory ailments. White pine's PCOs are active in boosting intracellular Vitamin C levels, decreasing capillary permeability and fragility, and inhibiting destruction of collagen. PCOs also prevent release of elements that promote inflammation and allergies, such as histamine, serine proteases, prostaglandins, and leukotrienes. Free radical scavenging ability decreases the chance of chronic degenerative diseases like heart disease, arthritis and cancer.
Safety Precautions: None in common use.
Synergy With Other Herbs: For a potent antioxidant combination, use with *vit. C (ascorbate) 120mg, bayberry bk., ginger rt., rose hips extr., white willow bk.,* and *capsicum.*

• **Wild Cherry Bark,** *Prunus serotina,* Family: *Rosaceae*
Common Names: choke cherry, black cherry and virginian prune (Am); cerisier de Virginie (Fr); virginianische traubenkirsche (Ge).
Traditional Use: Native Americans found wild cherry useful for colds, coughs, consumption, ague, fevers, measles, small pox, cholera, worms, diarrhea, bowel inflammations, bladder ailments, wounds, burns, cuts, sores, scrofula and as a tonic.
Medicinal Parts: bark and root
Preparation Forms: tincture, decoction, extract, tea, capsules, eyewash, syrup. Steep in cold water to retain cough-relieving properties. Dosage: tincture: 30-60 drops 3x daily; extract: $\frac{1}{2}$ to 1 tsp. 3x daily; tea: 6-oz. 3-4x daily; syrup: $\frac{1}{2}$ to 2 tsp. 3x daily.
Herbal Healing Actions: helps dry up excess mucous and stop diarrhea, and tension calming.
Nutrition Profile: the bark contains calcium, iron and potassium.

Cleansing Properties & Detox Activity: A specific for lung conditions such as tuberculosis, asthma, whooping cough, and colds with a cough. Its spring tonic qualities make it good for indigestion problems such as loss of appetite, diarrhea, gastritis and heartburn. Works as a restorative for nerves, lungs, heart and intestines helping to calm the nerves and heart, to relieve irritation of mucous membranes, stimulate and tonify digestion, and generate strength. The tea is especially helpful for children's coughs, colds, diarrhea and colic. Helps inflammations of the eye.

Safety Precautions: Not for use during pregnancy.

Synergy With Other Herbs: With *elecampane, cramp bark* and $^1/_4$ *part lobelia and ginger* in honey for an effective cough syrup. With *beet, milk thistle seed, Oregon grape, dandelion, wild yam, yellow dock, licorice, ginkgo biloba, barberry, gotu kola, ginger,* for a liver cleansing capsule combination.

- **Wormwood,** *Artemisia absinthium,* Family: *Compositae*

Common Names: madderwort, old woman, absinth (Eng); absinthe, herbe aux vers (Fr), elss, magenkraut, wurmkraut (Ge).

Traditional Use: An ancient herb and next to rue the most bitter in the herbal kingdom. Roman soldiers wore it in their sandals to relieve tiredness on long treks. Used to counteract mushroom and hemlock poisons. Strewn among furs to repel moths and insects. 18th century medics recommended wormwood to prevent kidney stones and gravel, and to relieve gout and strengthen digestion. It was the main ingredient in the banned alcoholic drink, absinthe.

Medicinal Parts: leaves and tops

Preparation Forms: tincture, capsules, tea, wash, compress oil (externally). Dosage: tincture: 10-30 drops 3x daily; powder: 15-20 grains 3x daily; tea: 2 cups daily.

Nutrition Profile: vitamins A and C, a bitters herb for bile stimulation and cholesterol reduction.

Herbal Healing Actions: vermifuge, alterative, astringent, stimulant, antiseptic, diuretic and tonic.

Cleansing Properties & Detox Activity: Wormwood's main use today is in formulas to expel intestinal worms and parasite infestations (both in people and animals), and as a poison antidote, especially for food poisoning. Small amounts may be used during acute illness to reduce fever and inflammation. As a bitters herb in small amounts, it stimulates enzyme secretions for better bile flow, reduces liver congestion and stimulates bowel peristalsis. Bitters herbs also encourage urination and drain fluid congestion. As a body cleanser, wormwood promotes menstruation, clears toxins and benefits the skin.

Wormwood may be used as a compress to relieve headaches, fevers, skin rashes, swellings, sprains and bruises, and to neutralize poisons from insect bites.

Safety Precautions: Not when pregnant or breast feeding as it is a uterine stimulant.

Synergy With Other Herbs: With *caraway seeds, peppermint* and *frangula bark* for a bitters tea with laxative and carminative action.

- **Yarrow,** *Achillea millefolium,* Family: *Compositae*

Common Names: thousandleaf, nosebleed, old man's pepper, soldier's woundwort, knight's milfoil, carpenter's weed, staunchweed (Eng); millefeuille, achillée, herbe aux charpentiers (Fr), garbenkraut (Ge).

Traditional Use: Used for centuries as a poultice to stop wound bleeding, particularly for soldiers in battle. Reputedly Achilles used it for dressing wounds, thus, its botanical name became Achillea. Gerard recommended it for toothaches; Culpeper said it was a good herb for cramps. Native Americans use yarrow for colds, coughs, headaches, fevers, ague, nausea, stomach ailments, diarrhea, kidney ailments, toothaches, wounds, sores, swellings, skin rashes, burns and blisters.

Medicinal Parts: the whole herb

Preparation Forms: tea, tincture, poultice, fresh juice, wash, essential oil. Dosage: tincture: 5-20 drops 3x daily, tea: 6-oz. 3-4x daily, powder: 30-60 grains 3x daily.

Herbal Healing Actions: hemostatic, expectorant, analgesic, carminative, diaphoretic, emmenagogic, anti-inflammatory, antipyretic, antiseptic and stomachic.

Nutrition Profile: Yarrow is high in chromium and potassium, selenium, vitamin B_1 and C, and contains significant amounts of calcium, magnesium, manganese, phosphorus, silicon, and sodium. Its amino acids include alanine, glutamic acid, histidine, leucine, and lysine.

Cleansing Properties & Detox Activity: Yarrow is used today as a hemostatic, antiseptic poultice to stop bleeding and reduce wound pain. Its cleansing properties restore the liver, stomach and spleen, reducing inflammation, clearing congestion, resolving intestinal mucous, stimulating liver activity and scouring the kidneys. It is effective as a urinary antiseptic for cystitis, urinary stones and bladder infections; its diuretic qualities help lower blood pressure. It has hormone stimulating properties for hormone imbalances, promoting cleansing, encouraging menstruation and removing pelvic congestion.

Yarrow is a powerful diaphoretic and antiseptic to induce sweating and lower fever during colds and flu. A good herb for childhood diseases like measles, chickenpox and diarrhea. Effective in cleansing for arthritis and rheumatism, gastroenteritis and colitis. Use externally for skin sores and hemorrhoids, it promotes tissue repair. Also effective as a compress for toothaches.

Safety Precautions: Not during pregnancy- strong astringent action may be abortive.

Synergy With Other Herbs: With *yucca, alfalfa, devil's claw, guggul resin, buckthorn bk., black cohosh, St. John's wort, burdock rt., licorice rt., dandelion, parsley, hydrangea, slippery elm, bilberry, ligusticum, poria mushroom, tumeric, rose hips, hawthorn* to neutralize acids and increase mobility against arthritis.

• **Yellow Dock Root**, *Rumex crispus*, Family: *Polygonaceae*

Common Names: curled dock, narrow dock, pharoms, sour dock, rumex, patience, parielle, rhubarbe sauvage, churelle, oreille de vache (Fr); grindampher, krauser ampfer, mengelwurz, (Ge).

Traditional Use: Called *Lapathon* by the ancient Greeks, meaning "to cleanse" and used for that purpose. Imported to North America by early settlers; used by Native Americans for jaundice, rheumatism, liver ailments, as a blood cleanser and tonic, for venereal disease, tumors, sores, ulcers, ringworm, dysentery and cancer.

Medicinal Parts: root

Preparation Forms: tea, capsules, decoction, extract, gargle, fomentation, wash, salve. Dosage: tincture: 5-30 drops 3x daily; powder: 30-60 grains 3x daily.

Nutrition Profile: A rich source of herbal iron. High in phosphorus and vitamin A, vitamin C, B_1 and B_2; high in calcium, iron, magnesium, selenium; contains significant amounts of manganese, potassium, silicon, sodium, and vitamin B_3, as well as trace amounts of chromium and zinc.

Herbal Healing Actions: alterative, bitter, hematonic, cholagogue, astringent, laxative.

Cleansing Properties & Detox Activity: Yellow dock is especially effective for liver congestion, gallbladder and spleen. Yellow dock increases liver ability to filter and purify the blood and promotes production of bile. A specific in treating anemia—blood building against iron deficiency. A lymphatic cleanser for swollen glands. Helpful in dissolving cancerous growths and tumors. A mild astringent for hemorrhoids and ulcers. A mild purgative for constipation and ridding the body of intestinal parasites. Specific ailments that benefit from yellow dock's detox properties include breast and uterine fibroids and vaginal infections. Helps reduce the pain and inflammation of gout, rheumatism and arthritis. Helps relieve and dissolve urinary stones, and gravel in the kidney and urethral areas. Important in herbal skin formulas for eczema, psoriasis and other inflammatory skin conditions.

Safety Precautions: Do not take during pregnancy or while breast-feeding. Not recommended for prolonged use (60 days) as it may cause laxative dependence.

Synergy With Other Herbs: With *dandelion, watercress, pau d' arco, hyssop, parsley, Oregon grape rt., red sage, licorice, milk thistle seed and hibiscus* for a liver flush tea. With *beet, milk thistle seed, Oregon grape, dandelion, wild yam, licorice, ginkgo biloba, barberry, gotu kola, ginger, wild cherry* for a liver

cleansing capsule. With *beet, alfalfa, dandelion, Siberian ginseng, parsley, nettles, burdock, dulse, bilberry* and *capsicum* for spleen and liver activity, blood building, mental clarity and disease resistance.

• **Yerba Santa,** *Eriodictyon californicum,* Family: *Hydrophyllaceae*

Common Names: mountain balm, bear's weed, consumptive's weed, gum bush, tarweed (America).

Traditional Use: Native Americans used the leaves as a poultice for rheumatism, swellings, sores and sprains. Internally, it was taken for colds, cough, sore throat, catarrh, stomach aches, vomiting and diarrhea.

Medicinal Parts: leaves

Preparation Forms: tea, wash, tincture, decoction, syrup. Dosage: tincture: 10-30 drops 3x daily; powder: 15-60 grains 3x daily; tea: 2-3-oz. 3x daily.

Herbal Healing Actions: astringent, stimulant, tonic, aromatic, carminative, alterative.

Nutrition Profile: Contains free formic acid and glycerides of fatty acids, phytosterols, resins, tannins that work on the bronchials, mucous membranes (useful in respiratory tract ailments), and urogenital areas. Also contains a mild amount of caffeine.

Cleansing Properties & Detox Activity: An expectorant herb with digestive cleansing properties. Used as part of a "spring cleansing" combination, especially for bladder and kidney. Used externally as an astringent antidote for poison oak rashes. Releases bronchitis phlegm and relieves coughing. Stimulates digestion and promotes the appetite. Reduces infection and opens the sinuses.

Safety Precautions: None in common use.

Synergy With Other Herbs: With *grindelia flowers* for an expectorant. With *red clover, hawthorn, pau d'arco, nettles, sage, alfalfa, horsetail, milk thistle seed, gotu kola, echinacea purpurea, blue malva* and *lemon grass* in a spring cleansing tea.

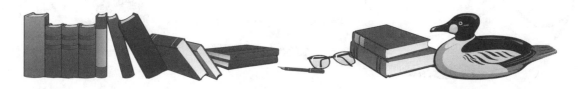

— Want more explanation of unusual, unfamiliar detox terms?

— Need clarification about detox techniques?

— Look it all up in this Quick Reference Glossary.

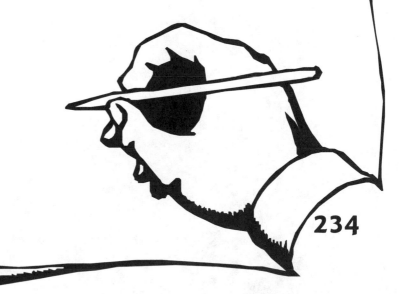

Quick Detox Reference

Detoxification and body cleansing rituals have been around for so many millennia that they have developed a language and terminology all their own. Many methods and techniques come to us from ancient times. This short chapter is an easy glossary of alternative medicine and herbal therapy with examples for detoxification.

• Absorbents: herbs used to produce absorption of diseased tissues. Examples of absorbents include *mullein* and *slippery elm.*

• Adaptogens: herbs that help normalize body chemistry and resistance to stress. Examples of adaptogens include *Siberian and panax ginseng, chlorella, astragalus* and *hawthorn.*

• Alkalizing enzyme cleanse: a good "spring cleaning" technique for liver, digestive and elimination system support. Balances and increases enzyme and systol/diastole activity, alkalizing an over-acid system. Used in spas in enzyme body wraps through herbal-infused gels applied to the skin for easy absorption. Examples of alkalizing, enzyme-stimulating herbs are *aloe vera, ginger, bladderwrack, spearmint* and *alfalfa.*

• Alteratives: tonifying herbs that restore proper body function and vitality by normalizing blood composition. Alteratives improve metabolism, increasing the body's ability to eliminate waste through the kidneys, liver, lungs or skin. Examples of alterative herbs include *echinacea, burdock, garlic, red clover, sarsaparilla, goldenseal, nettles* and *yellow dock.*

• Amino acids: cysteine, methionine, tyrosine and taurine support internal cleansing. Cysteine converts to glutathione, one of the most powerful natural detoxifiers of heavy metals, radiation, chemicals and drugs. Glutathione is found in *parsley* and *spinach.*

• Antacids: herbs which correct acidic conditions in the stomach, blood and bowels. Examples of antacids include *comfrey, flax seed, hops, mullein, raspberry* and *slippery elm.*

• Anthelmintics: herbs that help destroy or expel intestinal worms and parasites from the digestive system. (see also Vermifuge) Examples of anthelmintics include *wormwood, pumpkin seed, tansy, aloe vera, rue, black walnut hulls* and *garlic.*

• Anti-arthritics: herbs used to relieve and heal arthritic-type conditions. Examples of anti-arthritic herbs include *yucca, black cohosh, burdock, cayenne, chaparral, dandelion, Irish moss, sarsaparilla, scullcap, wintergreen* and *yellow dock.*

• Anti-bilious: herbs that help neutralize and remove excess bile, and overcome jaundice conditions. Examples of antibilious herbs include *barberry, dandelion root, goldenseal, wild yam* and *gentian.*

* **Anti-biotics (anti-bacterial):** herbs that kill and arrest the growth of harmful micro-organisms (see Anti-microbials). Examples of antibiotic herbs include *goldenseal root, echinacea, myrrh, marshmallow, St. John's wort, lomatium* **and** *garlic.*

* **Anti-catarrhal:** herbs that help remove excess mucous and congestion, particularly from sinus, bronchial and chest areas. Examples of anti-catarrhal herbs include *boneset, echinacea root, garlic, goldenseal, elecampane, marshmallow, mullein, sage* **and** *yarrow.*

* **Anti-emetic:** herbs that relieve nausea and vomiting, and upset stomach. Examples of anti-emetic herbs include *ginger root, cayenne, cloves, peppermint and spearmint, fennel, lemon balm, wild yam, alfalfa* **and** *dill.*

* **Anti-fungal:** herbs that destroys or prevents the growth of fungal infections. Examples of anti-fungal herbs include *black walnut hulls, tea tree oil, propolis, maitake mushroom, wormwood* **and** *garlic.*

* **Anti-hydropics:** herbs that eliminate excess body fluids or dropsy. Examples of anti-hydropic herbs include *anise, asparagus, barberry, black cohosh, burdock seeds and root, chamomile, carrot, celery, chaparral, dandelion, fennel, flaxseed, mullein* **and** *rosemary.*

* **Anti-inflammatory:** herbs that help reduce and overcome inflammation both externally and internally. Examples of anti-inflammatory herbs include *calendula, chamomile, devil's claw root, St. John's wort, feverfew* **and** *white willow.*

* **Anti-lithics:** herbs that help remove and prevent the formation of sediment, gravel and stones in the urinary/urethral area. Examples of anti-lithic herbs include *gravel root, hydrangea, stone root, cornsilk, buchu, uva ursi* **and** *parsley root.*

* **Anti-microbials:** herbs that help the body to destroy or resist pathogenic micro-organisms. Examples of anti-microbials include *myrrh, garlic, echinacea, calendula, elecampane, goldenseal* **and** *astragalus.*

* **Anti-neoplastics:** herbs that combat tumorous growth. Examples of anti-neoplastics include *calendula, red clover, burdock, dandelion, cleavers, mistletoe, guaiacum* **and** *echinacea.*

* **Anti-oxidants:** agents that unite with oxygen, protecting the cells and body constituents like enzymes from being destroyed or altered by oxidation. Although oxygen is vital to our body functions, the presence of either too much or too little oxygen creates toxic by-products called free radicals. These highly reactive substances can damage cell structures so badly that immunity is impaired and DNA codes are altered, resulting in degenerative disease and premature aging. Specifically, free radical attacks are the forerunners of heart attacks, cancer, and opportunistic diseases such as HIV infection or candidiasis. Anti-oxidants "quench" free radicals and render them harmless. Antioxidants are selective, acting against undesirable oxygen reactions but not against desirable oxygen activity. A poor diet, inadequate exercise, illness and emotional stress

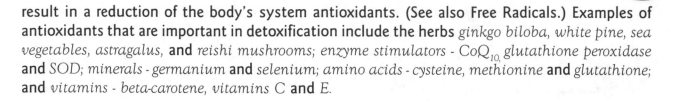

result in a reduction of the body's system antioxidants. (See also Free Radicals.) Examples of antioxidants that are important in detoxification include the herbs *ginkgo biloba, white pine, sea vegetables, astragalus,* **and** *reishi mushrooms; enzyme stimulators -* CoQ$_{10,}$ *glutathione peroxidase* **and** *SOD; minerals - germanium* **and** *selenium; amino acids - cysteine, methionine* **and** *glutathione;* **and** *vitamins - beta-carotene, vitamins C* **and** *E.*

* **Anti-carcinogens:** substances that prevent or delay tumor formation and development. Examples of anticarcinogens include *panax ginseng, garlic, echinacea, goldenseal, licorice, black cohosh, wild yam, sarsaparilla, maitake mushroom* **and** *cruciferous vegetables.*

* **Anti-parasitics:** Like viruses, parasites have adapted and become stronger in order to survive, developing defenses against the drugs designed to kill them. In fact, most drugs commonly used to treat parasites not only lose effectiveness against new parasitic strains, but also cause a number of unpleasant side effects in the host. Herbal remedies have been successfully used for centuries as living medicines against parasites, with little or no side effects. Antiparasitic herbs include *black walnut hulls, garlic, pumpkin seed, gentian root, wormwood, butternut bark, fennel seed, cascara, mugwort, slippery elm* **and** *false unicorn.*

* **Anti-phlogistics:** herbs that reduce inflammation or swelling (see Anti-inflammatories). Examples of anti-phlogistic herbs include *arnica (external), balm of Gilead, bayberry, black cohosh (nerves), blue cohosh (uterus), burdock root (external), cayenne, comfrey* **and** *licorice.*

* **Anti-pyretics:** herbs that help reduce fevers. (See Febrifuge.)

* **Anti-septics:** herbs that combat and neutralize pathogenic bacteria, and prevent infection. (See Anti-microbials and Anti-biotics.)

* **Anti-spasmodics:** muscle relaxant herbs that relieve cramping and spasms in a wide variety of uses, from hiatal hernias to PMS cramps, to lower back pain. Examples of anti-spasmodic herbs include *cramp bark, black haw, lady's slipper, motherwort, lobelia, scullcap, wild yam, chamomile* **and** *valerian.*

* **Anti-syphilitics:** herbs that help overcome venereal disease. Examples of anti-syphilitics include *sarsaparilla, black walnut, burdock, lobelia, white oak bark, goldenseal* **and** *myrrh.*

* **Anti-tussive:** herbs to prevent and relieve coughing. Examples of anti-tussive herbs include *licorice, horehound, comfrey, mullein, plantain, coltsfoot, wild cherry bark* **and** *valerian.*

* **Anti-venomous:** antidote herbs against poisons. Examples of anti-venomous herbs include *plantain (powerful), black cohosh, fennel, garlic, juniper berry, lobelia, marigold, olive oil, parsley, slippery elm* **and** *wormwood.*

* **Anti-virals:** herbs that combat and neutralize viruses. Examples of anti-virals include *echinacea, St. John's wort, lomatium dissectum, myrrh, goldenseal, astragalus and propolis.*

Aperients: herbs with mild, gentle laxative activity. Examples of aperients include *rhubarb root, flax seed, barberry, butternut root* **and** *cleavers.*

Aphrodisiacs: herbs that help impotency problems and strengthen sexual desire and vitality. Examples of aphrodisiacs include *yohimbe, gotu kola, kola nut, all the ginsengs, damiana, saw palmetto, muira pauma (potency wood)* **and** *dong quai.*

Aromatics: herbs with strong, pleasant odors, that stimulate digestion and well-being through both carminative activity and smell. Examples of aromatics include *anise seed, basil, peppermint, fennel, cinnamon, dill, rosemary, ginger, cloves, chamomile* **and** *coriander.*

Astringents: herbs that tighten tissue, reducing irritation, secretions and discharges. Examples of astringent herbs include *bayberry, St. Johns wort* **and** *white oak bark.*

Balsamics: herbs that soothe and heal skin inflammation. Examples of balsamics include *avocado leaves, balm of Gilead buds, clary sage, ox-eye daisy petals, poplar buds* **and** *spikenard.*

Bentonite: a natural clay used for internal cleansing and externally as a poultice.

Bitters: herbs with a bitter taste that stimulate the digestive system, producing healthful counteractive juices and bile secretions. Examples of bitters herbs include *gentian, angelica, wormwood, chamomile, barberry, goldenseal, dandelion* **and** *Oregon grape.*

Blood cleansing: ridding the blood, liver, kidneys and lymph glands of toxins while normalizing blood chemistry. Examples of blood cleansers include *echinacea, red clover, sarsaparilla* **and** *goldenseal.*

Brewer's Yeast: an excellent source of protein, B vitamins, amino acids and minerals. Chromium-rich brewer's yeast significantly improves blood sugar metabolism, and substantially reduces serum cholesterol, raising HDL's. Helps speed wound healing by increasing production of collagen. Antioxidant properties allow the tissues to take in more oxygen for healing. B vitamin and mineral content improve skin texture and heal blemishes. (I use it in a cleansing facial mask.) Brewer's yeast is not the same as *Candida albicans* yeast. It is one of the best immune-enhancing supplements available.

Calmatives: herbs that calm stress and nervous tension. Examples of calmatives include *peppermint, chamomile, scullcap, catnip, rosemary, hops* **and** *Siberian ginseng.*

Cardiotonics: herbs that strengthen and tonify heart and circulatory activity. Examples of cardiotonic herbs include *hawthorn, cayenne, motherwort* **and** *Siberian ginseng.*

Carminatives: herbs that normalize digestive system peristalsis to relieve gas. Examples of carminatives include *anise seed, cayenne, licorice, peppermint, ginger root, cinnamon, caraway, ginger* **and** *thyme.*

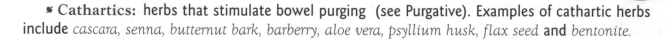

❧ Cathartics: herbs that stimulate bowel purging (see Purgative). Examples of cathartic herbs include *cascara, senna, butternut bark, barberry, aloe vera, psyllium husk, flax seed* **and** *bentonite.*

❧ Cell proliferants: herbs that promote rapid new cell growth. Examples of cell proliferants include *chlorella, spirulina, barley grass, horsetail, evening primrose, sea vegetables* **and** *ginsengs.*

❧ Charcoal, activated: a natural agent that relieves gas and diarrhea — an antidote for many poisons. An antacid, depurative and carminative that neutralizes and absorbs toxins allowing the kidneys to work more efficiently. Neutralizes acids and relieves flatulence in the stomach and intestinal tract. Helps normalize dysentery, diarrhea and constipation. Effective as a poultice for malodorous ulcers and wounds. An antidote for almost all poisons. *Note: For cases of severe poisoning, call the Poison Control Center 1-800-342-9293.*

❧ Chelation therapy: a safe intravenous therapy that increases blood flow and decreases excess plaque deposits in arteries and organs. EDTA, *(ethylenediamine tetra-acetic acid),* **used in** chelation therapy, removes toxic, clogging minerals from the circulatory system, particularly those that impair membrane function and contribute to free radical damage. EDTA puts these minerals into solution where they can be excreted by the kidneys.

❧ Cholagogue: herbs that stimulate bile secretion from the gall-bladder, engendering natural laxative activity and digestive improvement. **Examples of cholagogues include** *barberry bark, wild yam, dandelion rt., Oregon grape, calendula, golden seal, garlic* **and** *gentian root.*

❧ Clay, white, purified: absorbs and antidotes toxins to normalize intestinal inflammation. Used in formulas to relieve diarrhea and soothe the intestinal tract. Externally used as part of a poultice to disperse healing properties for skin ailments like eczema, boils, tumors and rashes.

❧ Colonic: a gentle, warm water cleansing of the colon. The procedure lasts approximately 45 minutes. A small nozzle or hose is inserted into the anus, allowing the water to flow in under gentle pressure and dislodge toxic wastes which are flushed out the rectum.

❧ Constipation: There are two types of constipation. One type happens when the feces are packed tight together. Another type happens when hardened feces stick to the walls of the colon and do not pass out during bowel movements.

❧ Colloidal silver: A universal antibiotic natural substance, pure metallic ionic silver is held in suspension by the minute electrical charge of each particle. Colloidal silver is tasteless, non-addictive and non-toxic. Many forms of bacteria, viruses and fungi utilize a specific enzyme for their metabolism. Colloidal silver acts as a catalyst to disable the enzyme. In fact, it proves toxic to most species of fungi, bacteria, parasites, even many viruses. Even more important, harmful organisms do not develop an immunity to silver as they do to chemical antibiotics.

❧ Cordials: tonic herbs that warm the stomach and stimulate cardiac activity. Examples of cordials include *ginger, ginsengs, cardamon, cinnamon, cloves* **and** *coriander.*

Dead Sea Salts: obtained from the Dead Sea in Israel - composed of potassium, chlorine, sodium, calcium and magnesium salts, and used in detoxifying baths.

Demulcents: soothing, coating mucilaginous herbs that protect irritated and inflamed tissue. Examples of demulcent herbs include *comfrey, marshmallow, milk thistle, slippery elm, flax seed, parsley root, Irish moss, aloe vera* **and** *mullein.*

Depurant: blood purifying herbs that stimulate elimination of toxins. Examples of depurants include *garlic, goldenseal, chlorella, barley grass, cranberry* **and** *sea plants.*

Diaphoretics: skin cleansing herbs that induce sweating, releasing body toxins through perspiration. Examples of diaphoretic herbs include *cayenne, elder, garlic, ginger, chamomile, boneset, angelica, bayberry, prickly ash, spikenard* **and** *buchu.*

Digestants: enzyme-containing herbs that promote digestion and nutrient assimilation. Examples of digestant herbs include *ginseng, chlorella, barley grass, spirulina, yellow dock, sea vegetables, papaya* **and** *garlic.*

Discutients: herbs that dissolve and remove tumors or abnormal growths. Effective in poultices and fomentations or taken internally as teas. Examples of discutients include *aloe vera, ginseng, pau d' arco, calendula, echinacea* **and** *sea plants.* **(See anti-neoplastics)**

Diuretics: herbs that stimulate kidney and bladder activity, and increase the flow of urine. Examples of diuretic herbs include *uva ursi, cleavers, dandelion leaf, buchu, couchgrass, juniper, yarrow, corn silk* **and** *gravel root.*

Electuary: a sweet paste, food or drink used to mask bitter or medicine-tasting herbs so they may be taken by children. Examples of electuaries include peanut butter, fruit juice, honey/ butter pastes, bread or cream cheese.

Emetics: herbs that in high doses cause vomiting to rid the body of toxic substances or excess mucous congestion. Examples of emetic herbs include *lobelia, elder flowers, boneset* **and** *ipecacuanha.*

Emmenagogues: herbs that stimulate and normalize menstrual flow. Examples of emmenagogues include *pennyroyal, blue cohosh, blessed thistle, motherwort, lovage, angelica, tansy* **and** *shepherd's purse.*

Emollient: externally applied, soothing herbs that smooth and soften the skin and reduce inflammatory skin conditions. Examples of emollient herbs include *slippery elm, marshmallow, plantain, comfrey, Irish moss, chickweed, borage, mullein* **and** *aloe vera.*

Essiac: an herbal tea formula of the Ojibway Indians, made famous by Rene Caisse for cleansing the body of cancer cells, has been rediscovered today. The name "Essiac" is actually an

anagram of her last name "Caisse." The formula consists of *sheep sorrel, burdock root, turkey rhubarb* and *slippery elm bark.*

• Expectorants: herbs that help remove mucous congestion from the chest and respiratory system. Examples of expectorant herbs include *licorice root, horehound, pleurisy root, coltsfoot, comfrey, anise seed, marshmallow* and *thyme.*

• Free radicals: unstable fragments of molecules produced from oxygen and fats in cell membranes when high energy chemical oxidation reactions in the body get out of control. Atoms and molecules consist of protons, neutrons and electrons, which normally come in pairs. Electron pairs form chemical bonds which hold all molecules together. A free radical contains an unpaired electron. In this unbalanced state, the free radical is stimulated to combine with other molecules, and in combination is capable of destroying an enzyme, a protein, or a complete cell. The destruction causes chain reactions that release thousands more free radicals and stimulate aging skin pigment, damage protein structures, and impair fat metabolizing enzymes. While the body normally produces some free radicals in its ordinary metabolic breakdown of organic compounds (like those released to fight bacteria during immune response) it also produces the necessary substances (like antioxidant enzymes) to deactivate them.

Free radical formation can be caused by:
—Infections from viruses, bacteria, or parasites.
—Trauma from surgery, injury, inflammation, burns and wounds.
—Smoking or passive exposure to cigarette smoke.
—Excessive alcohol and/or addictive drug intake.
—Exposure to toxic chemicals, like pesticide residues and household chemicals.
—Exposure to radiation, including excessive UV rays from sunlight.
—Cytotoxic drugs, such as the anticancer drug Adriamycin.
—Oxidant drugs that steal electrons, such as acetaminophen (Tylenol).
—Consumption of nitrites, nitrates and other food additives.
—A diet low in antioxidant foods; partially-hydrogenated fats in many snack and junk foods.

• Hemostatic: herbs that help stop bleeding (see Styptic). Examples of hemostatics include *shepherd's purse, comfrey, turmeric, plantain, witch hazel, cayenne, buckthorn* and *cranesbill.*

• Hemoglobin builder: A compound that aids absorption of iron and other minerals for red blood cell production. Examples of hemoglobin building herbs are *beet root, alfalfa, dandelion, Siberian ginseng, yellow dock root, parsley root, nettles, burdock root, dulse, capsicum.*

• Heavy metal poisoning: long term exposure to metals like lead, mercury, cadmium, arsenic, nickel and aluminum affects cell growth, behavior and immune response. Examples of herbs that help remove heavy metals are *bugleweed, bladderwrack, licorice root, astragalus, kelp.*

• Hepatics: herbs that support and stimulate the liver, gall bladder and spleen to increase bile flow. Examples of hepatics include *barberry, Oregon grape, beet root, dandelion, goldenseal, hyssop, wild yam, fennel* and *cleavers.*

* **Herbal wraps:** spas use herbal wraps as restorative body-conditioning techniques. Wraps are also body cleansing methods that may be used to elasticize, tone, alkalize and release body wastes quickly. For best results, use in conjunction with a short cleansing program, and 6 to 8 glasses of water a day to flush out loosened fats and toxins. Alkalizing enzyme wraps replace and balance minerals, enhance metabolism and alkalize the body.

* **Juice fasting:** a raw vegetable and fruit juice cleanse for 24 hours to 7 days for detoxification. Fruit juices promote cleansing; vegetable juices help build and regenerate.

* **Kidney flush:** ridding the kidneys of metabolic wastes such as ammonia and urea, allowing them to operate more efficiently. A purifying, kidney cleansing drink should have balancing potassium and other minerals, and naturally-occurring amino acids for protein synthesis. Examples of kidney flushing herbs are *juniper, dandelion leaf, uva ursi, cleavers.*

* **Lactobacillus:** beneficial bacteria, including *L. acidophilus, L. bifidus, L. caucassus, and L. bulgaricus,* that synthesize nutrients in the intestinal tract, counteract pathogenic microorganisms and maintain a healthy intestinal environment. Lactobacillus organisms are fragile flora readily destroyed by harmful chemicals and drugs, particularly chlorine and antibiotics. A single, long course of antibiotics can destroy most bowel flora, leading to an overgrowth of yeasty pathogens like *candida albicans,* which are resistant to antibiotics. Eating antibiotic-laced meats and dairy products leads to a decline of *Lactobacillus* organisms in the body. Skin disorders, chronic candidiasis, irritable bowel syndrome, intestinal disorders, hepatitis, lupus and heart disease are all associated with a *Lactobacillus* deficiency. Top food sources include *yogurt, kefir, miso, tempeh* **and** *cold-cooked sauerkraut.*

* **Laxatives:** herbs that promote evacuation of the bowels. Examples of laxative herbs include *cascara, senna, Oregon grape, rhubarb rt., butternut bark, buckthorn* **and** *barberry.*

* **Lithotropics:** herbs that dissolve and discharge urinary and gall bladder stones and gravel. Examples of lithotropics include *barberry, buchu, cascara, chaparral, cornsilk, dandelion, horsetail, juniper berry* **and** *parsley.*

* **Liver flush:** a liver flush releases wastes from the liver and surrounding organs, tones liver tissue and stimulates protein synthesis to increase production of new liver cells to replace damaged ones. Examples of liver flushing herbs include *dandelion and yellow dock roots, watercress, pau d'arco, hyssop, parsley, Oregon grape, red sage, licorice, milk thistle seed.*

* **Lymphatics:** herbs that stimulate and cleanse the lymph system. Examples of lymphatics include *black walnut, garlic, chaparral, dandelion, echinacea root, Oregon grape* **and** *yellow dock.*

* **Lymphatic massage:** a gentle, whole-body massage aimed at stimulating the lymphatic system to carry away excessive fluid in the loose connective tissue.

* **Mucilaginous:** herbs with high mucilage content that have soothing, demulcent action.

Examples of mucilaginous herbs include *comfrey, slippery elm, Irish moss, iceland moss, flax seed, psyllium, aloe vera* and *marshmallow root.*

❧ **Mucous cleanse:** releases excess mucous from the lungs, respiratory and digestive system allowing other body functions to operate more efficiently.

❧ **Nervines:** herbs that tone, relax and strengthen the nervous system. Examples of nervines include *lady's slipper, passionflowers, mistletoe, chamomile, oatstraw, lobelia, cramp bark, valerian* and *scullcap.*

❧ **Nutritives:** food supplement plants, rich in minerals, that nourish and promote growth. Examples of nutritive herbs include *chlorella, spirulina, barley grass, ginseng, wheat grass, sea vegetables, suma* and *astragalus.*

❧ **Parasiticides:** herbs that kill and remove parasites from the skin. Examples of parasiticide herbs include *black walnut, cinnamon and cajuput oils, chaparral, garlic, echinacea, rue, thyme, gentian* and *wood betony.*

❧ **Pectoral:** herbs that helps heal and strengthen the lung and respiratory system. Examples of pectorals include *comfrey, coltsfoot, goldenseal, elecampane, mullein, licorice, marshmallow, pleurisy root* and *hyssop.*

❧ **pH:** the scale used to measure acidity and alkalinity. H is hydrogen, or the "H" ion concentration of a solution. "p" stands for the power factor of the H ion. pH of a solution is measured on a scale of 14. A neutral solution, neither acidic nor alkaline, such as water, has a pH of 7. Acid is less than 7; alkaline is more than 7.

❧ **Pycnogenol:** a concentrated, highly active bioflavonoid extract from pine bark. A powerful antioxidant, 50 times stronger than vitamin E, 20 times stronger than vitamin C. Helps the body resist inflammation and blood vessel and skin damage caused by free radicals. Strengthens arteries and improves circulation. Reduces capillary fragility, develops skin smoothness and elasticity. Stimulates collagen-rich connective tissue against atherosclerosis and for joint flexibility in arthritis. Helps diabetic retinopathy, varicose veins and hemorrhoids. One of the few dietary antioxidants that easily crosses the blood-brain barrier to protect brain cells and aid memory.

❧ **Phytochemicals:** natural constituents in plants that have specific pharmacologic action. Also known as nutraceuticals, pharmafoods and phytonutrients, the best way for your body to utilize phytochemicals is to ingest the plant source in its whole form. Here are some phytochemicals that are of important interest to a cleansing balancing diet;
　— Anti-carcinogen phytochemicals prevent or delay tumor formation. Some herbs and foods with known anticarcinogens include *ginseng, soy foods, garlic, echinacea, goldenseal, licorice root, black cohosh, wild yam, maitake mushroom* and *cruciferous vegetables.*
　— Phytohormones contain substances with hormonal actions. Plant hormone chemicals are quite similar to human hormones and are capable of binding to human hormone receptor

sites. Unlike synthetic hormones, plant hormones show little or no adverse side effects. Some food plants and herbs that have phytohormone activity include *soy foods, licorice root, wild yam, sarsaparilla root, dong quai, damiana* **and** *black cohosh.*

— Phytoestrogens are plant estrogens remarkably similar to human estrogens. Important in inhibiting hormone-driven cancers, phytoestrogens bind to human estrogen receptor sites without the negative side effects of synthetic estrogens. Recent studies show phytoestrogens are essentially hormone balancers, inhibiting proliferation of both estrogen-receptor positive and negative breast tumor cells. Some plants with phytoestrogenic activity include *dong quai, panax ginseng, licorice, fennel, alfalfa* **and** *red clover.*

— Phytoprogesterones are plant hormones similar to human progesterone. Progesterone participates in almost every physiological process, biochemically providing material out of which other steroid hormones (cortisone, testosterone, estrogen and salt-regulating aldosterone) can be made. A precursor to estrogen, its tremendous increase during pregnancy serves to stabilizes hormone adjustment and growth of mother and child. When progesterone is deficient, there tends to be hypoglycemia, often combined with obesity. Some phyto-progesterone sources are *sarsaparilla, licorice root* **and** *wild yam.*

— Phyto-testosterone, or plant testosterone, is a similar substance to the androgen or male hormones found in both men and women. Testosterone determines sex drive in both sexes. Testosterone is essential for normal sexual behavior and the occurrence of male erections. *Ginseng* is an herb known to stimulate production of human testosterone.

⚘ **Probiotics:** beneficial microorganisms, including *Lactobacillus, Bifidobacteria,* **and** *Streptococcus termophilus,* that compete with disease-causing microorganisms in the gastrointestinal tract. Probiotics are responsible for the manufacture of B vitamins like biotin, niacin, folic acid and pyridoxine (B$_6$), improving digestion, combating vaginal yeast infections, killing harmful bacteria by normalizing acid/alkaline balance and depriving harmful bacteria of nutrients they need.

⚘ **Purgatives:** herbs that promote watery evacuation of the bowels (see Laxative).

⚘ **Rubefacient:** herbs that increase circulation and stimulate dilation of the capillaries. Examples of rubefacient herbs include *cayenne, ginger, horseradish, nettles, rosemary, peppermint oil, cloves, black pepper* **and** *garlic.*

⚘ **Sauna heat therapy:** a sauna is a way to use heat cleansing principles. A 20 to 30-minute sauna not only induces a healing, cleansing fever, but also causes profuse therapeutic sweating. The skin, in effect, acts as a "third kidney" to eliminate body wastes through perspiration. Native Americans used sweat lodges on much the same principle. Health benefits of a dry sauna include dramatic increase in the cleansing capacity of the skin, increased metabolism, a jump start for a weight loss program (especially for sugar cravers), gland and organ stimulation, enhanced immune response, and inhibition of virus replication. *Note: Although cleansing heat is a natural means of biological healing, supervision from a practitioner is recommended.*

⚘ **Sedatives:** herbs that calm the nerves and reduce stress and tension. Examples of sedatives are *valerian, scullcap, hops, black cohosh, black haw* **and** *passionflowers.*

❧ Stimulants: herbs that accelerate, enliven and vitalize body functions. Examples of stimulant herbs include *bayberry, cayenne, ginger root, horseradish, cardamom, peppermint, wild yam* and *ginsengs* of all kinds.

❧ Stomachics: agents that stimulate and strengthen the stomach, improving digestion and appetite. Examples of stomachics include *peppermint, wild yam, catnip, fennel* **and** *goldenseal.*

❧ Styptics: herbs to reduce and stop external bleeding (see Hemostatics and Astringents). Examples of styptics include *plantain, St. John's wort, witch hazel, yarrow, bayberry bark, cranesbill, white oak bark* **and** *cayenne.*

❧ Sudorifics: herbs that stimulate and increase perspiration. (see Diaphoretic)

❧ Tonics: herbs that strengthen and tone specific organs and body parts. Examples of tonic herbs include *ginsengs, hawthorn, black cohosh, dandelion, garlic, gotu kola, licorice rt.* **and** *damiana.*

❧ Toxins: toxic or poisonous compounds produced by microorganisms, that promote disease. Examples of toxins include heavy metals, environmental and chemical pollutants, chemical laced foods, tobacco smoke, drugs of all kinds, pesticides and food additives.

❧ Triphala: a detoxifying compound of three herbal fruits *terminalia chebula, terminalia bellerica* **and** *emblica officinalis.* Triphala has both laxative and tonic properties that regulate elimination, cleanse the digestive tract and colon, and revitalize the blood and liver. It is a specific for regulating bowel activity, constipation, diarrhea, biliousness, dyspepsia, and for headaches. Triphala regulates menstrual activity, helps weight control through cleansing, and is an effective eyewash to relieve redness and soreness.

❧ Vasodilators: herbs that relax and expand blood vessels. Examples of vasodilators include *ephedra, hawthorn, ginkgo biloba, feverfew* **and** *Siberian ginseng.*

❧ Vermifuge: herbs that help expel and/or destroy intestinal parasites (see Anthelmintics). Examples of vermifuge herbs include *thyme, black walnut hulls, chaparral, garlic, barberry, psyllium husks, tea tree oil, tansy* **and** *wormwood.*

Do you want
professional
help to
detoxify?

Pick an
American Spa
or Detox Center
that appeals
to you.

American Detox Centers and Spas

I believe the detox centers and spas listed here represent the best in America today. Many have long, successful histories with this type of healing technique; others have arisen more recently because of the enormous popularity of healing spa treatment in the U.S.

My associates and I have either been to the centers listed here or researched them extensively through conversations and letters about their programs and results. I have tried to give a short description of the essentials of each center in these pages, so that you can get an idea of which might be appealing to you. If you have further questions about a spa or center, please call the number listed under the center itself.

THE ANN WIGMORE FOUNDATION, P.O. Box 429, Rincon, Puerto Rico 00677, 787-868-6307 - located near the sea on the western side of the island. The new Ann Wigmore Foundation, P.O. Box 399, San Fidel, New Mexico 87049, 505-552-0595 and 617-267-9424.

One of the finest detoxification programs available, Dr. Ann Wigmore's "Living Foods Lifestyle" plan is a time-honored process for detoxifying your body, increasing energy and taking control of your health. Dr. Wigmore, the author of many books on body cleansing, has dedicated her life to educating the world about the transforming qualities of enzyme-rich, chlorophyll-rich living foods. I have personally attended seminars given by her staff and seen the results of her programs first hand.

The main elements of Dr. Wigmore's plan include fresh vegetables, young organic greens and fruits, sprouted foods, cultured vegetables (raw sauerkraut and Rejuvelac energy soup), smoothies and wheatgrass. Internal cleansing and colon care is an important part of the program.

There are a number of classes offered: How To Build A Healthy Diet; Good Food Combining; Food and Body Enzymes; Detoxification and Internal Cleansing; Reaching Ideal Weight; Morning Yoga by the Sea; Breathing and Relaxation Techniques; Mental and Emotional Balance and Communication; etc. Hands-on workshops include food preparation, indoor gardening skills, and facial, skin and body care. Highly recommended.

CANYON RANCH HEALTH RESORT, 8600 E. Rockcliff Road, Tuscon, AZ 85750, 520-749-9000.

Canyon Ranch is an internationally renowned health resort and three-time winner of the Best Spa Award in America. It is located on 70 lush desert acres, nestled in the foothills of the Santa Catalina mountains. The staff consists of a wide spectrum of health professionals — nutritionists, acupuncturists, medical doctors, psychologists and counselors, exercise physiologists, fitness instructors, movement therapists, tennis and racquetball pros, aesthetitians, massage, art and music therapists, hiking guides and support staff. Key programs include consultations and workshops in lifestyle changes, stress management, preventive health care guidance, smoking cessation and weight loss programs, spiritual awareness classes, yoga and meditation. There are 40 fitness classes daily, as well as tennis, hiking and biking. Group programs such as Living with Arthritis, Journey through Midlife and New Directions for Diabetes and a Healthy Heart are also offered.

Canyon Ranch is personally recommended by Zia Wesley Hosford, author of "Fifty and Fabulous," owner of Educated Beauty and advisory board member for the "Natural Healing Report."

☙ THE CHOPRA CENTER FOR WELL BEING, 7630 Fay Avenue, La Jolla, CA 92037, 619-551-7788.

This center, opened in August 1996, is located just north of San Diego. Programs are designed for guests who wish to achieve a higher level of physical, mental and spiritual well being. Dr. Deepak Chopra (author of a number of books and internationally recognized motivational speaker) has merged the concept of good health and self-knowledge by blending Western medicine with ancient Ayurvedic techniques of India. The center offers education and rejuvenating treatments through two programs: 1. Creating Health Program (which includes primordial sound meditation, mind/body education, Ayurvedic therapy, yoga and breathing techniques, seven laws of spiritual success, personal empowerment, and vegetarian meals); 2. Creating Health Ayurvedic Detoxification Program (includes all the classes mentioned above, a home preparation program, mind/body medical consultation, physician follow-up consultation, daily Ayurvedic purification therapies and Ayurvedic meals.

☙ OPTIMUM HEALTH INSTITUTE OF SAN DIEGO, 6970 Central Avenue, Lemon Grove, CA 91945, 619-464-3346 and the Optimum Health Institute of Austin, TX. R.R.1, Box 339-J, Cedar Creek, TX 78612, 512-303-4817.

These centers offer classes and hands on practical experience in cleansing your body of toxins and poisons, regaining a positive mental attitude, and releasing negative emotional issues that may be standing in your way of achieving optimal health. The programs are based on the principles from Dr. Ann Wigmore's work, offering a complete live foods diet, fresh greens and vegetables, enzyme-rich rejuvelac and seed sauces. The principles of proper food combining are taught for an efficient digestive system. The curriculum includes classes in understanding how your body works, diet and menu planning and advanced food preparation, sprouting, growing wheatgrass, fermented foods, mental and emotional detoxification, instant relaxation and pain control, boosting self-esteem, communication and daily exercise. There is at-home follow-up. I have personally attended this program. It is highly recommended.

☙ THE RAJ MAHARISHI AYURVEDA HEALTH CENTER, 1734 Jasmine Avenue, Fairfield, Iowa 52556, 800.248.9050.

The Raj is located in Fairfield, Iowa and is one of the leading centers for Ayurvedic Panchakarma treatment in the U. S. The Raj offers an ideal opportunity to experience transformation and rejuvenation in an atmosphere of quiet elegance. Three-Day, five-Day and one-week packages offer effective purification treatments to remove the damaging effects of stress and environmental pollutants, stimulating the body's natural rejuvenating abilities.

The Raj recommends a pre-treatment program at home before arriving at the center. Upon arrival you are evaluated by an Ayurvedic physician who designs a personalized Panchakarma program for your needs — including a doctor's consultation, two hours of Panchakarma treatments per day, health enhancement courses, and gourmet vegetarian meals. Extended meditation practice is available. A follow-up at home program includes specific recommendations for diet, exercise, herbal preparations, daily and seasonal routines, and stress management techniques.

The Raj also offers a "Beauty-From-Within Program," a detox program that recognizes that delicate skin tissues require treatments which are simultaneously cleansing and nourishing, replacing toxins and impurities with molecules of herbs, floral extracts and other products which support the structure of the skin. Many skin and hair problems are due to enviromental toxins, stress and aging. Beauty-from-Within transforms the internal functions of body physiology to create radiant beauty. The treatments include MD consultation and program design, herbal oil applications, steam treatments, milk elixir facial and mud applications, and milk baths.

☯ HEALTH REGENERATION INSTITUTE AT THE CIRCLE OF LIFE VILLAGE, 130 Biodome Dr., Waynesville, NC 28786, 704-926-2200.

The Health Regeneration Institute offers lifestyle therapy through the use of alternative and complementary healing modalities under supervision of doctors and other health care practitioners, and a lifestyle education program that addresses spiritual, mental, and practical approaches towards living. Individual programs are designed to help guests "discover and develop basic tools to meet the challenges of life."

Available services include detoxification programs, massage, osteopathic, chiropractic and other body work therapies, aromatherapy, steam baths, colonic irrigation, lymphatic detoxification and cold laser bio-stimulation. Treatment modalities include: Custom Designed Cleansing Programs; Living Foods and Sprouted Juices Cleansing & RegenerativeTherapy; ISIS Lymphatic Detox Therapy; Ozone Therapy with Colema, Bath and Steam; Live Blood Analysis Microscopy; Homeopathic Remedies; Chelation Therapy; Herbal and Chinese Medicines; Electronic Computer-mediated Acupuncture; Breath and Movement Classes; Kinesiology; Osteopathy and Chiropractic; Biologic Dentistry; Biofeedback; Direct Magnetic, Sound and Light Mediated therapies.

Individual programs include: medical evaluation and supervision; blood, urine and saliva tests; two tailor-made health service sessions per day; full participation in activities of your choice; accomodations for 6 nights; daily meals from the spa's organic gardens; wheat grass juice; and use of the center's facilities (i.e. swimming, riding, media lab, library, etc.).

☯ WESTGLOW SPA, P.O. Box 1083, Blowing Rock, NC 28605, 800-562-0807.

Westglow Spa is a full service European style spa nestled in the Blue Ridge Mountains. The spa offers a full range of life enhancing programs, including all the factors of good health, diet, physical activity, and emotional well being. Body treatments are provided by female and male therapists. Services include aromatherapy, upper back acne treatment, herbal body wrap, detoxification treatment and lymphatic drainage massage to decrease body toxins and promote tissue oxygenation. Personal counseling include fitness assessment and exercise prescription, nutrition assessment and diet consultation, acupressure, and personal stress management.

The Life Enhancement center was built to match the style and grace of the estate's mansion. The Center houses the latest in advanced fitness and therapeutic spa equipment— an indoor pool, whirlpools, wet/dry saunas, body treatment rooms, a hair and nail salon, cyber fitness equipment, cardiovascular conditioning center, testing clinic and poolside cafe.

☯ AMERICAN METABOLIC INSTITUTE, 555 Saturn Blvd. Building B,M/S 432, San Diego, Ca. 92154, 800-388-1083. Therapies provided in a hospital environment.

The American Metabolic Institute (AMI) and the St. Joseph Hospital (a health group) special-

ize in programs for treatment of degenerative diseases with a unique blend of alternative health care combined with conventional treatments. The AMI program focuses on restoring balance of body, mind and spirit. Every patient is given an individualized metabolic program which includes tests, detoxification, a catabolic diet and pH balancing. The program begins with a series of non-invasive tests to determine severity of disease and continues with ongoing tests throughout therapy determine efficacy of treatment.

American Metabolic Institute offers almost every known holistic approach, coupled with conventional methods when needed. Some of the holistic therapies include chelation, lymphatic congestion therapy, acupuncture, chiropractic, massage, oxygen therapies, immuno-therapy, colon therapy, rife frequency generator technology, cranial electro-stimulation, reflexology, colonics, colemas and enemas, mineral and herbal baths, shark cartilage treatments, saunas, clay, group therapy, nutritional counseling, writing programs, and positive thought therapy.

ⓢ **HOLISTIC MEDICAL CENTER,** 8264 Santa Monica Blvd., Los Angeles CA. 90046, 213-650-1789.

The Holistic Medical Center uses European methods for cleansing and detoxifying the body. Treatments include colon therapy, homeopathic treatments, viral and parasite treatments, and desensitization with homeopathic methods for environmental and food allergies.

ⓢ **ALTERNATIVE MEDICINE CENTER OF COLORADO,** 7601 E. Burning Tree Drive, Ste 100, Franktown CO., 80116, 303-688-1111.

The center offers improvement and restoration of the body's defenses, immune status assessment, herbal therapy, therapeutic nutrition, gastrointestinal cleansing and detoxification. Treatment lasts for 2-5 days at this outpatient facility.

ⓢ **BIO ETHICS MEDICAL CENTER,** 10752 North 78th Place #102, Scottsdale, AZ 85260, 602-860-0490.

The center treats chemically induced illnesses through detoxification and body balancing. Treatments rejuvenate the organs of detoxification such as the liver, gall bladder, kidneys and colon. Treatments offered include lymphatic drainage massage, herbs, nutrition, homeopathy for cancer, chemically induced illnesses, allergies, skin problems, chronic fatigue, gastrointestinal disorders and depression.

ⓢ **CENTER FOR GENERAL MEDICINE AND ACUPUNCTURE,** Avenue Ensenada #110, Tijuana, B.C. Mexico, 011-526-634-1412. Mailing address: P.O. Box 2757, Chula Vista, CA. 91912, 800-390-5610.

Located five minutes from the United States/ Mexico border, the clinic offers alternative treatments for cancer and other degenerative diseases. Emphasis is placed on strengthening and improving the immune system. Treatment includes complete body detoxification, diet and lifesytle changes, enzymes, immune therapy, chelation and colonics.

ⓢ **EUROPA INSTITUTE OF INTEGRATED MEDICINE,** Allen W. Lloyd Building Ste 201, 406 Avenue Paseo de tijuana, International Border Zone, Tijuana B.C. Mexico, 011-526-682-4902. In the U.S. P.O. Box 950, Twin Peaks, CA. 92391, 909-336-3671.

European Biological and Immunological Medicine encompasses treatment, research and education, with a commitment to the whole person. Europa Institute determines the roots of illness for each individual and changes the internal environment by helping to remove the toxins through various methods. Programs offered include detoxification and rejuvenation programs using chelation, hyperthermia, enzyme therapy, homeopathy, naturopathy, colon hydrotherapy, massage, heavy metals and dental neurotoxin removals and detoxification.

⊛ GERSON HEALING CENTERS OF AMERICA, P.O. Box 430, Bonita, CA. 91902, 619-585-7600.

The Gerson Therapy is an intensive, nutrition-based detoxifying medical treatment for cancer, heart disease, diabetes and other chronic, degenerative diseases. It works closely with nature to help a sick body rid itself of disease through the supportive effects of simple organic foods, juices, and non-toxic medication, coffee enemas, acupuncture, massage, mineral and enzyme therapies.

⊛ PREVENTIVE MEDICAL CENTER OF MARIN, 25 Mitchell Blvd. Ste 8, San Rafael CA. 94903, 415-472-7636.

The center uses a three level approach to therapy and prevention of further problems - lifestyle change, natural therapies and pharmaceutical treatment. The focus is to help each person understand the origins of the problem and to educate about treatment. Treatments include nutritional and herbal therapies, detoxification, acupuncture, Chinese herbal therapy and bodywork.

⊛ THE INNER BEAUTY INSTITUTE OF SAUSALITO, 3A Gate 5 Road, Sausalito, CA, 94965.

The Inner Beauty Institute combines sound guidance and treatment in restoring optimal health and well being. The Institute is owned by Helene Silver, author of "The Body Smart System", one of the leading information guides to the benefits of cleansing and detoxification. The Institute specializes in developing wellness programs tailored to suit personal health concerns, an approach that focuses on detoxifying, rejuvenating and revitalizing the body. The Institute uses colonic irrigations, full-body scrubs, lymphatic massage, and herbal steam baths, along with nutritional and stress reduction counseling.

Programs incorporate daily bodywork sessions with an eclectic synthesis of therapeutic styles. Daily yoga and fitness classes, mountain hikes, meditation, evening support series, nutritional counseling and much fresh air and relaxation are included in each three to seven day session. Special cleansing diets include vegetarian meals. Juice fasting is integrated into the program.

⊛ WE CARE HEALTH RETREAT, 18000 Long Canyon Rd., Desert Hot Springs Ca, 92241, 1-800-8882523.

We Care is located in Desert Hot Springs, Calif. near Palm Springs. The focus is body rejuvenation through cleansing techniques and exercise. We Care holistic health works with just eight guests at a time, ensuring individual guidance while cleansing body, mind, and spirit. The revitalization program offers the synergistic action of fasting, colon hygiene, lymphatic exercises, yoga and meditation, shiatsu, reflexology, facials, mud baths, herbal wraps and hot mineral waters.

Four different plans range from 1 day to 8 days. Basic plans include detoxing with juices, teas, and drinks, cleansing and rebuilding with green grasses, algae, sea veggies, minerals, colonics and

massages, yoga, nutrition classes, vegetarian cooking classes, walks in the desert, saunas and swimming. Colon hygiene, herbal glows, foot reflexology, facials with essential oils, salt rubs, iridology, scalp revitalization, ear cleaning, shiatsu, deep tissue massage, lymphatic body work and aromatherapy are available.

TAOS WELLNESS CENTER, P.O. Box 2843, Taos, N. M. 87571, 505-758-8900.

The Taos Wellness Center is located in Taos, New Mexico. The air quality is pristine and the environment amazingly beautiful. The center offers varied programs including health rejuvenation, personal transformation, wilderness retreats and holistic health care training. The health rejuvenation retreats are highly individualized programs developed for people experiencing high stress levels, chronic fatigue, executive burn-out, depression, recurrent illness, chronic illness, enviromental allergies and immune dysfunction, or for those who just need time to re-evaluate life situations and reach a depth of relaxation beyond the ordinary.

The program includes individual sessions for health assessment, nutritional and lifestyle evaluation, constitutional homeopathic interview, physical exam and personalized treatment plan. Monitored cleansing diets are offered to facilitate the rejuvenation process. The healing process is supported with a full range of services — naturopathic medicine, massage, guided imagery, counseling, polarity therapy and wellness education. Chronic fatigue intervention includes daily bio-magnetic treatments to interrupt replication of the viruses that contribute to CFS. Retreats are one week sessions accommodating six participants only.

ABUNDA LIFE, Holistic Healing Retreat Prevenative Medicine Through Body-Fat Weight Loss. 208 Third Ave., Asbury Park, NJ 07712, 908-775-4141.

The approach is a no nonsense body-fat weight loss program based on the idea that effective and permanent weight loss can only be achieved through effective detoxification and cleansing in combination with proper nutrition and lifestyle changes. Abunda Life believes that toxicity is the common denominator of most disease, over weight and energy problems experienced by humans.

The program includes fasting with health drinks - raw juices, potassium broths, amino acid drinks, green drinks, fiber drinks and superfood drinks. Vitamins, minerals, herbs and enzymes are included. Bodywork includes ozone baths, skin brushing, colon hydrotherapy, massage, thalassotherapy, herbs, overheating therapy, ocean bathing, walking and special supervised exercise.

LOTUS HOLISTIC HEALTH INSTITUTE, 4145 Clares Street, Suite D, Capitola, CA 95010, 408-479-1667.

The center offers Pancha Karma (PK) treatment for detoxification, cleansing and rejuvenation. PK treatments restore individual balance by improving digestion and body system function to allow the body's natural healing processes to operate at full capacity. PK therapy addresses the root cause of imbalance instead of the symptoms themselves, eliminating the underlying toxins which, lodged in the tissues, result in physical symptoms. Treatments begin with a hot herbal oil massage and herbal steams that promote the extraction of deeply set toxins. Other PK treatments are chosen from your individual Ayurvedic consultation. Enemas, nasal cleansing and gland stimulation promote deep relaxation. Special herbs and diet help body detoxification and rejuvenation. Also available are Ayurvedic herbs, oils and the massage clinic offering Swedish, shiatsu, deep tissue, Ayurvedic (body and facial), aromatherapy, polarity and energy balancing massage.

⊗ **GLOBAL FITNESS ADVENTURES,** P.O. Box 1390, Aspen, CO 81612, 800-488-TRIP; 970-972-9583.

Global Fitness Adventures takes the idea of spa pampering and combines it with fitness, adventure and exotic locale to create a body and mind cleansing, stress reducing vacation aimed at the active individual. It's a traveling spa, or "Spa-Fari." The trips are 6 day to 3 week group adventures to places like Aspen, Sedona, AZ, Santa Barbara, CA, Lake Como, Italy, Bali, Bhutan, Nepal, Peru or Dominica in the Caribbean. Private groups may arrange for other locations.

Benefits include nutrition education for energy, clearer thinking, weight loss if desired, stress management, a higher level of fitness and esteem, a personalized daily home exercise routine and more. Meals are designed around an organic, whole-food program geared to detoxification and cleansing — no sugar, caffeine, alcohol or animal fats.

⊗ **HIPPOCRATES HEALTH INSTITUTE,** 1443 Palmdale Court, West, Palm Beach, FL 3341, 407-471-8876 800-842-2125.

Located in West Palm Beach, Florida, the institute is housed in an expansive hacienda with comfortable cottages for guests. The institute is operated by Brian and Anna Maria Clement, both of whom have nearly 20 years of experience in alternative health care.

The institute offers personalized health and nutritional programs for recovery and prevention of degenerative disease. Benefits include more alertness, clear, fresh complexion, emotional stability for better relationships, healthy blood cholesterol or triglyceride levels, reversal of degenerative diseases, improved digestion, painless back, muscular flexibilty and strength, cell oxygenation, tension release and zesty youthfulness.

Exercise classes and personal fitness training, tai chi and yoga, Thai massage, shiatsu, and other body work are aimed at eliminating and correcting physical problems. Nutritional counseling and gourmet food preparation classes are offered for lifestyle changes. Other therapies include saunas, ozonated mineral pools, vibrational medicines, electromagnetic therapies, polarity, reflexology, homeopathy and herbal treatments. The staff includes an M.D. for consultation and blood testing, a psychologist for counseling and massage and alignment therapists.

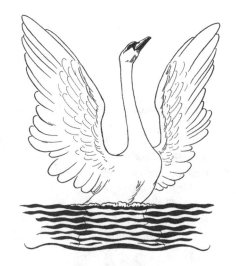

Recommended Products

The following listing is included for your convenience in obtaining products recommended in this detoxification book.

The list is unsolicited by the companies named. We contact each company and review in person and with a test group the quality and effectiveness of each product. While we know there are many other fine companies and products not listed here, you can have every confidence in the products included

Allergy Research Group, 30806 Santana Street, Hayward, CA 94544, 800-545-9960 / 510-487-8526
All One, 719 East Haley St., Santa Barbara, CA 93103, 800-235-5727
Aloe Life International, 4822 Santa Monica Ave. #231, San Diego, CA 92107, 800-414-2563
Alta Health Products, Inc., 1979 E. Locust Street, Pasadena, CA 91107, 626-796-1047
American Biologics, 1180 Walnut Ave., Chula Vista, CA 91911, 800-227-4473
Arise & Shine, P.O. Box 1439, Mt. Shasta, CA 96067, 800-688-2444
Barleans Organic Oils, 4936 Lake Terrell Rd., Fern Dale, WA 98248, 800-445-3529
Beehive Botanicals, Route 8, Box 8257, Hayward, WI 54843, 800-233-4483
Bio-Tech Foods Ltd., 250 S. Hotel St., Ste. 200, Honolulu, HI 96813-2869, 800-468-7578
Body Ecology, 6515 Aldrich Road, Bellingham, WA 98226, 800-511-2660 / 360-384-1238
Boericke & Tafel Inc., 2381 Circadian Way, Santa Rosa, CA95407, 800-876-9505
Burt's Bees, 2050 Greenway Ave., Charlotte, NC 28204, 704-370-6671
CamoCare/Abkit, Inc., 207 East 94th St.., New York, NY 10128, 800-226-6227
Country Life, 28300 B Industrial Blvd., Hayward, CA 94545, 510-785-1196
Creations Garden, 25269 The Old Road, Suite B, Newhall, CA 91381, 805-254-3222
Crystal Star Herbal Nutrition, 6305 Wedgeway Ct., Earth City, MO, 800-736-6015
Diamond/Herpanacine Associates,138 Stout Rd., P.O. Box 544, Ambler, PA 19002, 215-542-2981
Earth Therapeutics, 30 Sagamore Hill Dr., Port Washington, NY 11050, 800-453-4503
Eidon Silica Products, 9988, Hibert St. #104, San Diego, CA 92131, 800-700-1169
Enzymatic Therapy, Dept. L, P.O. Box 22310, Green Bay, WI 54305, 800-783-2286
Ethical Nutrients, 971 Calle Negocio, San Clemente, CA 92673, 714-366-0818
Flora, Inc., 805 East Badger Road, P.O. Box 73, Lynden, WA 98264, 800-446-2110, (Info.) 604-451-8232
Frontier Natural Products, P.O. Box 299, Norway, IA 52318, 800-669-3275
Futurebiotics, 145 Ricefield Lane, Hauppauge, NY 11788, 800-367-5433
Gaia Herbs, Inc., 12 Lancaster County Road, Harvard, MA 01451, 800-831-7780
Golden Pride, 1501 Northpoint Pkwy., Suite 100, West Palm Beach, FL 33407, 561-640-5700
Green Foods Corp., 320 North Graves Ave., Oxnard, CA 93030 800-777-4430
Green Kamut Corp., 1542 Seabright Ave., Long Beach, CA 90813, 800-452-6884
Hayestown Assoc.,123 Bank Ave., New Iberia, LA 70560, 318-365-1553
Healthy Tek, Inc., 2502 S. Broadway, Yorktown, IN 47396, 800-937-1104
Heart Foods Company, Inc., 2235 East 38th Street, Minneapolis, MN 55407, 612-724-5266
Herbal Answers, Inc. P.O. Box 1110, Saratoga Springs, NY 12866, 888-256-3367
Herbal Magic, Inc. P.O. Box 70, Forest Knowlls, CA 94933, 415-488-9488
Herbal Products & Development, P.O. Box 1084, Aptos, CA 95001, 831-688-8706
Herbs Etc., 1340 Rufina Circle, Santa Fe, NM 87505, 505-471-6488
HSU's Ginseng Enterprises, Inc. T6819 Cty Hwy W, P.O. Box 509, Wausau, WI 54402-0509, 715-675-2326
Institute of HeartMath, P.O. 1463, 14700 West Park Ave., Boulder Creek, CA 95006, 800-450-9111
Jarrow Formulas, 1824 South Robertson Blvd., Los Angeles, CA 90035, 310-204-6936
Jean's Greens, 119 Sulphur springs Road, Norway, NY 13416, 315-845-6500
Klamath Blue Green, Inc, P.O. Box 1626, Mt. Shasta, CA 96067, 800-327-1956
Live Food Products, Inc. Box 7, Santa Barbara, CA 93102, 800-446-1990
Maine Coast Sea Vegetables, RR1 Box 78, Franklin, Maine 04634, 207-565-2907

Matrix Health Products, 8400 Magnolia Ave., Ste. N, Santee, CA 92071, 800-736-5609

M.D. Labs, 1719 W. University, Suite 187, Tempe, AZ 85281, 800-255-2690

Mendocino Sea Vegetable Co., P.O. Box 1265, Mendocino, CA 95460, 707-937-2050

Motherlove Herbal Co., P.O. Box 101, Laporte, CO 80535, 970-493-2892

MRI (Medical Research Institute), 2160 Pacific Ave., Suite 61, San Francisco CA 94115, 888-448-4246

National Enzyme Company, Hwy. 160, P.O. Box 128, Forsyth, MO 65653, 800-825-8545

Natural Balance (Pep Products), 3130 N. Commerce Ct., Castle Rock, CO 80104-8002, 303-688-6633

Natural Labs Corporation (Deva Flowers), P.O. Box 20037, Sedona, AZ86341-0037, 800-233-0810

Nature's Answer, 320 Oser Avenue, Hauppauge, NY 11788, 800-439-2324

Nature's Apothecary, 6350 Gunpark Drive #500, Boulder, CO 80301, 800-999-7422

Nature's Herbs, 600 E. Quality Drive, American Fork, UT 84003, 800-437-2257

Nature's Path, P.O. Box 7862, Venice, FL 34287, 800-326-5772

Nature's Plus, 548 Broadhollow Road, Melville, NY 11747-3708, 516-293-0030

Nature's Secret/Irwin Naturals, 10549 West Jefferson Blvd., Culver City, CA 90232, 310-253-5305

Nature's Way, 10 Mountain Springs Parkway, Springville, UT 84663, 800-962-8873

Nelson Bach, Wilmington Technology Park, 100Research Drive, Wilmington MA 01887-4406, 800-319-9151

New Chapter, P.O. Box 1947, Brattleboro, VT 05302, 800-543-7279

North American Herb & Spice Co., P.O. Box 4885, Buffalo Grove, IL 60089, 800-243-5242

Nova Homeopathic Therapeutics, Inc. 5600 McLeod NE. Suite F, Albuquerque, NM 87109, 800-225-8094

NutriCology, 30806 Santana Street, Hayward, CA 94544, 800-545-9960 / 510-487-8526

Peruvian Rainforest Botanicals, 212 N. U.S. Hwy. One, Suite 17, Tequesta, FL 33469, 800-742-2529

Planetary Formulas, P.O. Box 533 Soquel, CA 95073. 800-606-6226

Premier Labs, 27475 Ynez Rd. Suite 305, Temecula, CA 92591, 800-887-5227

Prevail Corporation, 2204-8 NW Birdsdale, Gresham, Or 97030, 800-248-0885

Professional Nutrition, 811 Cliff Dr. , Suite C-1, Santa Barbara, CA 93109, 800-336-9301

Prozyme Products, LTD., 6600 N. Lincoln Ave., Suite 312, Lincolnwood, IL. 60645, 800-522-5537

Rainbow Light, P.O. Box 600, Santa Cruz, CA 95061, 800-635-1233

Rejuvenative Foods, P.O. Box 8464, Santa Cruz, CA 95061, 800-805-7957

Sage Woman Herbs Ltd, 2211 W. Colorado Ave., Colorado Springs, CO 80904, 719-473-9702

Schiff, 2002 South 5070 West, Salt Lake City, UT 84104-4726, 800-526-6251

Seeds of Change, Inc., P.O. Box 15700, Santa Fe, NM 87506, 888-762-7333

Solaray, Inc., 1104 Country Hills Dr., Suite 300, Ogden, UT 84403, 800-669-8877

Solgar, 500 Willow Tree Rd., Leonia, NJ 07605, 800-645-2246

Sonne's Organic Foods, Inc., P.O.Box 2160, Cottonwood, CA 96022, 800-544-8147

Source Naturals Inc. 23 Janis Way, Scotts Valley, CA 95066, 800-777-5677

Spectrum Essentials, 133 Copeland St., Petaluma, CA 94952, 707-778-8900

Sun Wellness, 4025 Spencer St. #104, Torrance, CA 90503, 800-829-2828

Trace Minerals Research, 1990 West 3300 South, Ogden, UT 84401, 800-624-7145

Transformation Enzyme Corporation, 2900 Wilcrest, Suite 220, Houston, TX, 800-777-1474

Transitions For Health, 621 SW Alder, Suite 900, Portland, OR 97205, 800-888-6814

Traditional Medicinals Inc., 4515 Ross Rd., Sebastopol, CA 95472, 707-823-8911

Triple Leaf Tea, Inc. 434 N. Canal Street, Unit 5, So. San Francisco, CA 94080, 800-552-7448

Twin Laboratories, Inc., 2120 Smithtown Ave., Ronkonkoma, NY 11779, 516-467-3140

Vale Enterprises, Inc., 820 S. Monaco Parkway, Suite 261, Denver, CO 80224, 800-488-8253

Vibrant Health, 432 Lime Rock Rd., Lakeville, CT 06039, 800-242-1835

Wakunaga of America Co., Ltd., 23501 Madero, Mission Viejo, CA 92691-2764, 800-421-2998 / 800-825-7888

Wyndmere Naturals, Inc., 153 Ashley Road, Hopkins, MN 55343, 800-207-8538

Y.S. Royal Jelly & Organic Bee Farm, RT. 1, Box 91-A, Sheridan IL 60551, 800-654-4593

Zand Herbal Formulas, P.O. Box 5312, Santa Monica, CA 90409, 310-822-0500

Note: For your convenience, you can order any of the products listed in this book. Just call The Healthy House @ 888-447-2939.

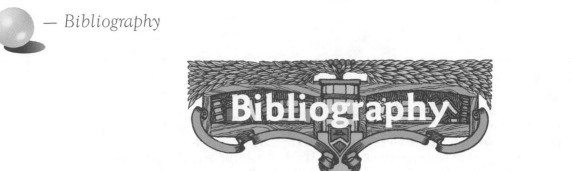

Anderson, Dr. Richard, N.D., N.M.D. Cleanse & Purify Thyself. 1994

Anderson, Nina & Dr. Howard Peiper. *Crystalloid Electrolytes - Our Body's Energy Source for the New Millen nium.* 1997

Arvigo, Rosita & Michael Balick. *Rainforest Remedies - 100 Healing Herbs of Belize.* Twin Lakes: Lotus Press, 1993.

Baker, Elizabeth & Dr. Elton. *The Uncook Book.* 1983

Baranowski, Zane, C.N. *Living Ecology.* 1997

Bauman, Edward, Ph. D. "Immune Boosting Foods and Herbal Tonics." 1994

Bensky, Dan; Gamble, Andrew (translators), *Materia Medica - Chinese Herbal Medicine.* Seattle: Eastland Press, 1993

Buchman, Dian Dincin, *Herbal Medicine.* New York, Gramercy Publishing Company, 1980.

Calbom, Cherie, MS, CN; Keane, Maureen, MS, CN. *Juicing For Life.* Garden City Park: Avery Publishing Group, 1992.

Carper, Jean, *Food - Your Miracle Medicine.* New York, Harper Collins Publishers, 1993.

Chen, Ze-lin, M.D. and Mei-fang Chen, M.D. *A Comprehensive Guide to Chinese Herbal Medicine.* Long Beach: Ojai Press, 1992.

Childre, Doc Lew. Fast Action Stress Relief - Freeze Frame.1994

Cichoke, Anthony J., D.C. *Enzymes & Enzyme Therapy - How To Jump Start Your Way To Lifelong Good Health.* 1994

Crayhon, Robert. Health Benefits Of FOS (Fructooligosaccharides). 1995

Davis, F. A. Taber's Cyclopedic Medical Dictionary. 1989

DiPasquale, Anthony. "Detox Products - Helping Your Customers Survive The Chemical Revolution," Whole Foods. Jan. 1996

Duke, James, PhD. Vasquez, Rodolfo, Amazonian Ethnobotanical Dictionary. Boca Raton: CRC Press, 1994.

Duke, James, PhD. *Handbook of Medicinal Herbs.* Boca Raton: CRC Press, 1985.

Duke, James, PhD. *Handbook of Northeastern Indian Medicinal Plants.* Lincoln: Quaterman Publications, 1986

"Efficacy of Buffered Ascorbate Compound In Detoxification & Aftercare of Clients Involved In Opiate and Stimulant Abuse," Product Research Survey Developed & Funded by Allergy Research Group. Nov. 1987.

Felter, Harvey, M.D.; J. Lloyd, Phr. M., PhD. *King's American Dispensatory.* Sandy: Eclectic Medical Publ., 1983.

Foster, Steven, *Herbal Renaissance.* Salt Lake City: Gibbs-Smith Publisher, 1984.

Gates, Donna. *The Body Ecology Diet.* 1996

Grieve, Mrs. M. *A Modern Herbal.* New York: Dover Publications, 1971.

Haas, Elson M., M.D. *The Detox Diet.* 1996.

Harrison, Lewis. *30 - Day Body Purification. How To Cleanse Your Inner Body & Experience the Joys of Toxin-Free Health.* 1995

"Health and Longevity: The Probiotic Revolution," Health/Science Newsletter. 1997

Hoffman, David. *The Herbal Handbook.* Rochester: Healing Arts Press, 1988.

Holmes, Peter. *The Energetics of Western Herbs Vol. I & II.* Berkeley: NatTrop Publshing, 1993.

Howard, Judy. *Bach Flower Remedies for Women.* 1992

Howard, Judy. *The Bach Flower Remedies Step By Step.* 1994

Hsu, Hong-Yen Dr. *How to Treat Yourself With Chinese Herbs.* New Canaan: Keats Publishing, 1993.

Hsu, Hong-Yen Dr. *Oriental Materia Medica.* Long Beach: Oriental Healing Arts Institute, 1986.

Hutchens, Alma R. *Indian Herbalogy of North America.* Boston: Shambhala Publications, 1973.

Institute of HeartMath. Research Overview - Exploring the Role of the Heart in Human Performance. 1997

Jensen, Bernard, D.C. *Tissue Cleansing Through Bowel Management.* 1981

Jensen, Bernard, Ph. D. Chlorella, Jewel Of The Far East. 1992

Kaminski, Patricia and Richard Katz. Flower Essence Repertory. 1994

Kapoor, L.D. CRC *Handbook of Ayurvedic Medicinal Plants.* Boca Raton: CRC Press. 1990.

Keith, Velma J.; Gordon, Monteen, *The How To Herb Book.* Pleasant Grove: Mayfield Publishing, 1987.

Kennedy, David C. DDS, June, 18, 1998 Letter & Paper (Addressing Fluoride's Relationship to Dental Fluorosis, Hip Fracture, Cancer, & Tooth Decay Costs Savings).

Keuneke, Robin. *Total Breast Health - The Power Food Solution for Protection & Wellness.* 1998

Kuwaki, Takahide, M.D. *Chinese Herbal Therapy.* Long Beach: Oriental Healing Arts Institute, 1990.

Levine, Stephen A., Ph.D. "Food Addiction, Food Allergy and Overweight," Bestways. Nov. 1988.

Levine, Stephen A., Ph.D. "More About Allergy and Addiction," April 1988.

Lewallen, Eleanor and John. *Sea Vegetable Gourmet Cookbook & Wildcrafter's Guild.* 1996.

Martlew, Gillian, N.D. *Electrolytes The Spark Of Life - The Key To Longevity & Quality of Life.* 1998

Markowitz, Elysa. *Living With Green Power - A Gourmet Collection of Living Food Recipes.* 1997.

Millspaugh, Charles F. *American Medicinal Plants.* New York: Dover Publications, 1974.

Mowrey, Daniel B., Ph.D. *Next Generation Herbal Medicine.* New Canaan: Keats Publishing, 1990.

Mowrey, Daniel B., Ph.D., *The Scientific Validation of Herbal Medicine.* New Canaan: Keats Publishing, Inc. 1986.

Murray, Michael, N.D. and Joseph Pizzorno, N.D. *Encyclopedia of Natural Medicine.* Prima Publishing, 1998.

Nadkarni, K.M., DR., *Indian Materia Medica.* Bombay: Popular Prakashan, 1982.

Ody, Penelope, *The Complete Medicinal Herbal.* London-New York-Stuttgart: Dorling Kindersley, 1993.

Olarsch, I. Gerald, N.D. Electrolytes - Your Body's Strongest Health Link! 1998

Page, Linda R. *Healthy Healing* - Tenth Edition. 1997

Page, Linda R. *Detoxification & Body Cleansing.* 1997

Page, Linda R. *Renewing Female Balance.* 1997

Page, Linda R. *How To Be Your Own Herbal Pharmacist.* 1997

Pedersen, Mark, *Nutritional Herbology Vol. I & II.* Pedersen Publishing, 1987.

Pitchford, Paul. *Healing with Whole Foods.* 1993

Price, Shirley. *Practical Aromatherapy - How to Use Essential Oils to Restore Vitality.* 1987

"Probiotics = Proactive Health Care," Whole Foods. Dec. 1997

Rose, Jeanne, *Herbs & Things.* New York: Perigee Books, 1972.

Royal, Penny C. *Herbally Yours.* Provo: Sound Nutrition, 1982.

Salome, Richard. Hippocrates Health Institute Health Manual. 1993

Santillo, Humbart, B.S., M.H., *Natural Healing with Herbs.* Prescott: Holm Press, 1991.

Schauss, Alexander G., Ph.D. "An analysis of colloidal mineral claims," Health Counselor. Feb/Mar 1997

Scheer, James F., "Acidophilus Nature's Antibiotic," Better Nutrition. Aug. 1993

Schroeder, Henry A., M.D. The Trace Elements and Man. 1973

Steenblock, Dr. David, B.S., M.Sc., D.O. Chlorella - Natural Medicinal Algae. 1987

Studer, William H. *American Ginseng In America*. Brooklyn: American Ginseng Society, 1993.

Swann, Denise. *Light Vegetarian Recipes for Higher Energy*. 1993.

Tenney, Louise. *Today's Herbal Health*. Provo: Woodland Books, 1992.

Tierra, Dr. Michael, C.A., N.D., O.M.D. *Planetary Herbology*. Twin Lakes: Lotus Press. 1988.

Tierra, Dr. Michael, C.A., N.D. *The Way of Herbs* NY: Pocket Books. 1990.

Tisserand, Robert. *Aromatherapy - To Heal and Tend the Body*. 1988

Transformational Enterprise Corporation. Enzymes - The Life Force Within Us. 1991

Trattler, Ross, Dr. Better Health Through Natural Healing. N.Y.: McGraw-Hill Book Company, 1985.

Tunella, Kim, C.D.C. "Changing American Dietary Patterns." 1994 .

Turner, Kristina. *The Self - Healing Cookbook*. 1989

Turner, Lisa. "Probiotics - The Good, The Bad and The Friendly," Health Foods Business. Feb. 1997

Tyler, Varro E., Ph.D., Sc.D., *Herbs Of Choice*. New York-London-Norwood: Pharmaceutical Products Press, 1994.

Tyler, Varro E., Ph.D.; Brady, Lynn R., Ph.D.; Robbers, James E., Ph.D. *Pharmacognosy*. Philadelphia: Lea & Febiger, 1988.

Uphof, J.C. Th., *Dictionary Of Economic Plants*. J. Cramer: Publisher In Lehre, 1968.

Valnet, Jean, M.D. *The Practice of Aromatherapy - A Classic Compendium of Plant Medicines & Their Healing Properties*. 1990

Walker, N.W. D. Sci. *Raw Vegetable Juices*. New York: Jove Books, 1987.

Weiss, Rudolf Fritz, M.D. *Herbal Medicine*. Beaconsfield: Beaconsfield Publishers LTD, 1988.

Wigmore, Ann. *Recipes for Longer Life*. 1978

Wren, R.C., F.L.S. *Potter's New Cyclopaedia of Botanical Drugs and Preparations*. Saffron Walden: C.W. Daniel Company Limited, 1989.

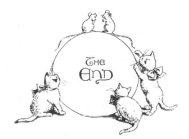

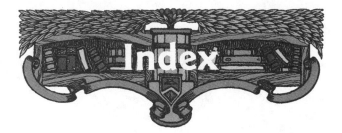

Index

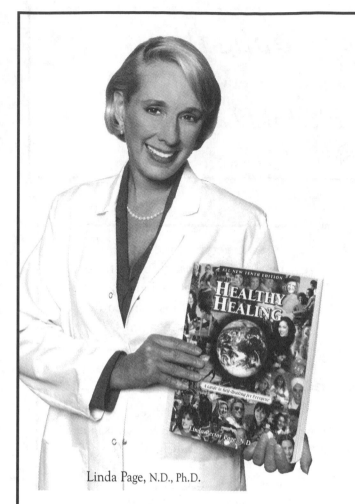

Linda Page, N.D., Ph.D.

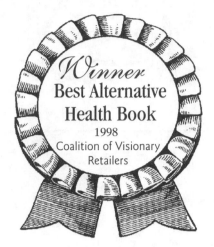

Winner
**Best Alternative
Health Book**
1998
Coalition of Visionary
Retailers

*Over
One-half Million
Sold!*

Healthy Healing, by Linda Page, N.D., Ph.D.
Named Best Alternative Health Book

When first compiled 13 years ago, <u>this book was the only one of its kind.</u>

"I worked in a health food store, and there was no information to answer people's questions," says Dr. Linda Page, author of *Healthy Healing.* "That was before DSHEA (Dietary Supplement Health and Education Act), and the FDA placed restrictions on books and other information about using supplements and natural therapies to maintain health. I felt that the lack of information created a dangerous situation for people who chose to use natural therapies."

Healthy Healing - A Guide To Self Healing For Everyone has been the "health bible" of the natural health industry and is used by people around the world. Now in its 10th edition, *Healthy Healing* is complete and concise. It has the latest information on preventative therapies and natural healing, and features an alphabetical listing of over 150 health complaints with easy-to-use four point healing programs for each ailment: diets and superfood; herbal; supplements; lifestyle support.

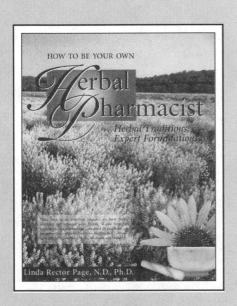

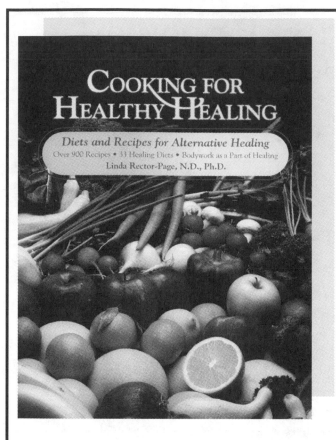

Cooking For Healthy Healing
by Linda Page, N.D., Ph.D,

Good food is good medicine. It is the primary factor for changing the body, chemically and psychologically, and is the foundation element for human life. The food you eat changes your weight, your mood, the texture of your hair and skin, your outlook on life... literally your entire universe! In this book Dr. Page teaches how to use food as a natural pharmacy.

The food therapy sections include cleansing, rebuilding, and maintenance diets and recipe programs. The accompanying recipe and menu suggestions can be used as an initial healing course, as a complete guide or as a start-off point for individual needs.

Party Lights
by Linda Page, N.D., Ph.D.
and Doug Vanderberg

From its imaginative suggestions of party themes to its easy-to-follow decorating instructions and user-friendly recipes, *Party Lights* is your guide to affordable, low-fat, high fun celebrations! It is the encyclopedia of home entertaining that puts you at ease with the planning and preparation of your dream party.

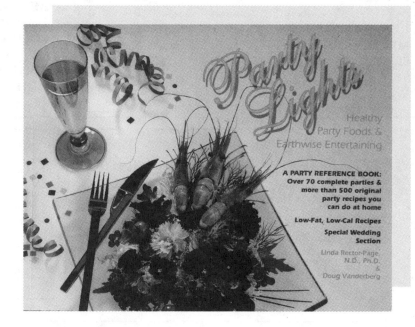

Whether you are giving a romantic dinner for two or a costume party for 200, *Party Lights* provides you with a step-by-step guide to creating the kind of event that will bring praise from your guests.

Party Lights includes complete plans, menus and recipes for anniversaries, holiday celebrations, children's parties, weddings, bridal or baby showers, fund-raisers and more!

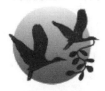

HEALTHY HEALING PUBLICATIONS
Books

(Book availability and prices subject to change.)

HEALTHY HEALING - *Tenth Edition, A Guide to Self Healing for Everyone* - by Dr. Linda Page, N.D., Ph.D. - A 500 page alternative healing reference used by professors, students, health care professionals and private individuals. $28.95 - ISBN# 1-884334-85-7

COOKING FOR HEALTHY HEALING - *Diets and Recipes for Alternative Healing* - by Dr. Linda Page, N.D., Ph.D. - Over 900 recipes and 33 separate diet and healing programs. 698 pages $29.95 - ISBN# 1-884334-56-3

HOW TO BE YOUR OWN HERBAL PHARMACIST - *Herbal Traditions, Expert Formulations* - by Dr. Linda Page, N.D., Ph.D. A complete reference guide for herbal formulations and preparations. 256 pages $18.95 - ISBN# 1-884334-78-4

DETOXIFICATION - *All You Need to Know to Recharge, Renew and Rejuvenate Your Body, Mind and Spirit!* - by Dr. Linda Page, N.D., Ph.D. - A complete encyclopedia-guide of detailed instructions for detoxification and cleansing. 264 pages $19.95 - ISBN# 1-884334-54-7

PARTY LIGHTS - *Healthy Party Foods & Earthwise Entertaining* - by Dr. Linda Page. N.D., Ph.D., and Doug Vanderberg - A party reference book with over 70 parties and more than 500 original recipes you can prepare at home. 358 pages $19.95 - ISBN# 1-884334-53-9

THE BODY SMART SYSTEM - *The Complete Guide to Cleansing & Rejuvenation* - by Helene Silver - A complete 21 day regimen and guide that includes diet, relaxation techniques, massage and bath, exercise programs and recipes. 242 pages $19.95 - ISBN# 1-884334-60-1

NEW EXPANDED LIBRARY SERIES
by Dr. Linda Page, N.D., Ph.D.
ISBN#'s - 1884334 -

36-9 **CANCER 96 pages - $8.95**
14-8 **FATIGUE SYNDROMES 46 pages - $3.95**
64-4 **RENEWING FEMALE BALANCE 48 pages - $4.50**
65-2 **MENOPAUSE & OSTEOPOROSIS 64 pages - $5.95**
15-6 **SEXUALITY 96 pages - $8.95**
67-9 **STRESS & ENERGY 96 pages - $8.95**
66-0 **WEIGHT LOSS** & Cellulite Control **96 pages - $8.95**

THE HEALTHY HEALING LIBRARY SERIES
by Dr. Linda Page, N.D., Ph.D. - **32 pages, $3.50 each.**
ISBN#'s - 1884334 -

35-0 **ALLERGY CONTROL & MANAGEMENT**
13-X **REVEALING THE SECRETS OF ANTI-AGING**
27-X **DO YOU WANT TO HAVE A BABY?**
47-4 **COLDS, FLU & YOU** - Building Optimum Immunity
49-0 **DETOXIFICATION & BODY CLEANSING**
34-2 **BOOSTING IMMUNITY WITH POWER PLANTS**
29-6 **FIGHTING INFECTIONS WITH HERBS**
30-X **RENEWING MALE HEALTH & ENERGY**

Continental U.S. shipping info: $4.50 each for books, $1.00 each for Library Series Booklets.

NAME_____ADDRESS_____

CITY_____ STATE_____ ZIP_____ PHONE_____

☐Check (Make payable to Healthy Healing) ☐Visa   ☐Mastercard   ☐American Express   ☐Discover

CARD #_____EXP. DATE_____SIGNATURE_____

QTY.	BOOK	PRICE	SHIPPING	TOTAL
	CA Residents add 7.25% tax			

Mail to: Healthy Healing Publications, P.O. Box 436, Carmel Valley, CA 93924.   **TOTAL** _____
Or, fax your order to: 831-659-4044. Or, Call 1-800-811-8725.
Or order on-line @ www.healthyhealing.com.

Code: DTX: 1-99